Current Techniques in Arthroscopy

Current Techniques in Arthroscopy

Second Edition

Edited by

J. Serge Parisien, MD

Chief, Arthroscopic Surgery Service
Hospital for Joint Diseases Orthopaedic Institute
Associate Clinical Professor
Orthopaedic Surgery
New York University Medical School
New York City, New York USA

With 30 Contributors

CM CURRENT MEDICINE

Philadelphia

Current Medicine

400 Market Street
Suite 700
Philadelphia, PA 19106

MANAGING EDITOR: .... Lori J. Bainbridge
DEVELOPMENTAL EDITOR: .... Charlene French
ART DIRECTOR: .... Paul Fennessy
DESIGNER: .... Jerilyn Bockorick
ILLUSTRATION DIRECTOR: .... Ann Saydlowski
ILLUSTRATORS: .... Marie Dean, Wiesia Langenfeld,
Jim Perkins, Ann Saydlowski, Beth Starkey, Larry Ward, Gary Welch
INDEXER: .... Ellen Murray
TYPESETTING DIRECTOR: .... Colleen Ward
PRODUCTION: .... David Myers and Wendy Feinstein

Printed in Hong Kong
by Imago

1 3 5 4 2

ISBN:1-878132-63-6
ISSN:1068-4107

Contributors

STEPHEN P. ABELOW, MD
Director, Lake Tahoe Sports Medicine Center
South Lake Tahoe, California, USA
President, Orthopedic Laser Society of North America
Medical Director, US Professional Ski Racing Tour

LTC ROBERT A. ARCIERO, MD
Head Team Physician
Director, US Army Joint and Soft Tissue Fellowship (Sports Medicine)
Keller Army Hospital
West Point, New York, USA

BERNARD R. BACH, JR., MD
Associate Professor
Department of Orthopedic Surgery
Director
Sports Medicine Section
Rush-Presbyterian-St. Luke's Medical Center
Chicago, Illinois, USA

CHAMP L. BAKER, JR., MD
Clinical Assistant Professor
Department of Orthpaedics
Tulane University School of Medicine
New Orleans, Louisiana, USA
President and Staff Physician
The Hughston Clinic
Columbus, Georgia, USA

JOHN P. BELZER, MD
Associate Professor
Department of Orthopedics
University of California
San Francisco, California, USA

EDWARD S. BITTAR, MD, PhD
Associate Professor of Clinical Orthopedics
Department of Orthopedics
University of Florida
Gainsville, Florida, USA

ANDREW A. BROOKS, MD
Fellow in Sports Medicine
The Hughston Clinic
Columbus, Georgia, USA

WILLIAM W. COLMAN, MD
Resident in Orthopedics
Columbia Presbyterian University
New York City, New York, USA

PAUL C. DELL, MD
Professor and Chief
Hand and Microsurgery
Department of Orthopedics
University of Florida
Gainsville, Florida, USA

JAMES C. ESCH, MD
Assistant Clinical Professor
Department of Orthopaedics
University of California
San Diego, California, USA

ALEXANDER I. GLOGAU, MD
Associated Orthopedics & Sports Medicine
Plano, Texas, USA

E. MARLOWE GOBLE, MD
Associate Clinical Professor
University of Utah
Salt Lake City, Utah, USA
Western Surgery Center
Logan, Utah, USA

RONALD P. GRELSAMER, MD
Chief of Hip and Knee Reconstruction
Maimonides Medical Center
Attending Surgeon
Hospital for Joint Diseases
and Beth Israel North
New York City, New York, USA

JEFFREY L. HALBRECHT, MD
Orthopedic Surgery and Sports Medicine
California Pacific Medical Center
San Francisco, California, USA

CHERIE A. HOLMES, MD
Fellow, Section of Sports Medicine
Rush-Presbyterian-St. Luke's Medical Center
Chicago, Illinois, USA

DOUGLAS W. JACKSON, MD
Medical Director
Southern California Center for Sports Medicine
Long Beach, California, USA

ROGER V. LARSON, MD
Associate Professor
Department of Orthopaedic Surgery
University of Washington
Seattle, Washington, USA

CHRISTOPHER D. MILLER, MD
Mississippi Sports Medicine
and Orthopaedic Center
Jackson, Mississippi, USA

CLAUDE T. MOORMAN III, MD
Assistant Clinical Professor
Duke University Medical Center
Department of Orthopedic Surgery
Durham, North Carolina, USA
Triangle Orthopaedic Associates
Durham, North Carolina, USA

J. SERGE PARISIEN, MD
Associate Clinical Professor
Orthopaedic Surgery
New York University Medical School
New York City, New York, USA
Chief, Arthroscopic Surgery Service
Hospital for Joint Diseases Orthopaedic Institute

THOMAS J. PAZIK, MD
Attending Orthopedic Surgeon
Greeley Orthopedic Associates
Greeley, Colorado, USA

JOSHUA PORT, MD
Blair Orthopedic Associates
Altoona, Pennsylvania, USA

DONALD J. ROSE, MD
Clinical Assistant Professor
New York University School of Medicine
New York City, New York, USA
Attending Orthopedic Surgeon
Shoulder Service
Hospital for Joint Diseases
Orthopedic Institute
New York City, New York, USA

THOMAS D. ROSENBERG, MD
The Orthopedic Specialty Hospital
Co-director
Orthopedic Biomechanics Institute
Salt Lake City, Utah, USA

FELIX H. SAVOIE III, MD
Mississippi Sports Medicine and Orthopaedic Center
Jackson, Mississippi, USA

NEAL C. SMALL, MD
Associated Orthopaedics & Sports Medicine
Plano, Texas, USA
Associate Professor of Orthopedics
South West Medical School
Dallas, Texas, USA

STEPHEN J. SNYDER, MD
Director, Southern California Orthopedic Research and Education
Van Nuys, California, USA

KEVIN P. SPEER, MD
Assistant Professor
Shoulder and Elbow Service
Duke University Medical Center
Durham, North Carolina, USA

RONALD B. STARON, MD
Assistant Professor of Radiology
Columbia Presbyterian University
New York City, New York, USA

RUSSELL F. WARREN, MD
Surgeon-in-chief
Hospital for Special Surgery
Cornell University Medical Center
New York City, New York, USA

Preface

This is the second edition in the *Current Techniques in Arthroscopy* series. Although I have continued to focus on established arthroscopic techniques, I have also invited experienced surgeons to present new and promising techniques in their field of expertise. This is particularly important as it pertains to shoulder surgery, where an increasing number of procedures are being done arthroscopically.

Separate chapters are devoted to arthroscopic shoulder stabilization and the treatment of frozen shoulder. Other chapters include office arthroscopy, techniques for meniscal reimplantation, patellar realignment, laser meniscectomy, and endoscopic carpal tunnel release. The role of magnetic resonance imaging, the usefulness of the infusion pump, and the role of arthroscopy in some procedures on the ankle joint are also discussed.

Each author has done an outstanding job. They have fulfilled the goal of this book with the timeliness and clarity of their presentations. To them and their co-authors, I express my deepest gratitude. I am most appreciative of the invaluable assistance of Charlene French, developmental editor, who worked so diligently to produce this new volume. I would also like to thank Elizabeth Howard, developmental editor, and the staff at Current Medicine who deserve full credit for the immense success of the first edition.

J. Serge Parisien, MD, *New York City, New York*

Contents

CHAPTER 1 The Use and Misuse of Magnetic Resonance Imaging of the Knee
Ronald P. Grelsamer, William W. Colman, and Ronald B. Staron

Meniscal tears 1
Meniscal cysts 2
Patella malalignment 3
Tibial plateau fracture 4
Osteochondritis dissecans in unusual locations 4
Osteonecrosis avascular necrosis 5
Synovitis 6
Tumors 6
Intra-articular scar and adhesions 7
Vascular conditions 7
The cruciate ligaments 7
Future directions 8

CHAPTER 2 Office Arthroscopy
Jeffrey L. Halbrecht

What is office arthroscopy? 11
History and indications 12
Technique 13
Postoperative care 15
Complications 15
Conclusion 16

CHAPTER 3 The Use of Infusion Pumps in Arthroscopic Surgery
J. Serge Parisien

Advantages and disadvantages 19
Technique 19
Complications 26
Conclusions 27

CHAPTER 4 **The Use of Lasers in Arthroscopic Meniscal Surgery**
Stephen P. Abelow

The Holmium laser 30
The 1.44 Neodymium:YAG laser 32
The 1.06 Neodymium:YAG laser 33
Meniscal repair 33
Future of lasers 33
Conclusion 34

CHAPTER 5 **Meniscal Allograft Reconstruction in Arthroscopic Surgical Technique**
E. Marlowe Goble

Medial meniscus allograft technique 36
Lateral meniscal allograft technique 40

CHAPTER 6 **Arthroscopically Assisted Proximal Extensor Mechanism Realignment of the Knee**
Neal C. Small and Alexander I. Glogau

Case I: patellar fracture dislocation 45
Case II: acute patellar subluxation 46
Surgical procedure 46
Postoperative care 47

CHAPTER 7 **The Use of Hamstring Tendons in Anterior Cruciate Ligament Surgery**
Roger V. Larson

Technique for reconstruction with double loops of semitendinosus and gracilis tendons 53
Rehabilitation 61
Discussion 61

CHAPTER 8 **Two-Incision Arthroscopy-Assisted ACL Reconstruction Using Patellar Tendon Substitution**
Cherie A. Holmes and Bernard R. Bach, Jr.

Preliminary technique 66
Diagnostic arthroscopy 66
Intercondylar notch preparation 66
Notchplasty 67
Graft harvest 67
Supracondylar femur preparation 68
Femoral drill hole placement 68
Tibial hole placement 69
Alternative method of femoral tunnel placement 71
Isometry testing 72
Graft placement 72
Summary 74

CHAPTER 9 Anterior Cruciate Ligament Reconstruction With Quadrupled Semitendinosus Autograft
Thomas D. Rosenberg and Thomas J. Pazik

Technique. 79
Femoral bisocket technique. 84
Postoperative rehabilitation. 85

CHAPTER 10 Posterior Cruciate Ligament Arthroscopic Techniques
Joshua Port and Douglas W. Jackson

Anatomy 90
Biomechanics. 92
Clinical evaluation 93
Treatment. 94
Surgical technique 96
Selection of isometric points 97
Placement and fixation of the graft 100
Graft selection 101
Autografts 102
Allografts 102
Artificial ligaments. 103
Complications following cruciate reconstructions. 103
Conclusions 103

CHAPTER 11 The Frozen Shoulder
James C. Esch

History 107
Clinical presentation 108
Natural history. 108
Differential diagnosis 108
Pathology 109
Arthroscopic observations 109
Patient selection for manipulation or surgery 111
Surgical treatment 112
Postmanipulation exercises 114
Results 115

CHAPTER 12 Arthroscopic Stabilization of Acute, Initial Anterior Shoulder Dislocations
Robert A. Arciero

Technique 118
Results 121
Discussion 123

CHAPTER 13 **Arthroscopic Shoulder Stabilization Using the Bioabsorbable Tack**
Claude T. Moorman III, Kevin P. Speer, and Russell F. Warren

The bioabsorbable tack 125
Indications 126
Technique of tack stabilization 127
Postoperative care 130
Complications 131
Summary 132

CHAPTER 14 **Technique of Capsulorrhaphy (Caspari Technique)**
Felix H. Savoie III and Christopher D. Miller

Arthroscopic techniques 134
Pathology of anterior instability 134
Arthroscopic capsulorrhaphy 135
Results 139
Conclusions 140

CHAPTER 15 **Shoulder Capsulorrhaphy Using Suture Anchors and Nonabsorbable Sutures**
Stephen J. Snyder and John P. Belzer

Pathophysiology 144
History 145
Surgical indications 145
Technique 145
Surgical technique 147
Surgical technique for anterior stabilization 149
Postoperative care and rehabilitation 154
Southern California Orthopedic Institute results 155
Conclusion 156

CHAPTER 16 **Arthroscopic Transglenoid Suture Capsulorrhaphy for Anterior Shoulder Instability**
Donald J. Rose

Surgical technique 160
Postoperative management 167
Complications and pitfalls 167
Variations of pathology 168
Results 170
Discussion 171
Conclusions 172

CHAPTER 17 Arthroscopic Surgery for Soft-Tissue Lesions of the Ankle
J. Serge Parisien

Types of synovial lesions 173
Arthroscopic technique 178

CHAPTER 18 Arthroscopically Assisted Ankle Arthrodesis
Champ L. Baker, Jr. and Andrew A. Brooks

Technique 186
Fixation 189
Results 190
Conclusion 191

CHAPTER 19 Avoiding Possible Complications Associated with Ankle Arthroscopy
J. Serge Parisien

Complications associated with technique 194
Complications associated with specific procedures 201
Conclusions 204

CHAPTER 20 Endoscopic Carpal Tunnel Release
Edward S. Bittar and Paul C. Dell

Techniques 206
Discussion 213

INDEX 217

1

CHAPTER

The Use and Misuse of Magnetic Resonance Imaging of the Knee

RONALD P. GRELSAMER, WILLIAM W. COLMAN,
RONALD B. STARON

The ability of magnetic resonance (MR) imaging to visualize the bony and soft-tissue structures about the knee is unmatched by any other modality. Not surprisingly then, MR imaging studies are being ordered in spectacular numbers. Patients expect them. Even primary care doctors order them in anticipation of a consultation with the orthopedic specialist. However, because of the high cost of MR imaging, every effort should be made to order it when there is a reasonable chance that it will affect treatment. MR imaging was never designed to replace the history and physical examination. Finally, MR imaging is not a perfect science. The limitations of MR imaging and difficult-to-explain concepts like *false-positive* and *false-negative* need to be discussed with the patient. On the positive side, MR imaging can often confirm or rule out a suspected diagnosis, detect an unsuspected condition, or quantify the extent of a known problem.

MENISCAL TEARS

One of the common reasons for ordering MR imaging is to determine the presence of a meniscal tear [1–6]. Unfortunately, it is also one of the areas most prone to misinterpretation. The natural aging process is accompanied by changes in MR appearance of the meniscus, and thus most older patients will exhibit some signal changes. Moreover, as of this writing MR imaging will not reliably detect small, early stage (but possibly painful) articular cartilage damage. Thus, the patient over 60 years with chronically achy knees from a probable combination of degenerative menisci and scattered arthritic lesions is probably not the best candidate for MR imaging.

Meniscal abnormalities are read as grade I, II, or III intrameniscal signal abnormalities. Grade I changes involve globular intrameniscal signal abnormalities that do not reach an articular surface of the meniscus. Grade II signals are linear changes that do not reach an articular surface, and grade III signals involve either the femoral or tibial meniscal articular surface. Grade III can be further subdivided into IIIA for linear changes and IIIB for complex changes. Figure 1-1 is an example of a medial meniscus with a grade III signal.

Interestingly, meniscal changes are sometimes referred to in radiology reports as grade I, II, or III *tears*. Such nomenclature sends a signal to the patient that there is something definitely wrong that needs fixing. The unfortunate orthopedist is then obligated to perform an arthroscopy. On the other hand, in planning an anterior cruciate ligament (ACL) reconstruction, knowledge that a significant meniscal tear exists can significantly alter the informed consent. The surgeon may indeed wish to discuss the issue of a meniscal repair. A patient with a torn medial collateral ligament may also have a torn meniscus. For the average patient, a "wait-and-see" attitude may be most reasonable, but for very active patients, ordering MR imaging may be more cost-effective.

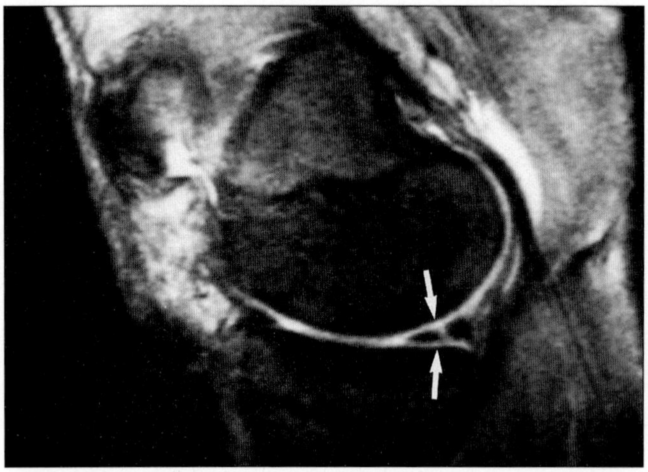

Figure 1-1. Magnetic resonance imaging shows grade III signal within the posterior horn of the medial meniscus, which apparently was not found to represent a meniscal tear during careful arthroscopic examination at another institution. This sagittal gradient-echo image (repetition time and echo time 813 and 32; 30°flip angle) demonstrates a vertical line of grade III signal that contacts both superior and inferior articular surfaces of the posterior horn of the medial meniscus (*arrows*).

The sensitivity, specificity, and accuracy of MR imaging for meniscal tears have been amply reported and are thought to be approximately 90%, with a somewhat lesser sensitivity for the lateral meniscus [7•]. For practical purposes, the patient can be told that, with respect to the menisci, the MR imaging will be correct nine out of 10 times, and that overreading a tear is as much of an issue as is underreading (missing) a tear.

The discoid meniscus represents a special problem because the meniscus is not normal to begin with. It is thicker than the normal meniscus, and it appears on more MR cuts because of its greater surface area. Discoid menisci are usually lateral, although they have also been found on the medial side [8–12]. It is considered complete when there is no central opening and the posterior horn can be relatively attached or detached. In the latter case (Wrisberg type), the posterior horn is attached to bone via only the meniscofemoral ligament of Wrisberg. An association with osteochondritis dissecans of the lateral femoral condyle has been reported. Treatment of the torn discoid meniscus remains controversial, especially for the Wrisberg type. Figure 1-2 shows an example of a torn discoid lateral meniscus in a pediatric patient.

Meniscal Cysts

Patients who present localized swelling at the joint line may have a meniscal cyst, the major differential being a ganglion that is not an intra-articular lesion [13–16]. Preoperative knowledge of this intra-articular pathology will greatly aid the preoperative planning because this pathology can be addressed arthroscopically (Fig. 1-3).

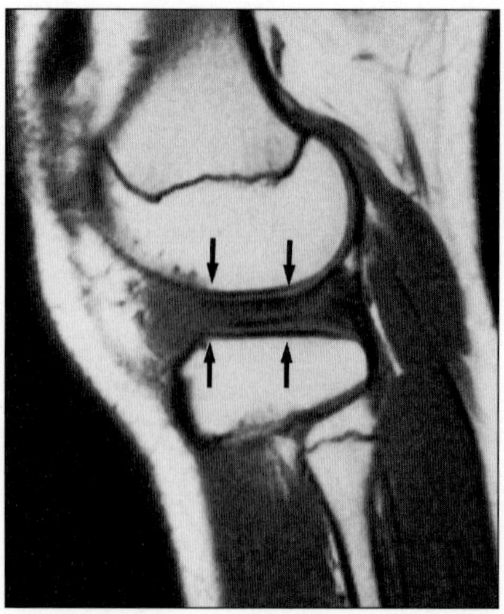

Figure 1-2. Sagittal T_1-weighted spin-echo image (repetition time and echo time, 535 and 15) demonstrates the magnetic resonance imaging appearance of a torn discoid lateral meniscus. Abnormal intermediate signal intensity material, indicating a meniscal tear, is seen within the low-signal intensity band of the larger-than-normal lateral meniscus (*arrows*).

PATELLA MALALIGNMENT

Subluxation

MR imaging of the patella has been studied by various authors [17–21]. The patella can follow a somewhat wobbly path down the trochlea, a path that can vary from patient to patient. The position of the patella near extension is controversial, in part, because the terms *full extension* and *zero* (neutral) *extension* have been erroneously used interchangeably. In full extension (maximal quadriceps contraction), a number of patients exhibit an element of recurvatum. It is possible that in this degree of extension it is normal for the patella to be laterally positioned. However, MR imaging is not carried out in full extension. It is carried out at 0° of extension or slight flexion. In a study of 60 patients without clinical or radiologic signs of patellar pathology, the MR image revealed the patella to be centered over the underlying femur-trochlea in 59 of the 60 cases (Grelsamer and Newton, Unpublished data). It is our opinion that on routing MR scanning a laterally positioned patella should not be summarily dismissed as normal. Figure 1-4 shows a laterally subluxated patella.

Tilt

Laurin [22] was one of the first to bring up the issue of patellar tilt on diagnostic imaging. He described a *lateral patellofemoral angle* that reflects the tilt of the patella as seen on plain radiographs. Grelsamer and coworkers [23] have further developed the concept. Schutzer and coworkers [24,25] carried the concept over to computerized imaging. In their 1986 study, they found that when the knee is flexed 15°, the tilt angle should be more than 7°. In this particular case, the tilt angle is defined as an angle subtended by a line drawn across the posterior condyles and a line drawn along the bony portion of the lateral facet. The tilt angle, when defined in this manner, decreases as the actual tilt of the patella increases. This was already the case with Laurin's angle.

Of great significance is the issue of whether axial views should be included in routine MR scanning of the knee. A significant percentage of MR studies currently carried out do not include such views. It is our opinion that this is an error. Patella malalignment is the source of much knee pain in the young, and in the older population we know that the patella is a main cause of total knee failure.

Chondromalacia

The detection of true chondromalacia, *ie*, cartilage softening and cartilage lesions, remains a weak area of MR imaging. Large, late-stage lesions can be easily detected on fat-suppressed, T_2-weighted imaging, but smaller, early-stage (yet no less painful) lesions can still escape detection. When possible, this is best explained to the patient prior to any surgical procedures.

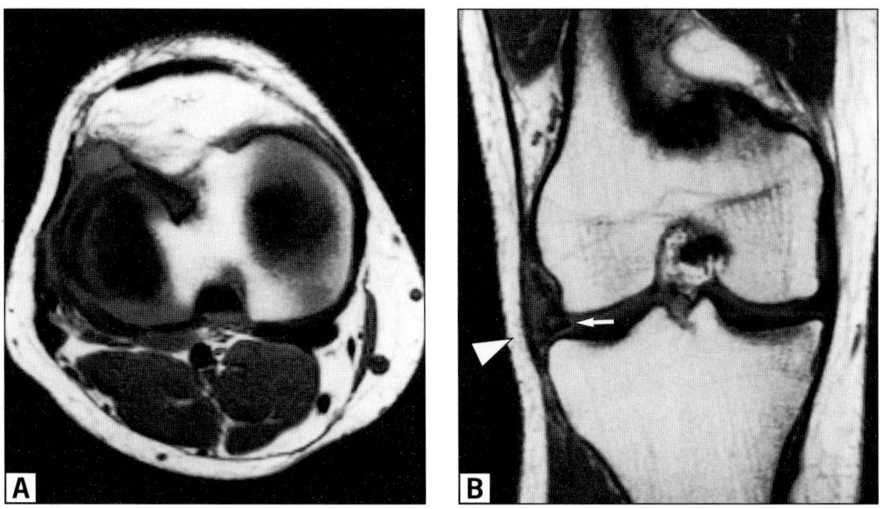

Figure 1-3. Magnetic resonance imaging appearance of a lateral meniscal cyst. **A**, Axial T_1-weighted spin-echo (image repetition time [TR] and echo time [TE], 535 and 15) demonstrates intermediate signal intensity material lateral to, and immediately anterior to, the lateral meniscus. This material is a meniscal cyst wrapping around the capsular margin of the meniscus, with its thickest portion located anteriorly. **B**, Coronal T_1-weighted spin-echo image (TR and TE, 535 and 15) demonstrates the meniscal cyst (*arrowhead*) just lateral to the body of the lateral meniscus. The meniscus contains a grade III signal abnormality indicative of a meniscal tear (*white arrow*).

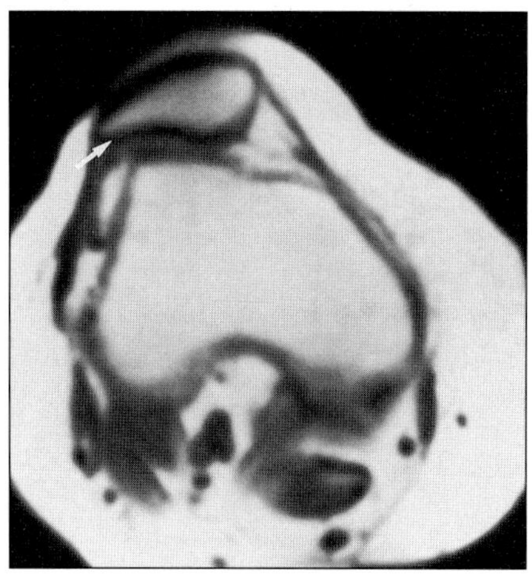

Figure 1-4. Axial T_1-weighted spin-echo image (repetition time and echo time, 500 and 30) demonstrates lateral subluxation of the patella (*arrow*).

TIBIAL PLATEAU FRACTURE

Consider the following scenario: a knee injury, severe pain, and a negative radiograph. If the pain seems to be greater than what would be expected from a soft-tissue injury, the patient may have an occult fracture. Missing it can have medical or legal consequences. MR imaging can be helpful in a number of respects. It is accurate enough with respect to the diagnosis of a fracture that a negative MR image effectively rules out the condition (high negative predictive value). If there is depression of a plateau, it can be specifically localized and the degree of depression can be quantified. A fracture will appear as a linear dark signal on T_1 images or a bright signal on T_2 images (Fig. 1-5).

Similarly, MR imaging will detect a tibial or femoral *bone bruise*—a bone injury not severe enough to be a fracture but severe enough to cause *marrow edema, ie,* a gray (intermediate signal) area on T_1, fat-suppressed images, and a bright area on T_2-weighted, fat-suppressed images. The presence of such a bruise may turn out to be of predictive value with respect to long-term arthritic changes following an ACL injury [26–29].

OSTEOCHONDRITIS DISSECANS IN UNUSUAL LOCATIONS

Usually located on the lateral (central) aspect of the medial femoral condyle, osteochondritis dissecans (OCD) represents a localized osteochondral separation from the underlying bony bed. The bony portion of the fragment is mostly avascular, is grossly dense and brittle, and appears as a moderately low-intensity signal on T_1-weighted MR images (Fig. 1-6) [30•,31]. The fragment is surrounded by fibrous tissue of even lower signal intensity. Its appearance is similar to a long bone nonunion, and lends some credence to the "traumatic origin" theory of OCD.

The separation of the fragment can range from mild to complete. At one extreme, the cartilaginous surface can remain unbroken, in which case the MR image will show an absence of fluid (absence of high-signal intensity on a T_2-weighted image) between the OCD fragment and the bony bed. At the other extreme, the fragment can become a loose body. By determining the amount of separation between the lesion and the femur, MR can be of great assistance in staging the lesion and can help with respect to the preoperative planning and informed consent. There is still controversy with regard to the etiologic role of trauma, the role of the tibial spines, and the role of intrinsic vascular changes.

Osteochondritis dissecans can theoretically occur anywhere, in any joint. In the knee, it occurs most frequently on the lateral aspect of the medial femoral condyle, but it can occur on the central, weight-bearing portion of either the medial or lateral condyle, or more rarely on the trochlear portion of the lateral femoral condyle [32]. It has been reported on the patella [33]. Lesions of the lateral condyle are usually larger and carry a worse prognosis than their medial counterparts. Adolescent OCD is far more likely to heal

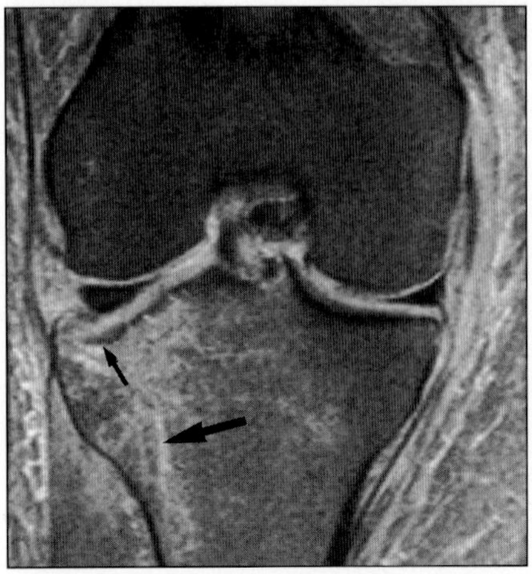

Figure 1-5. Coronal spectral inversion recovery image (repetition time and echo time, 1300 and 20) demonstrates a depressed lateral tibial plateau fracture (*small arrow*) with a vertical fracture line extending inferiorly (*large arrow*). The streaks of high signal intensity within the soft tissues around the knee indicate soft-tissue injury.

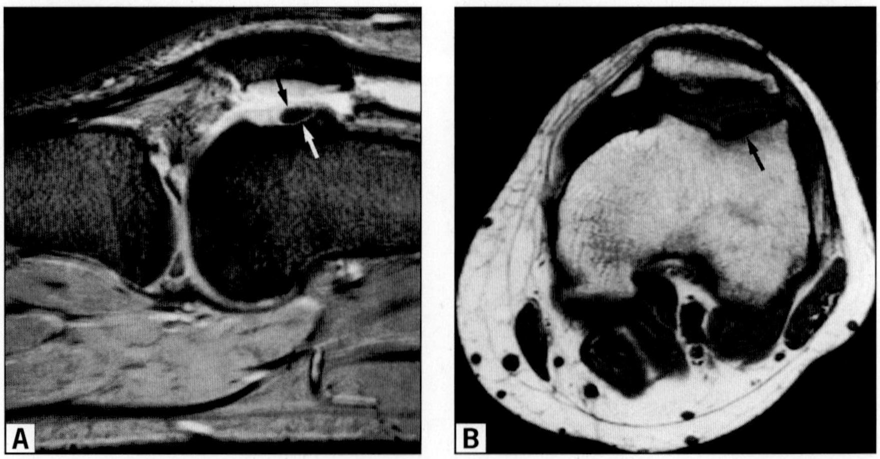

Figure 1-6. Magnetic resonance imaging appearance of osteochondritis dissecans involving the anterior aspect of the lateral femoral condyle. **A**, Sagittal fast field echo imaging (repetition time [TR] and echo time [TE], 660 and 15; 30° flip angle) through the lateral femoral condyle demonstrates an osteochondral defect anteriorly containing a small osteochondral fragment (*arrows*). **B**, Axial T_1-weighted spin-echo image (TR and TE, 535 and 15) demonstrates the osteochondral defect containing the dark osteochondral fragment (*arrow*).

spontaneously than the adult form. Age 15 is thought by some to be the approximate cut-off [30•,34–35].

OSTEONECROSIS AVASCULAR NECROSIS

The prototypical healthy patient with avascular necrosis (AVN) is a woman in her 60s who develops sudden, severe pain in the knee. As with other joints, AVN can also occur in a steroid-taking person of any age, and as with other joints, radiograph findings can initially be negative [36,37]. It is now quite clear that of all the readily available modalities, MR imaging is the most likely to detect a roentgenographically silent lesion. It is therefore the modality of choice in someone whose AVN must be documented, *ie*, a patient whose knee pain has not responded to basic, nonoperative measures. AVN can be readily seen on both T_1 and T_2 images. On T_2 images, there is sometimes a peripheral rim that can be subdivided into a dark band and an adjacent bright band, the *double rim sign*. Early AVN can present on MR imaging as marrow edema, but there is controversy as to whether the presence of such marrow changes by themselves automatically constitute early AVN. Transient edema patterns have been described that clinically and radiologically resolve spontaneously. Figure 1-7 and 1-8 illustrate early spontaneous osteonecrosis and multiple bony infarcts, respectively.

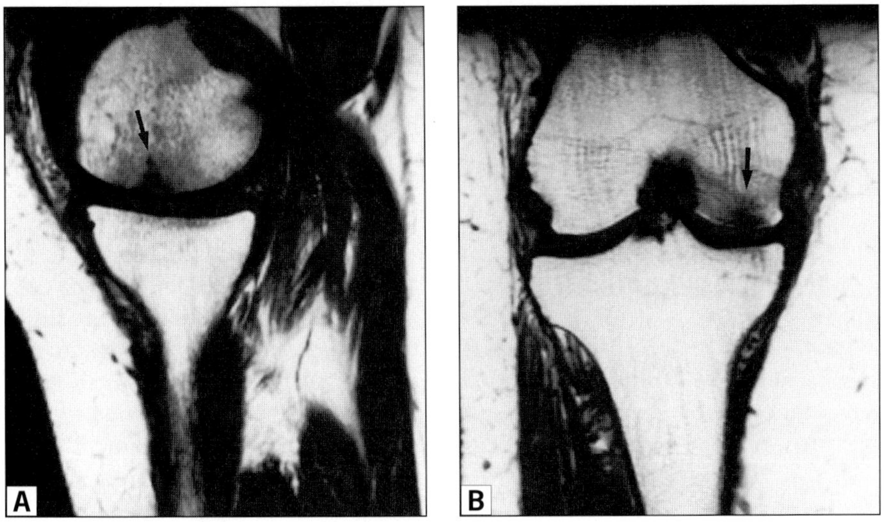

Figure 1-7. Magnetic resonance imaging appearance of early spontaneous osteonecrosis of the medial femoral condyle. **A**, Sagittal T_1-weighted spin-echo image (repetition time [TR] and echo time [TE], 525 and 20) demonstrates a focal area of low signal, representing spontaneous osteonecrosis, in the subchondral region of the medial femoral condyle (*arrow*). The overlying articular cartilage is intact. **B**, Coronal T_1-weighted spin-echo image (TR and TE, 525 and 20) demonstrates the area of osteonecrosis in the subchondral region of the medical femoral condyle (*arrow*). At the time of magnetic resonance imaging, the radiographs of the knee appeared normal.

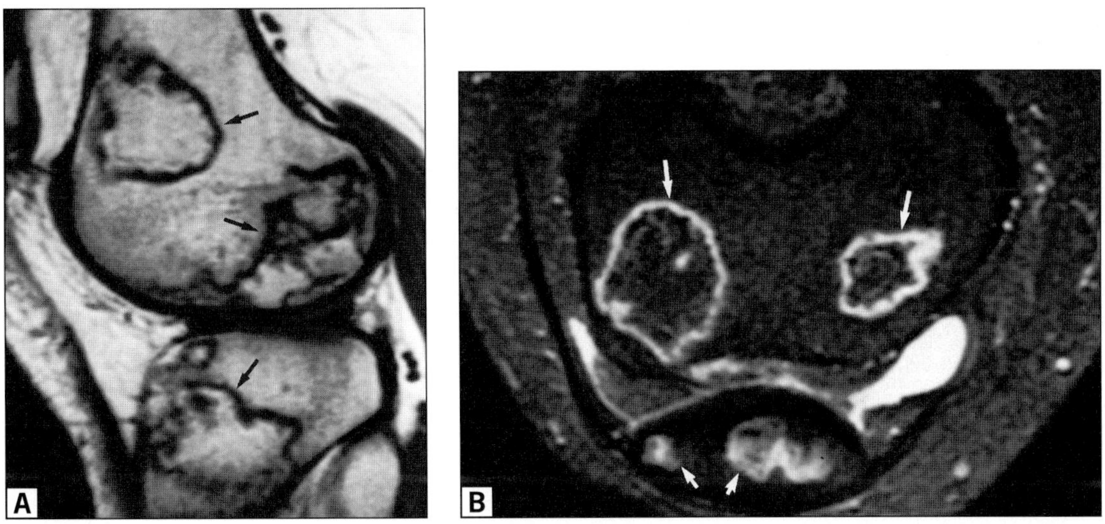

Figure 1-8. Magnetic resonance imaging appearance of multiple bone infarcts. **A**, Sagittal T_1-weighted spin-echo image (repetition time [TR] and echo time [TE], 600 and 13) demonstrates multiple areas of osteonecrosis outlined by irregularly shaped low intensity rims (*arrows*). **B**, Axial fast spin-echo image (TR and TE, 5300 and 54) demonstrates multiple areas of osteonecrosis (*arrows*) within the femur and patella. Each osteonecrotic region is outlined by a high-intensity rim in this T_2-weighted image.

SYNOVITIS

Tuberculosis

The prevalence of tuberculosis is on the increase. Symptoms can be quite nonspecific, and in the right setting, the clinician must remain leery of this notorious "great impersonator." Often, the knee will exhibit a boggy synovitis not necessarily different from other types of synovitis [38]. Such synovitis is apparent on both T_1 and T_2 imaging. Figure 1-9 shows an example of the boggy synovitis usually associated with tuberculosis of the knee.

Pigmented Villonodular Synovitis

Pigmented villonodular synovitis is a monoarticular condition most commonly involving the knee (80% of cases). The patient usually presents with pain, stiffness, swelling, and warmth over the affected joint. Joint aspiration will usually reveal either a bloody effusion or the classic chocolate brown effusion. The condition actually encompasses a number of histologic and clinical subsets. There is a localized form that is easier to treat (local excision) than the diffuse form (synovectomy), which is traditionally believed to recur with significant frequency (30%—50%). Recently, certain investigators have noted a very low recurrence rate with a total, open synovectomy, and they have postulated that recurrences may in fact represent incomplete resection of the lesion [39]. The MR findings are influenced by the presence of hemosiderin, which tends to produce a low signal in T_1 and even lower signal in T_2-weighted images. The differential includes the other synovitides [40–45].

Synovial Chondromatosis

Synovial chondromatosis is another monoarticular synovial condition. It is characterized by synovial metaplasia with formation of multiple cartilaginous loose bodies. Again, the condition can be focal or generalized. Pain and stiffness are the clinical hallmarks, plain radiographs are negative. If the cartilaginous loose bodies are small enough, they can be missed on MR imaging, and the synovial metaplasia may produce nonspecific MR signals [41,46–49].

TUMORS

Although tumors are infrequently encountered by orthopedists, the clinician must keep in mind that the knee is one of the most common areas for musculoskeletal tumors, both benign and malignant [50–52]. Symptoms can begin after an injury, and early on radiographs can be negative. This can mislead the doctor into thinking that the patient has a common soft-tissue injury. Medications, prolonged physical therapy, and even arthroscopy can be prescribed before the tumor is eventually discovered. Conversely, the fear of missing a tumor can lead many doctors to order a knee MR study for the slightest injury. Surely a happy medium exists, but to define this happy medium one must necessarily conjure up not just medical but legal, ethical, and economic issues beyond the scope of this chapter. Until specific guidelines are established, each practitioner must judge both his patient and the setting of his or her practice in deciding on the timing of MR imaging.

Giant-cell tumors are among the most common tumors encountered about the knee, and likewise the

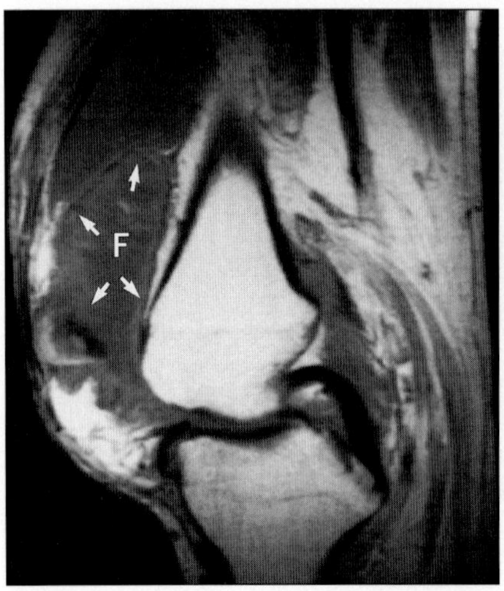

Figure 1-9. Magnetic resonance imaging appearance of tuberculosis synovitis. This sagittal T_1-weighted spin-echo image (repetition time and echo time, 900 and 30) demonstrates a large knee joint effusion (*F*) surrounded by a thickened rim of synovium (*arrows*) with slightly higher signal intensity than the effusion. This is the typical appearance of synovitis on T_1-weighted images without gadolinium enhancement. The contrast in signal intensities between the fluid and the hypertrophied synovium is increased by the use of intravenous gadolinium.

knee is one of the more common sites for giant-cell tumors. Typically, there is a sharp demarcation between tumor and healthy bone, but there is no dark rim of reactive bone on either T_1- or T_2-weighted images. There can be areas of fluid and fluid-fluid levels within the tumor that represent foci of aneurysmal bone cystlike changes that are commonly seen in giant-cell tumors (Fig 1-10).

INTRA-ARTICULAR SCAR AND ADHESIONS

Intra-articular scar tissue and adhesions from either previous surgery or arthrofibrosis can reveal impressive intra-articular whorls (T_1 or T_2) suggestive of inflammatory synovitis, infection, or tumor. These conditions share a number of features on MR imaging, and as of this writing, the surgeon may have no choice but to perform a biopsy on the tissue if this is warranted by the clinical picture.

VASCULAR CONDITIONS

Not all knee pain has an intra-articular origin. The popliteal space is host to a number of structures that can be diseased and painful. Examination of the patient in the prone position can reveal tender swelling. This swelling is usually medial and reflects a Baker's cyst, but on rare occasions can represent a synovial or neurologic neoplasm, or a vascular condition (injury or malformation) [53,54]. MR imaging can clearly detect a vascular condition. Where there is doubt, an MR angiogram can be performed. Figure 1-11 is an example of an MR image of a popliteal aneurysm.

THE CRUCIATE LIGAMENTS

In the chronic setting, a number of clinical signs are available to suggest a cruciate tear, but in the acute setting, pain, spasm, and swelling make these signs less practical [41,55–59]. MR imaging can shed light on the subject with a sensitivity and a specificity reported to be in the range of 70% to 95% for ACL tears. Positioning of the leg is a significant factor as the ACL does not lie squarely in the sagittal plane. External rotation of the leg by 15° is recommended to improve the accuracy of ACL imaging. Continuity, contour, and signal are the parameters by which ligament integrity is assessed: the ligament should be straight (rather than sagging) and the signal should be homogeneous. When the ligament is outright missing from the picture, this is highly suggestive of a complete tear.

In addition to assessing the ligament itself, imaging of the posterior cruciate ligament (PCL) can also be used to infer the integrity of the ACL. The PCL normally appears straight or curved, loosely approximating the letter "C." A sigmoid or "S" shaped PCL correlates with a rupture of the ACL [41,60•].

Another study has concluded that there is a correlation between the curvature of PCL and the integrity

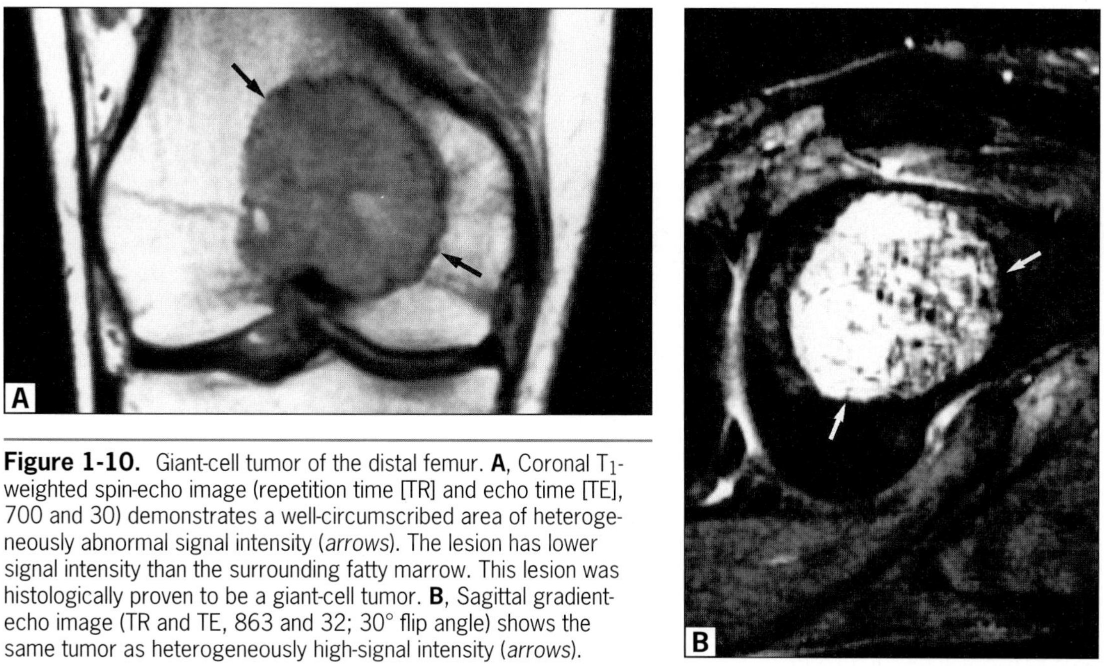

Figure 1-10. Giant-cell tumor of the distal femur. **A**, Coronal T_1-weighted spin-echo image (repetition time [TR] and echo time [TE], 700 and 30) demonstrates a well-circumscribed area of heterogeneously abnormal signal intensity (*arrows*). The lesion has lower signal intensity than the surrounding fatty marrow. This lesion was histologically proven to be a giant-cell tumor. **B**, Sagittal gradient-echo image (TR and TE, 863 and 32; 30° flip angle) shows the same tumor as heterogeneously high-signal intensity (*arrows*).

of the ACL: the greater the curvature, the greater the chances of an ACL rupture [61].

Detection of a torn PCL is more straightforward to the extent that the ligament lies in the sagittal plane (Fig. 1-12).

FUTURE DIRECTIONS

For a number of select areas, current, routine MR imaging remains suboptimal. For example, on a routine basis, T_2-weighted fat suppression techniques are well-suited for the detection of articular cartilage lesions. However, articular cartilage lesions are not automatically detected, especially if they are small and not accompanied by bony changes. This can lead to surprises at the time of surgery, surprises that the patient may have difficulty accepting if they have had a preoperative MR imaging report that did not mention such lesions. In the future, the sensitivity of MR imaging with respect to such lesions will most likely improve [62•].

Evaluation of the repaired or transplanted meniscus remains problematic because the "healed" area will still present an area of abnormality. Gadolinium has been investigated for such cases, but ideally one would like to evaluate the healing of such menisci without having to resort to techniques that are invasive and add further expense to MR imaging.

Considering the tremendous progress that has taken place in MR imaging technology in just a few years, there is every reason to believe that the above issues will be addressed in the not-too-distant future.

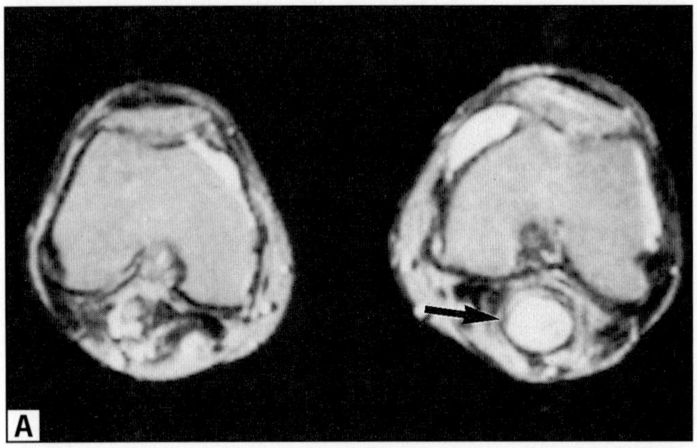

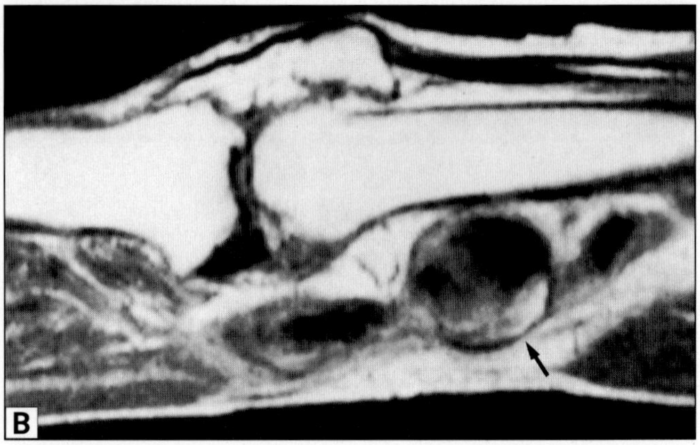

Figure 1-11. Popliteal artery aneurysm. **A**, Axial T_2-weighted spin-echo image (repetition time [TR] and echo time [TE], 2233 and 100) demonstrates a left popliteal artery aneurysm (*arrow*) containing high-signal intensity blood. **B**, Sagittal T_1-weighted spin-echo image (TR and TE, 866 and 30) demonstrates the elongated popliteal artery aneurysm. The largest area of dilatation is indicated by the *arrow*. Areas of flowing blood are visible as low-signal intensity (*dark*) regions.

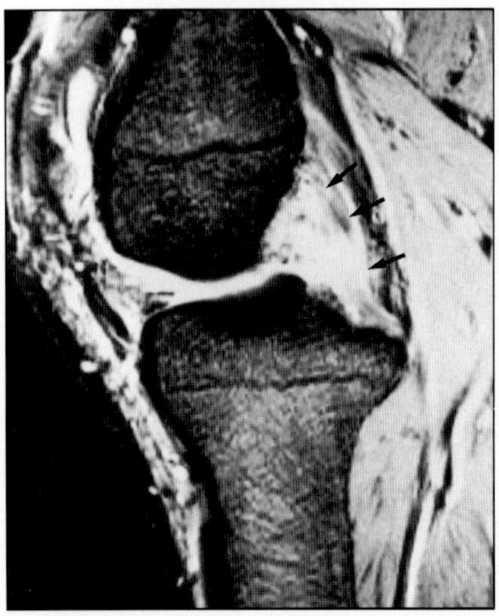

Figure 1-12. Sagittal fast field echo image (repetition time and echo time, 722 and 15; 30° flip angle) demonstrates the magnetic resonance imaging appearance of a torn posterior cruciate ligament. The absence of the normal dark band of the posterior cruciate ligament (*arrows*) indicates a tear of the ligament. Bright signal within this region reflects the presence of fluid and inflammation resulting from the injury.

References and Recommended Reading

Papers of interest, published recently, have been highlighted as:

- • Of interest
- •• Of outstanding interest

1. Singson RD, Feldman F, Staron R, *et al.*: MR imaging of displaced bucket-handle tear of the medial meniscus. *Am J Roentgenol* 1991, 157:1126–1127.

2. Hassine D, Feron JM, Henry Feugeas MC, *et al.*: The meniscofemoral ligaments: Magnetic resonance imaging and anatomic correlations. *Surg Radiol Anat* 1992, 14:59–63.

3. Bronstein R, Kirk P, Hurley J: The usefulness of MRI in evaluating menisci after meniscus repair. *Orthopedics* 1992, 15:149–152.

4. Evancho AM, Fajman WA, Stiles RG, *et al.*: Magnetic resonance imaging of knee menisci: Comparison of spin echo pulse sequences. *Invest Radiol* 1990, 25:1224–1227.

5. Haramati N, Staron RB, Rubin S, *et al.*: The flipped meniscus sign. *Skeletal Radiol* 1993, 22:273–277.

6. Kelly MA, Flock TJ, Kimmel JA, *et al.*: MR imaging of the knee: Clarification of its role. *Arthroscopy* 1991, 7:78–85.

7.• Cannon WD: Problems of the menisci and their treatment. In *The Knee*. Edited by Larson RL, Grana WA. Philadelphia: WB Saunders; 1993:429–470.

Thorough review of the current status of meniscal pathology and treatment.

8. Silverman JM, Mink JH, Deutsch AL: Discoid menisci of the knee: MR imaging appearance. *Radiology* 1989, 173:351–354.

9. Hayashi LK, Yamaga H, Ida K, *et al.*: Arthroscopic meniscectomy for discoid lateral meniscus in children. *J Bone Joint Surg* 1988-A, 70:1495–1500.

10. Araki Y, Ootani M, Furukawa T, *et al.*: MRI of discoid lateral meniscus. *Nippon Igaku Hoshasen Gakkai Zasshi* 1991, 51:1189–1194.

11. Aichroth PM, Patel DV, Marx CL: Congenital discoid lateral meniscus in children: A follow-up study and evolution of management. *J Bone Joint Surg* 1991, 73-B:932–936.

12. Woods GW, Whelan JM: Discoid meniscus. *Clin Sports Med* 1990, 9:695–706.

13. Parisien JS: Arthroscopic treatment of cysts of the menisci. A preliminary report. *Clin Orthop* 1990, 257:154–158.

14. Fielding JR, Franklin D, Kustan J: Popliteal cysts: A reassessment using magnetic resonance imaging. *Skeletal Radiol* 1991, 20:433–435.

15. Lantz B, Singer KM: Meniscal cysts. *Clin Sports Med* 1990, 9:707–725.

16. Coral A, van Holsbeeck M, Adler RS: Imaging of meniscal cyst of the knee in three cases. *Skeletal Radiol* 1989, 18:451–455.

17. Kujala UM, Jaakkola LH, Koskinen SK, *et al.*: Scoring of patellofemoral disorders. *Arthroscopy* 1993, 9:159–163.

18. Koskinen SK, Hurme M, Kujala UM: Restoration of patellofemoral congruity by combined lateral release and tibial tuberosity transposition as assessed by MRI analysis. *Int Orthop* 1991, 15:363–366.

19. Koskinen SK, Hurme M, Kujala UM, *et al.*: Effect of lateral release on patellar motion in chondromalacia: An MRI study of 11 knees. *Acta Orthop Scand* 1990, 61:311–312.

20. Nakanishi K, Inoue M, Harada K, *et al.*: MRI evaluation of the patellar articular cartilage in patients with subluxation of the patella. *Nippon Igaku Hoshasen Gakkai Zasshi* 1991, 51:387–393.

21. Shellock FG: Patellofemoral joint abnormalities in athletes: evaluation by kinematic magnetic resonance imaging. *Top Magn Reson Imaging* 1991, 3:71–95.

22. Laurin CA, Lévesque HP, Dussault R, *et al.*: The abnormal lateral patellofemoral angle: a diagnostic roentgenographic sign of recurrent patellar subluxation. *J Bone Joint Surg* [Am] 1978, 60A:55–60.

23. Grelsamer RP, Bazos AN, Proctor CS: Radiographic analysis of patellar tilt. *J Bone Joint Surg* 1993, 75B: 822–824.

24. Schutzer SF, Ramsby GR, Fulkerson JP: Computed tomographic classification of patellofemoral pain patients. *Orthop Clin North Am* 1986, 17:235–248.

25. Fulkerson JP, Hungerford DS: *Disorders of the Patellofemoral Joint*. Baltimore: Williams and Wilkins; 1990.

26. Masciocchi C, Barile A, Simonetti C, *et al.*: Intra-osseus hidden fractures of the knee in athletes: assessment with magnetic resonance imaging. *Radiol Med* 1993, 85:378–383.

27. Berger E, Ofstein RA, Jackson DW, *et al.*: MRI demonstration of radiographically occult fractures: what have we been missing? *Radiographics* 1989, 9:407–436.

28. Jensen DB, Johansen TP, Bjerg Nielson A, *et al.*: Magnetic resonance imaging in the evaluation of sequelae after tibial plateau fractures. *Skeletal Radiol* 1990, 19:127–129.

29. Resnick D, Niwayama G, eds.: *Diagnosis of Bone and Joint Disorders*, 2nd ed. Philadelphia: W.B. Saunders Co; 1988:2756–3008.

30.• Garrett JC: Osteochondritis Dissecans. In *The Knee*, Edited by Larson RL, Grana WA. Philadelphia: W.B. Saunders Co; 1993:471–488.

Thorough review and description of allograft technique.

31. Milgram JW: Radiological and pathological manifestations of osteochondritis dissecans of the distal femur: a study of 50 cases. *Radiology* 1978, 126:305–331.

32. Aichroth P: Osteochondritis dissecans of the knee. *J Bone Joint Surg* 1971, 53-B:440–447.

33. Desai SS, Patel MR, Michelli LJ, *et al.*: Osteochondritis dissecans of the patella. *J Bone Joint Surg* 1987, 69-B:320–325.

34. Pfeiffer WH, Gross ML, Seeger LL: Osteochondritis dissecans of the patella. MRI evaluation and a case report. *Clin Orthop* 1991, 271:207–211.

35. Garrett JC: Osteochondritis dissecans. *Clin Sports Med* 1991, 10:569–593.

36. al Rowaih A, Bjorkengren A, Willen H, *et al.*: Primary osteonecrosis in the knee evaluated by histopathology and specimen scintimetry related to clinical radiography, scintimetry and MR. *Chir Organi Mov* 1992, 77:257–269.

37. Dey HM, Jaros RH, Swan CS II, *et al.*: Spontaneous femoral osteonecrosis: correlation with MRI. *Clin Nucl Med* 1988, 13:756–758.

38. Singson RD, Zalduondo FM: Value of unenhanced spin-echo MR imaging in distinguishing between synovitis and effusion of the knee. *Am J of Roentgenol* 1992, 159:569–571.

39. Flandry FC, Hughston JC, Jacobson KE, *et al.*: Surgical treatment of diffuse pigmented villonodular synovitis of the knee. *Clin Orthop* 1994, 300:183–192.

40. Mink JH, Reicher MA, Crues JV: *Magnetic Resonance Imaging of the Knee.* New York: Raven Press; 1987:126–127.

41. Mink JH, Deutsch AL: *MRI of the Musculoskeletal System: a Teaching File.* edn 2. New York: Raven Press; 1990:253–311.

42. Steinbach LS, Neumann CH, Stoller DW, *et al.*: MRI of the knee in diffuse pigmented villonodular synovitis. *Clin Imaging* 1989, 13:305–316.

43. Bessette R, Cooley A, Johnson RP, *et al.*: Gadolinium enhanced MRI of pigmented villonodular synovitis of the knee. *J Comput Assist Tomogr* 1992, 16:992–994.

44. Goldman AB, DiCarlo EF: Pigmented villonodular synovitis. Diagnosis and differential diagnosis. *Radiol Clin North Am* 1988, 26:1327–1347.

45. Poletti SC, Gates HS, Martinez SM, *et al.*: The use of magnetic resonance imaging in the diagnosis of pigmented villonodular synovitis. *Orthopedics* 1990, 13:185–190.

46. Abdelwahab IF, Klein MJ, Lewis MM: Case report 817: synovial chondrosarcoma secondary to synovial chondromatosis. *Skeletal Radiol* 1993, 22:623–626.

47. Abraham JH, Canoso JJ: Tumors of soft tissues and bone. *Curr Opin Rheumatol* 1993, 5:193–198.

48. Rosenbaum DH, Hay RM, Adkison DP, *et al.*: Imaging rounds: synovial chondromatosis. *Orthop Rev* 1992, 21:621–628.

49. Osburn AW, Bassett LW, Seeger LL, *et al.*: Case report 609: synovial (osteo) chondromatosis. *Skeletal Radiol* 1990, 19:237–241.

50. Manaster BJ, Doyle AJ: Giant cell tumors of bone. Imaging of bone and soft tissue tumors. *Radiol Clin North Am* 1993, 31:299–323.

51. Herman SD, Mesgarzadeh M, Bonakdarpour A, *et al.*: The role of magnetic resonance imaging in giant cell tumor of bone. *Skeletal Radiol* 1987, 16:635–643.

52. Aoki J, Moriya K, Yamashita K, *et al.*: Giant cell tumors of bone containing large amounts of hemosiderin: MR-pathologic correlation. *J Comput Assist Tomogr* 1991, 15:1024–1027.

53. Abrams HL: *Angiography: Vascular and Interventional Radiology*, edn 3. Boston: Little, Brown & Co.; 1983.

54. Neiman H, Yao JST, Silver TM: Grey-scale ultrasound diagnosis of peripheral arterial aneurysms. *Radiology* 1979, 130:413–416.

55. Victor J, Gielen J, Martens M, *et al.*: Correlation between magnetic resonance imaging and arthroscopy in the diagnosis of anterior cruciate ligament and meniscus lesions. *Acta Orthop Belg* 1991, 57:56–61.

56. Ekelund L, Bjornebrink J, Elmqvist LG: Ultra low field magnetic resonance imaging of acute cruciate ligament tears. *Magn Reson Imaging* 1991, 9:179–185.

57. Rosen MA, Jackson DW, Berger E: Occult osseous lesions documented by magnetic resonance imaging associated with anterior cruciate ligament ruptures. *Arthroscopy* 1991, 7:45–51.

58. Saragaglia D, Rose Pittet L, Lebas JF, *et al.*: Magnetic resonance imaging in studying injuries of the ligaments and menisci of the knee. 85 cases controlled by arthroscopy. *Rev Chir Orthop* 1989, 75:452–458.

59. Tehranzadeh J, Kerr R, Amster J: Magnetic resonance imaging of tendon and ligament abnormalities. Part II: Pelvis and lower extremities. *Skeletal Radiol* 1992, 21:79–86.

60.• Boeree NR, Ackroyd CE: Magnetic resonance imaging of anterior cruciate ligament rupture. *J Bone Joint Surg* 1992, 74B:614–616.

Describes buckling of the posterior cruciate ligament in 60 certain anterior cruciate ligament tears.

61. Liu SH, Osti L, Dorey F, Yao L: Anterior cruciate ligament tear. A new diagnostic index on magnetic resonance imaging. *Clin Orthop* 1994, 302:147–150.

62.• Deutsch AL, Shellock FG, Mink JH: Imaging of the patellofemoral joint: emphasis on advanced techniques. In *The Patellofemoral Joint.* Edited by Fox JM, DelPizzo W. New York: McGraw-Hill; 1993:75–104.

All-inclusive text on the patella.

2

CHAPTER

Office Arthroscopy

JEFFREY L. HALBRECHT

There has been a general trend in the past few years to move procedures out of the expensive environment of the hospital and into ambulatory surgery settings or even into the practitioner's office. Many specialists, including oral surgeons, plastic surgeons, and podiatrists, have been performing surgery in the office setting for decades. In orthopedics, the limiting factor has been—until recently—the expense and cumbersome size of the equipment. Recent advances in arthroscopic technology have now made in-office arthroscopy a viable option.

We have been performing office-based arthroscopy for almost 5 years. Initial indications were for diagnostic evaluation of the knee joint only. Currently, office arthroscopy is being performed for the knee, shoulder, and ankle and includes surgical as well as diagnostic indications.

WHAT IS OFFICE ARTHROSCOPY?

Office arthroscopy is simply the performance of arthroscopic procedures in the office setting. For most practitioners, this involves using small-diameter arthroscopes under local anesthetic in a routine examination room. A few surgeons have taken this concept one step further and have created true ambulatory surgery suites in their offices using intravenous anesthesia and large-diameter arthroscopes for their office procedures. The set-up costs and risks of this latter option are obviously much higher and so far have been limited to a few practices.

History and Indications

The initial stimulus to perform office arthroscopy came from a dissatisfaction with the accuracy of magnetic resonance (MR) imaging. Despite the reported accuracy of this test, many false-negatives and false-positives seem to occur in the clinical practice setting. With the introduction of a flexible fiber optic small-diameter mini arthroscope (Medical Dynamics, Santa Rosa, CA), we undertook a study to compare the accuracy of office arthroscopy of the knee with MR imaging [1]. In a study of 20 patients with knee symptoms, office arthroscopy was found to be significantly more accurate for chondromalacia and meniscal tears, particularly in the postoperative knee (Fig. 2-1). Patients undergoing office arthroscopy experienced no complications and greatly preferred the office arthroscopy to the MR imaging.

Office arthroscopy has become the diagnostic procedure of choice for us in patients with enigmatic complaints about the knee, postoperative complaints, or patients with previously performed equivocal MR imaging scans. Irrigation and debridement of the arthritic knee and shaving chondroplasty of the patella can be quite successful in the office setting using a mini shaving system. An additional indication includes preoperative surgical planning for the early arthritic knee (high tibial osteotomy, unicondylar knee replacement, total knee replacement, or meniscal allograft). The office arthroscope is also extremely useful for evaluating the integrity of a meniscal repair, ligament reconstruction, to help plan a return to sports activities, or for follow-up studies. Therapeutic irrigation and debridement of the degenerative knee is also beneficial. Localized shaving chondroplasty and partial meniscectomies can be performed at the time of the diagnostic procedure under local anesthetic. With the use of supplementary intravenous anesthesia, difficult posterior horn meniscectomies and even lateral releases can be routinely performed [2].

With our success in the knee, it was only natural that we would expand our use of the office arthroscope to other joints. We performed a second study, this time comparing office arthroscopy of the shoulder with MR imaging. In a group of 20 patients, office arthroscopy proved to be more accurate for the evaluation of partial tears of the rotator cuff, for labral tears, for lesions of the biceps, and for articular cartilage lesions [3].

Office arthroscopy of the shoulder is more challenging than its counterpart in the knee. Small-diameter flexible arthroscopes are not rigid enough for manipulation around the soft-tissue bulk of the shoulder and more length is necessary. The performance of shoulder arthroscopy in the office has led us back to more rigid and somewhat larger arthroscopes. We now use a 2.7-mm rigid rod arthroscope for all of our procedures (Fig. 2-2).

We have found fewer indications for office arthroscopy of the shoulder than for the knee. Current indications include patients with an equivocal MR image or an MR imaging finding that does not match the clinical symptoms, patients with painful clicking to evaluate the labrum, symptomatic postop-

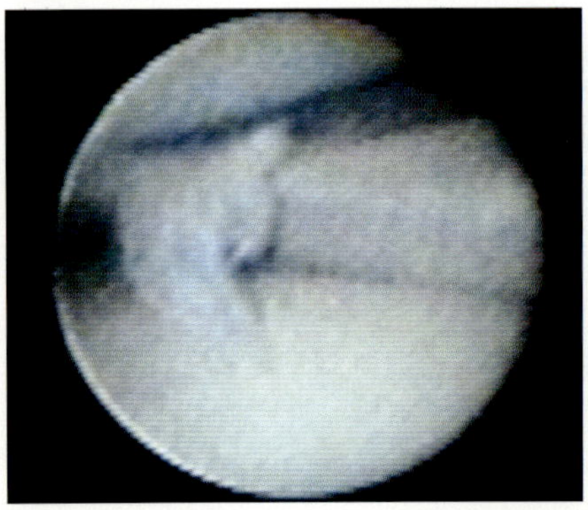

Figure 2-1. Meniscal tear missed by magnetic resonance imaging, as seen by office arthroscopy.

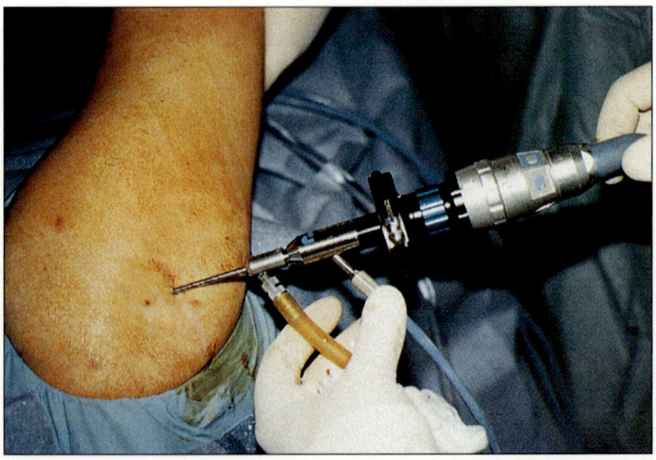

Figure 2-2. A 2.7-mm rigid rod arthroscope is used for office arthroscopy.

erative patients to evaluate the integrity of a rotator cuff repair or Bankart reconstruction, and patients with suspected degenerative arthritis for evaluation and irrigation. Patients with impingement syndrome can also be easily evaluated for rotator cuff tears. Office arthroscopy is particularly helpful for differentiating partial-thickness from full-thickness tears. Shoulder arthroscopy is technically more challenging to perform in the office and we have found fewer indications for performing it than for the knee (almost a 10:1 ratio).

TECHNIQUE

Patients are brought into the office as though for a routine examination (Fig. 2-3). Gowns are provided for shoulder surgery; patients usually wear shorts for knee surgery. A routine consent is obtained. Insurance authorization is obtained prior to the procedure and has not been a problem to date.

Anesthetic

Injection is performed with 30 cm^3 of a 1:1 combination of 0.25% bupivacaine hydrochloride with epinephrine and 1% lidocaine. For the knee, anteromedial and anterolateral portal sites are injected as well as the intra-articular space. On occasion, a superolateral portal is injected as well if dynamic patella tracking is to be evaluated from above. In the shoulder, a posterior portal is injected using an 18-gauge spinal needle to ensure adequate penetration into the glenohumeral joint and the subacromial space. We have found that it is easier to perform the shoulder injection with the patient in the lateral decubitus position with the arm in traction (Fig. 2-4).

In our practice, patients are not given an intravenous line or any additional sedation on a routine basis. At the surgeon's discretion, anxious patients may be offered an oral sedative one half hour prior to the procedure.

When intravenous sedation is being used, the surgeon administers midazolam hydrochloride (0.025 to 0.05 mg/kg) and fentanyl citrate (2 mg/kg) prior to initiating the procedure. Naloxone hydrochloride is kept handy for reversal of both of these anesthetic agents if necessary [2]. When intravenous sedation is used, monitoring becomes essential. Recommendations are to use a blood pressure monitor, pulse oximeter, and electrocardiogram. Resuscitation equipment should be available regardless of what type of anesthesia is used and should include oxygen, endotracheal tubes, a laryngoscope, an ambu bag, and possibly even a defibrillator. Surgeons currently using intravenous sedation often have a nurse anesthetist monitoring the patient during the procedure. In our practice, using local anesthetic only, we have not found it necessary to monitor the patients thus far, although we keep an emergency resuscitation kit available at all times, and have personnel trained in cardiopulmonary resuscitation.

Equipment

Many systems are currently available for office arthroscopy. They range from disposable to flexible to scaled-down rigid rod systems. The disadvantage of the flexible rod system is the 0° angle of view, some-

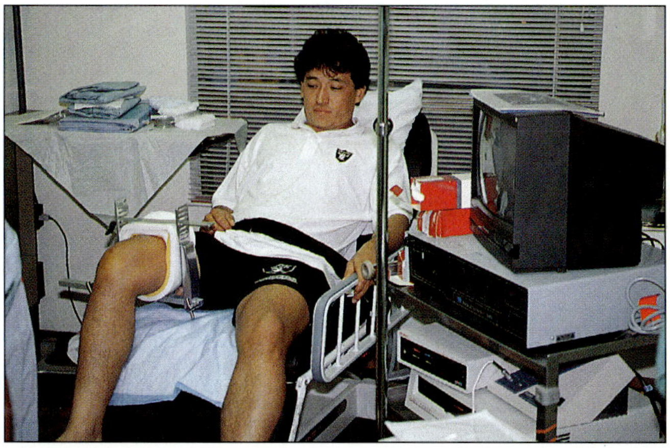

Figure 2-3. A routine examination room can be used to perform office arthroscopy.

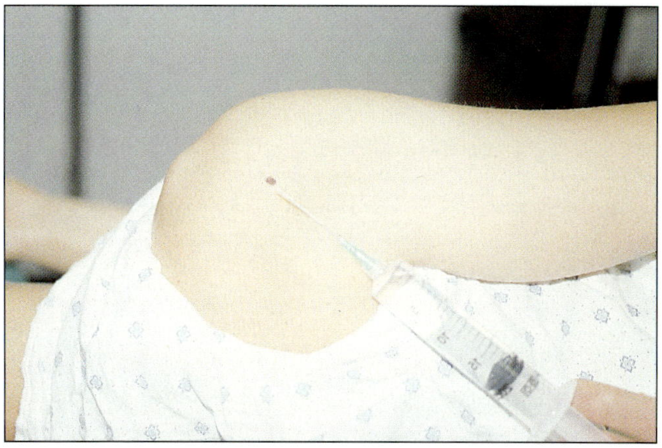

Figure 2-4. Shoulder injections for local anesthesia are given in the lateral decubitus position.

what inferior optics, and the lack of rigidity for use in the shoulder. Its advantage is ease of use and greater resilience. The disadvantage of the disposable system is inferior optics and flow characteristics as well as lack of rigidity. A number of companies now make scaled-down versions of hospital-based rigid rod lens systems for use in the office (Fig. 2-5). The key features necessary for a dependable system are quality of optics, ease of set-up and use, adequate flow for intraoperative irrigation, a 30° angle, and of course, reasonable cost. A good system can be had for somewhere between $10 000 and $20 000 for the arthroscopy equipment alone. Total set-up costs for in-office arthroscopy can range from $25 000 to $100 000 including all equipment and facility improvements.

We have also found it indispensable to have an operating room type table for the performance of office arthroscopy. This table should have a surgical bar for attachment of a leg holder or post and a shoulder traction bar. We initially performed our knee arthroscopies without a thigh holder and have noted a tremendous improvement in the ease of the procedure since adding this option. (Fig. 2-6). In a similar fashion, shoulder arthroscopies were initially performed in the sitting position. However, this position increases the risk of vasovagal reaction and was not as well tolerated as the lateral decubitus position (Fig. 2-7).

The surgical table we currently use is on locking casters and can be easily moved to any position necessary in the examination room to accommodate the procedure and side to be operated on. The chair is pneumatic and goes from the seated or knee arthroscopy position to the supine shoulder arthroscopy position and can be placed in Trendelenburg if necessary (Fig. 2-8). Table height can also be adjusted easily.

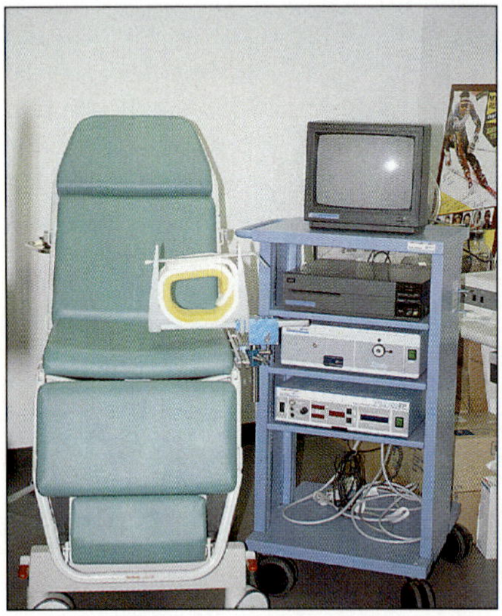

Figure 2-5. Scaled-down versions of standard arthroscopy equipment is available for office use.

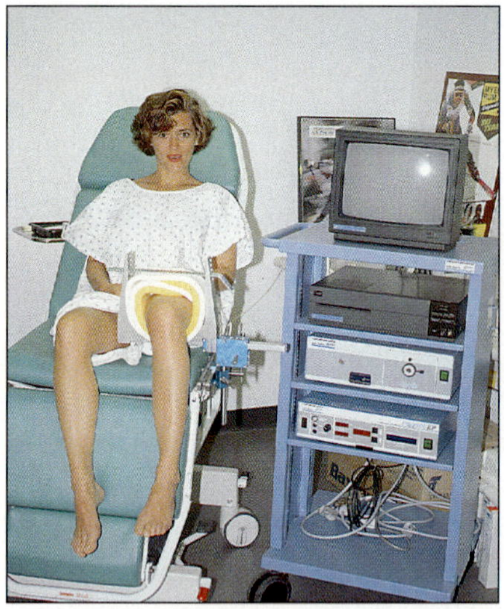

Figure 2-6. A thigh holder is extremely helpful for stabilizing the knee and eliminating the need for an assistant.

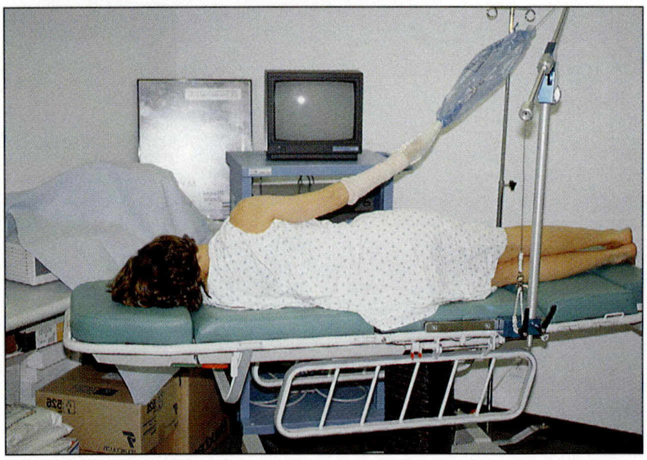

Figure 2-7. Office shoulder arthroscopies are best performed in the lateral decubitus position.

Knee Arthroscopy

The patient is anesthetized a minimum of 15 min prior to the actual incision and placed in a leg holder on the surgical table. An assistant prepares the patient and set-up for the procedure. Instruments are soaked in Cidex (Johnson and Johnson Medical, Arlington, TX) for 20 min and washed with sterile water. The knee is painted with chlorhexidine gluconate or povidone-iodine, and an extremity drape and stockinette is applied. The surgeon and the assistant then dress in gowns and gloves without scrubbing. Instruments required for diagnostic arthroscopy are a 2.7-mm arthroscope, arthroscopic camera and light cord, an arthroscopic sheath, sharp and blunt trocars, a #11 blade, cystoscopy tubing, a 60-cm^3 syringe, intravenous extension tubing, a 1-L bag of lactated Ringer's solution, a sterile basin, and some 4 x 4-in gauze sponges. An 18-gauge spinal needle or a temporomandibular joint mini probe is used for probing.

The smallest portal incision possible is used. Irrigation is performed through gravity with syringe assistance as necessary. Gravity-assist devices are available and have been used on occasion.

For surgical arthroscopy in the office, small baskets and a mini shaver system are used. Suction is provided by a portable suction unit.

For knee arthroscopy, the only discomfort occasionally felt is thigh pain on applying valgus force to the knee against the thigh post. It is important to pad the thigh well. The leg holder we currently use has a thick Velcro thigh pad that works very well (Fig. 2-6).

Shoulder Arthroscopy

For shoulder arthroscopy, the only additional equipment required is a shoulder traction device (Figs. 2-7 and 2-8). Ten to 15 lbs of traction are applied using an arm gauntlet. Patients do experience discomfort after 30 min in this position, so the practitioner performing office shoulder arthroscopy must be skilled and efficient. The average procedure time in our series for diagnostic shoulder arthroscopy was approximately 12 min. The practitioner should be comfortable performing routine bursoscopy and glenohumeral arthroscopy before attempting shoulder arthroscopy in the office.

Recently, we have been performing shaving of partial-thickness rotator cuff tears, flap tears of the labrum, and bursectomies under local anesthesia. Preliminary results have been very promising.

Postoperative Care

Patients are given bandages for their portal sites. No analgesics have been necessary following the use of a local anesthetic. Patients are advised to shower and change their bandages daily. Activities are limited for the first few days. Most patients are able to return to work within 2 days. Sports activities are restricted for 1 week.

Complications

To date, we are aware of very few complications related to office arthroscopic procedures. We have had one patient suffer a vasovagal reaction to the initial

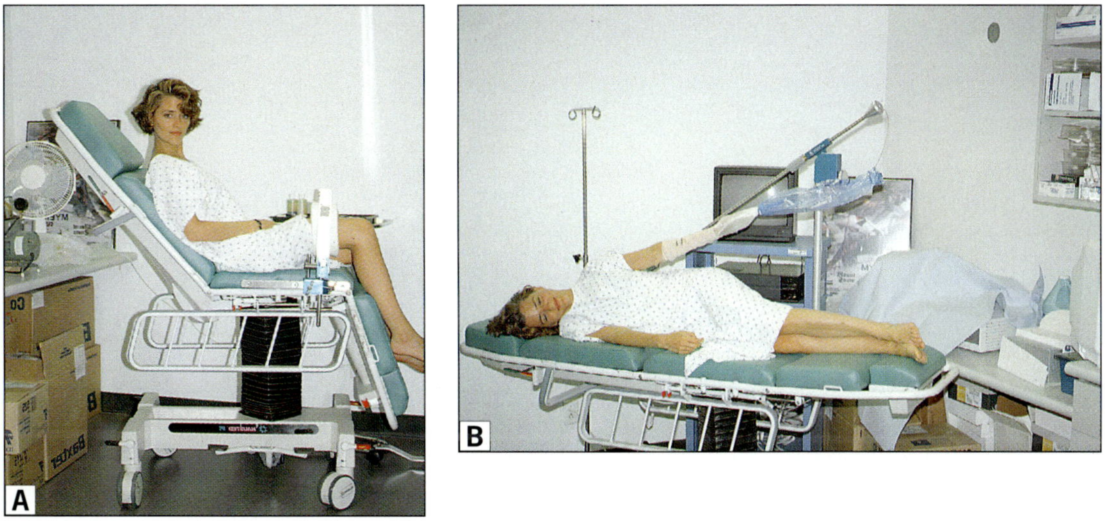

Figure 2-8. A versatile light-weight surgical chair is extremely helpful. This particular chair can go from **A**, a seated position, to **B**, a supine position, has surgical side rails for attachment of traction and leg holder devices, and is on casters for easy mobilization.

anesthetic injection and have had one superficial cellulitis of a portal site out of over 100 cases. We are also aware of one case of seizure following what appears to be a reaction to an overdose of local anesthetic given by another physician in our community.

CONCLUSION

Office arthroscopy is becoming an increasingly attractive option in today's healthcare environment. Diagnostic office arthroscopy is currently the most practical option for most practitioners. Limited surgical office arthroscopy is possible under local anesthesia. However, for complete surgical capabilities, intravenous anesthesia is necessary and requires a significantly greater cost as well as risk. As healthcare reform pushes us to perform more of our surgery in an outpatient and even an office setting, office arthroscopy will become an increasingly attractive option.

REFERENCES AND RECOMMENDED READING

Papers of interest, published recently, have been highlighted as
- • Of special interest
- •• Of outstanding interest

1. Halbrecht JL, Jackson DW: Office arthroscopy: a diagnostic alternative. *Arthroscopy* 1992, 3:320–326.

2.•• Small NC: *Office Operative Arthroscopy*. New York: Raven Press; 1994.

Comprehensive review of all aspects of office arthroscopy, including cost issues and reimbursement.

3.•• Halbrecht JL, Wolf EM: Office arthroscopy of the shoulder. *Orthop Clin N Am* 1993, 24:193–200.

Compares diagnostic accuracy of office arthroscopy to magnetic resonance imaging for the shoulder.

3

CHAPTER

The Use of Infusion Pumps in Arthroscopic Surgery

J. SERGE PARISIEN

The successful outcome of any arthroscopic procedure depends primarily on perfect visualization of the intra-articular structures. This visualization depends on the availability of a good optic and video camera system and adequate joint distention. Proper joint distention by a medium such as gas or fluid [1] enables the arthroscopic surgeon to accurately provide a diagnosis and to safely manipulate the fine microsurgical instruments.

Currently, most surgeons prefer to use a fluid medium such as normal saline or Ringer's solution [2]. The latter is advocated by some because it is a more physiologic solution for the articular cartilage. The methods of delivering the fluid medium into the joint vary. For many years, joint irrigation was achieved through a gravity system in which 3- or 6-L bags were hung 1 or 2 m above the operating table (Fig. 3-1). The flow obtained through the arthroscope follows Poiseuille's formula [3]:

Flow = Pressure/Resistance.

Inflow can be obtained through the arthroscopic sheath or through a separate cannula placed in the suprapatellar pouch. When obtained through the arthroscope sheath, the high resistance from the spigot and water canal must be considered. However, this can be compensated for by elevating the bags of fluid or by using inflow lines with a large inner diameter. Also, most arthroscopic cannulas now are capable of delivering 200 cm^3 per min through the water canal [4]. Although the inflow is quicker, it will slow down when the intra-articular pressure from capsular distention approaches the pressure by gravity from the suspended bag. The rate of inflow will also vary with the outflow speed and requires meticulous clamping and unclamping of the outflow tubing by the assistant.

When the inflow is through a separate cannula, as advocated by Johnson [5], a very strong suction may be necessary through the arthroscope. The disadvantage of such a system is the possibility of clouding due to the exit of joint debris through the visual field.

An elevated intra-articular pressure is important to control intra-articular bleeding as well. The minimal pressure necessary for good visualization has been found to be around 28 mm Hg [6,7]. Good capsular distention requires 70 mm Hg according to Ewing and coworkers [7]. The knee position also affects the intra-articular pressure. Noyes and coworkers reported pressures of 150 mm Hg by flexing the knee from 30° to 80° in a closed fluid system (Noyes and coworkers, Paper presented at the Annual Meeting of the AANA, Houston, 1987). In contrast, Ewing and coworkers [7] reported high transient values of 750 mm Hg in a closed fluid system and values of 140 mm Hg in an open fluid system.

Increases in pressure in the suprapatellar pouch (up to 400 mm Hg) and in the posteromedial compartment (up to 300 mm Hg) have also been reported by Dolk and Augustini [8] in their comparison of three irrigation systems for motorized arthroscopic surgery.

Mastering the control of both flow and pressure with the gravity system may not be easy even for the most dedicated team of assistants and circulating nurses.

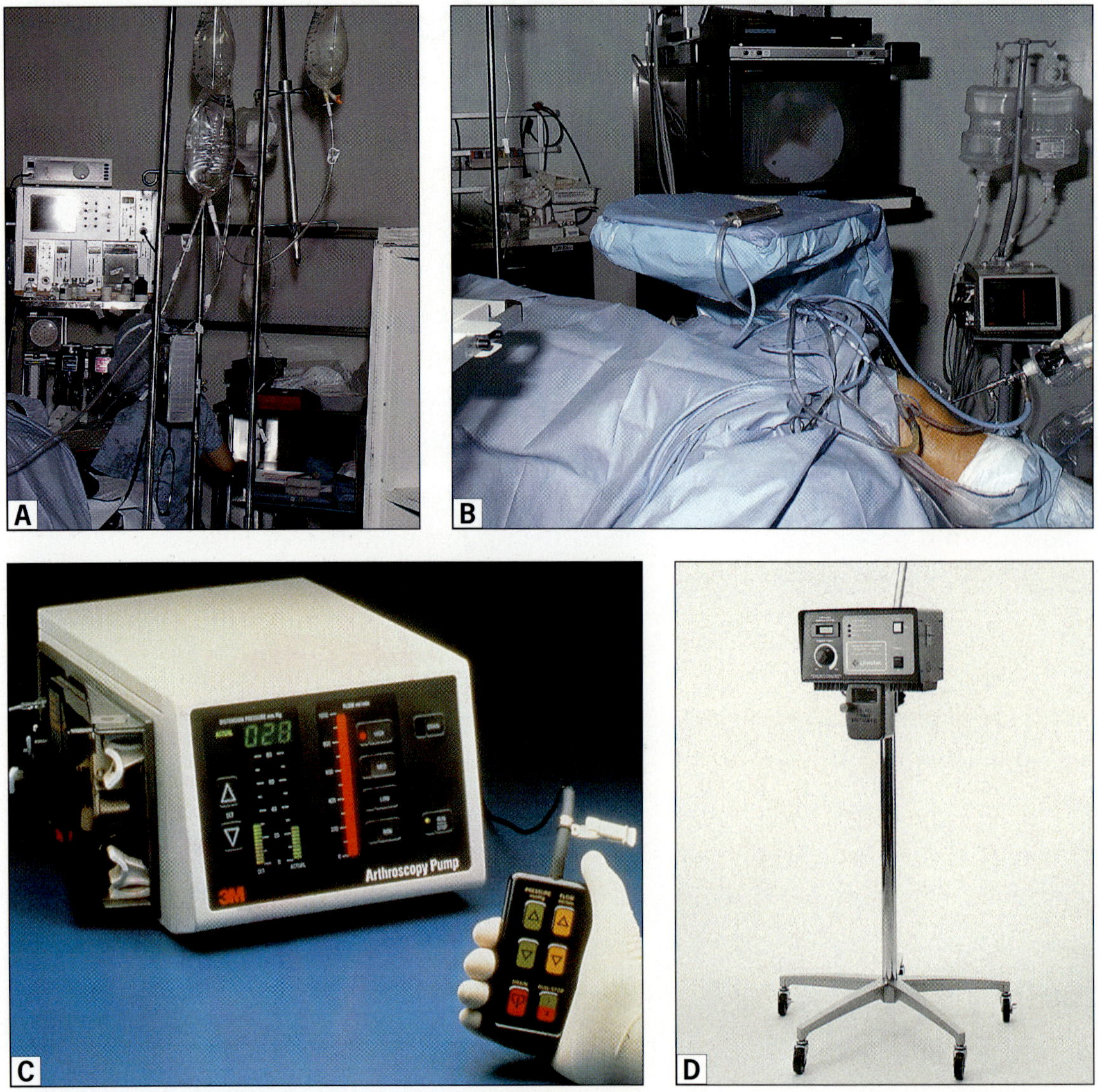

Figure 3-1. Infusion pumps. **A**, Gravity system for irrigation. **B**, Knee positioning for arthroscopic surgery with video camera and infusion pump next to the knee. **C**, Commercial infusion pump (Photo courtesy of 3M, St. Paul, MN). **D**, Commercial infusion pump (Photo courtesy of Linvatec Corp., Largo, FL).

The addition of the mechanical irrigation system to the armamentarium has allowed for better control of flow and pressure inside the joint cavity. This control can be performed by gravity outflow drainage, as it was used in Sweden for years, [3,9] or as it is more commonly done now by the use of pressure-sensing monitors. The latter can automatically shut down the pumps when the preset pressure levels are lost and control the flow and pressure independently. A special hand touch pad control allows the surgeon to control flow rates and pressure levels. With flow rates of 45 cm^3 per min, Bergstrom and Gillquist [9] reported that pressures between 40 and 60 mm Hg obtained with a pump gave good visualization. Modern pumps can offer various flow rates ranging from 0 to 1000 mL per min and pressures up to 100 mm Hg. Flow rates of up to 1500 mL per min have been noted with the Arthro-Flo, High Flow Irrigator (Davol, Cranston, RI).

Advantages and Disadvantages

The advantages of the infusion pump are numerous. The ideal pump should not only be capable of delivering constant intra-articular pressure to cause tamponade of small, intra-articular vessels, but it should regulate the flow rate on demand and include a safety device to avoid very high intra-articular pressure.

The disadvantages of the mechanical pump are the high cost and the complexity of the multitube set-up system that can be confusing to operating room personnel.

Technique

Presently, infusion pumps are being used successfully for various areas of the body, *eg*, the knee, glenohumeral joint, subacromial space, ankle, elbow, wrist, and hip joints.

Knee

The patient is placed supine with the foot of the table bent 90° (Fig. 3-1). The opposite lower extremity may be positioned in a well leg support.

Superomedially, approximately 1 cm above the superomedial pole of the patella, an incision is made for the introduction of the pump cannula with its sensing device, making sure that the cannula is placed distal to any suprapatellar plica that may be present (Fig. 3-2).

The joint is infused with a few cm^3 of fluid. The arthroscope is then placed through the inferolateral portal in order to check the position of the pump cannula (Fig. 3-3). The inflow is then switched to the arthroscope and the suction tubing to the outflow cannula (Fig. 3-4).

Diagnostic examinations can be performed using low flow and a pressure of 40 mm Hg. The flow can be adjusted to clear away the blood and articular debris from the field of view, and the pressure can be adjusted to maintain distention when power equipment is being used.

To prevent extravasation of fluid, large capsular incisions should be avoided and all fenestrations of the cannula system must be located inside the joint. A sensory arthroscope sheath system is also available that allows simultaneous viewing through the arthroscope, fluid inflow, and monitoring of the intra-articular pressure at the operative site (Fig. 3-5).

Shoulder

Arthroscopic procedures for the shoulder can be performed with the patient in the lateral decubitus position or in the sitting position (Fig. 3-6). Various portals are available: posterior, superior, anterosuperior, and anteroinferior (Fig. 3-7). The posterior

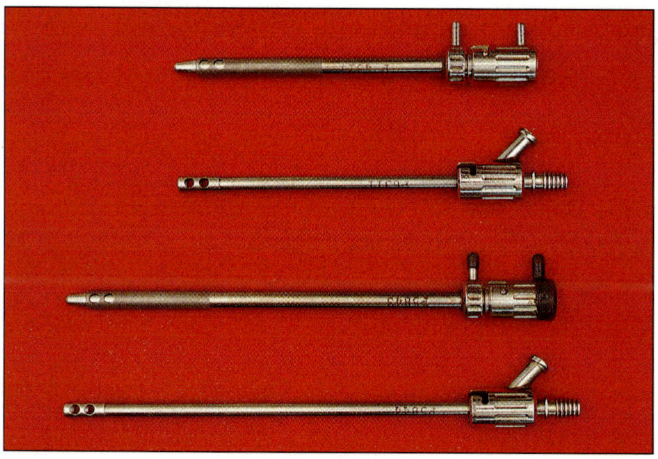

Figure 3-2. Combination cannula with inflow-outflow and pressure gauge.

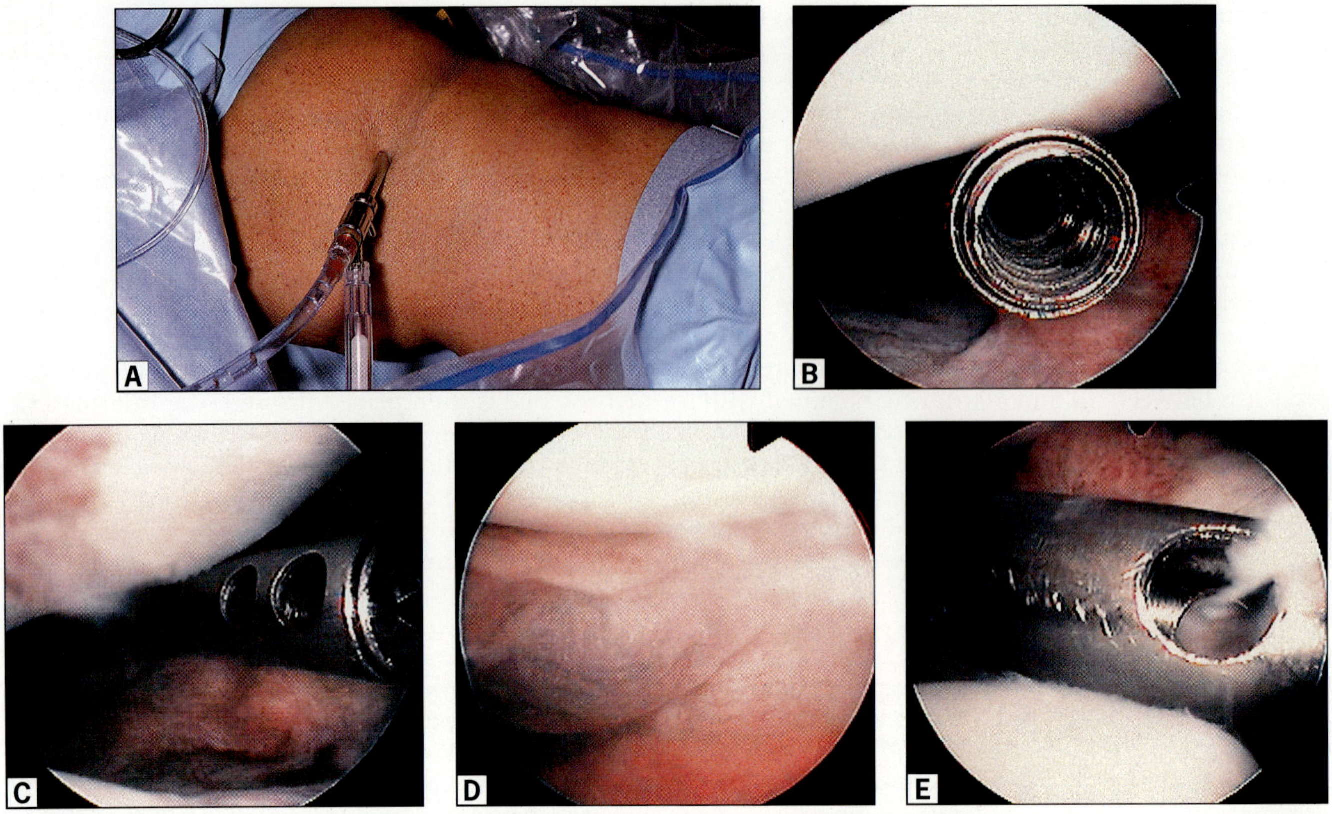

Figure 3-3. Placement of the infusion pump for knee surgery. **A,** After an incision is made at the superomedial aspect of the patella for the introduction of the pump cannula, the inflow tubing is attached to the pump cannula so that the joint cavity can be distended with some fluid. **B**, Intra-articular placement of the cannula. **C**, Fenestrations of the cannula are seen without obstruction. **D**, If the cannula is placed above an existing complete suprapatellar plica, extravasation of fluid above the plica can collapse the suprapatellar pouch. **E**, The cannula is redirected below the plica into the joint cavity.

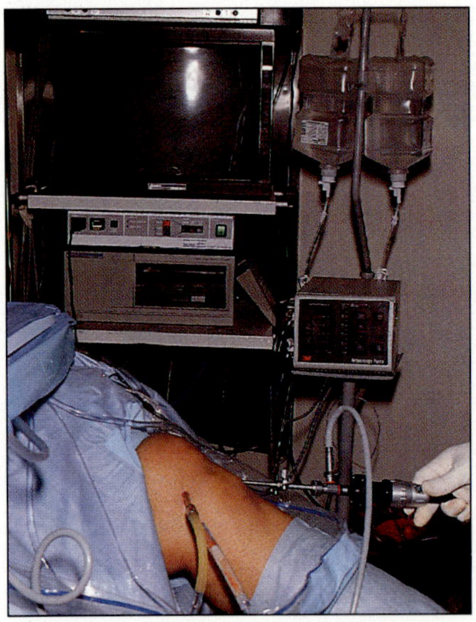

Figure 3-4. Inflow is switched to the arthroscope with the outflow attached to the pump cannula.

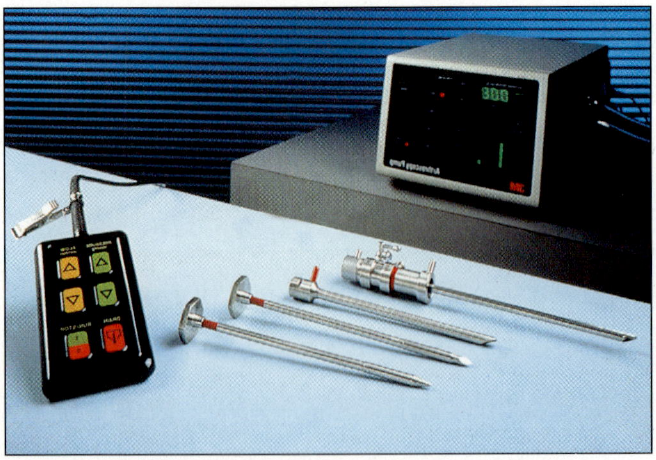

Figure 3-5. The sensory scope sheath system for the arthroscope. Note the fluid inflow and pressure gauge.

portal, which is the entrance portal for the arthroscope, is developed approximately 2 cm below and 1 cm medial to the posterior tip of the acromion. Some authors prefer not to distend the joint with fluid prior to portal placement in order to better identify the landmarks of the posterior aspect of the shoulder [10]. The superior portal can be used for the combination cannula and is located in the space between the distal clavicle and the scapular spine (Fig. 3-8). Pressure of 40 to 60 mm Hg can control bleeding by tamponade of the capillaries.

For subacromial decompression, the same posterior and anterosuperior portals used for the glenohumeral joint can be utilized. A lateral portal (Fig. 3-9), developed approximately 2 to 3 cm below and lateral to the anterolateral corner of the acromion, is necessary as well. The combination cannula can be placed through the anterior portal with the arthroscope and the

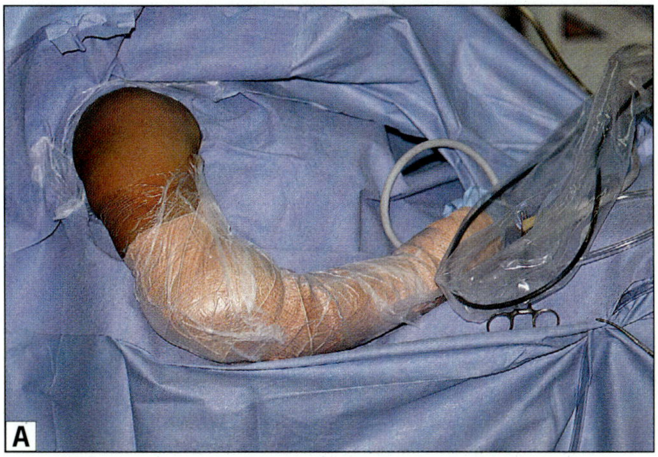

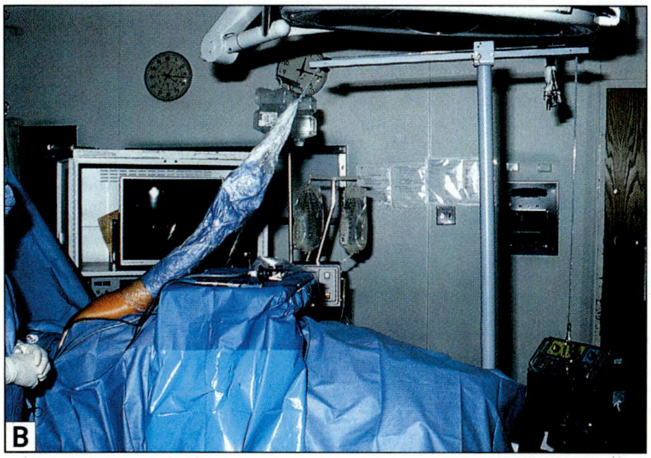

Figure 3-6. A, The sitting position and **B**, lateral position for shoulder arthroscopy.

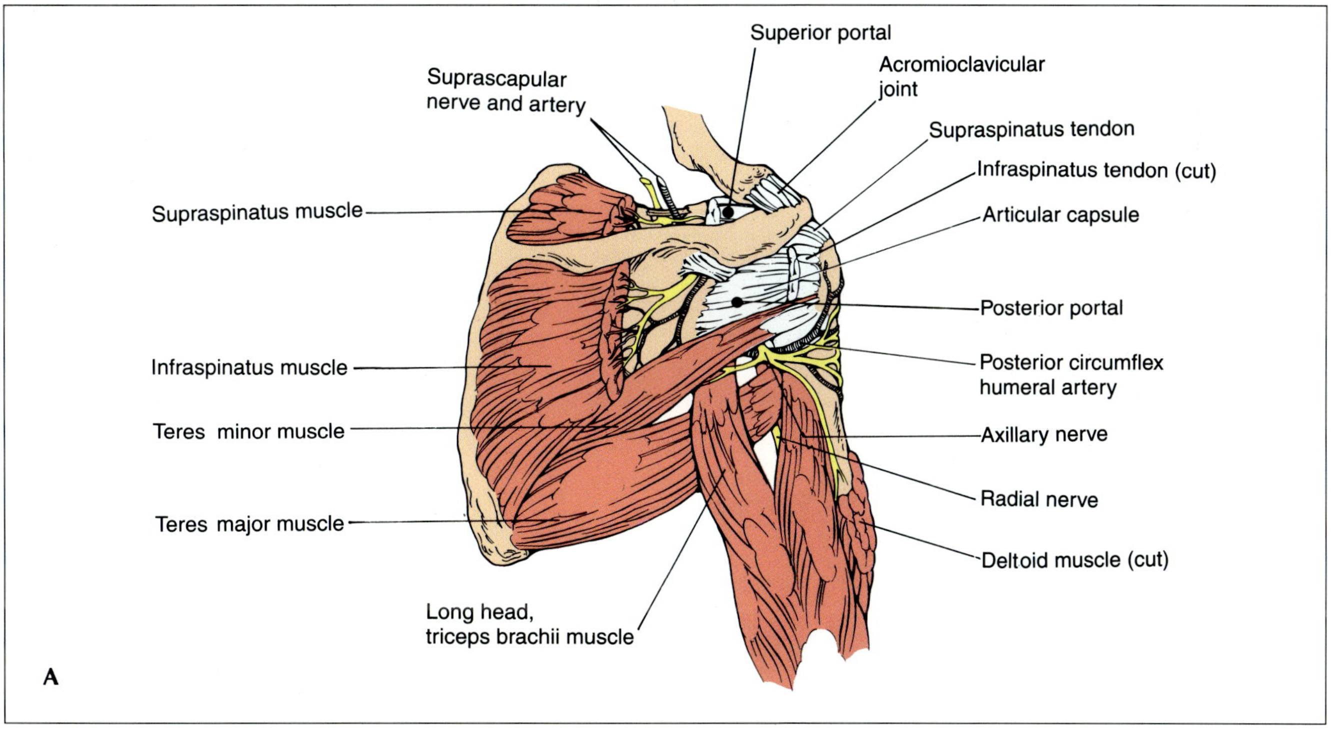

Figure 3-7. Arthroscopic positioning for shoulder surgery. **A**, Posterior view of the shoulder with posterior and superior portals. *(continued)*

motorized instrument placed through the posterior and lateral portals interchangeably.

Ankle

Two anterior portals—the anteromedial and anterolateral—are commonly used for ankle arthroscopy. The posterolateral portal may be used for placement of the inflow cannula when the gravity system is preferred (Fig. 3-10).

With the infusion pump, it is preferable to use the combination cannula anteriorly to have it under constant observation—especially if mechanical distraction (invasive or noninvasive) is not used. This cannula can be placed through an accessory medial portal by using a snug incision (Fig. 3-11).

A small joint cannula fluid control system is available for small joints such as the ankle, elbow, and wrist. It uses a specially designed tube set that diminishes the volume of flow delivered into the joint (Fig. 3-12).

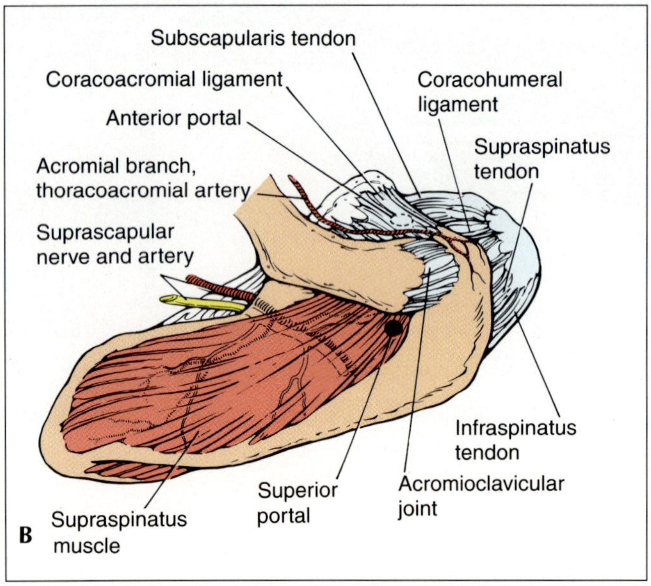

Figure 3-7. (*continued*) **B**, Superior view of the shoulder with superior and anterior portals.

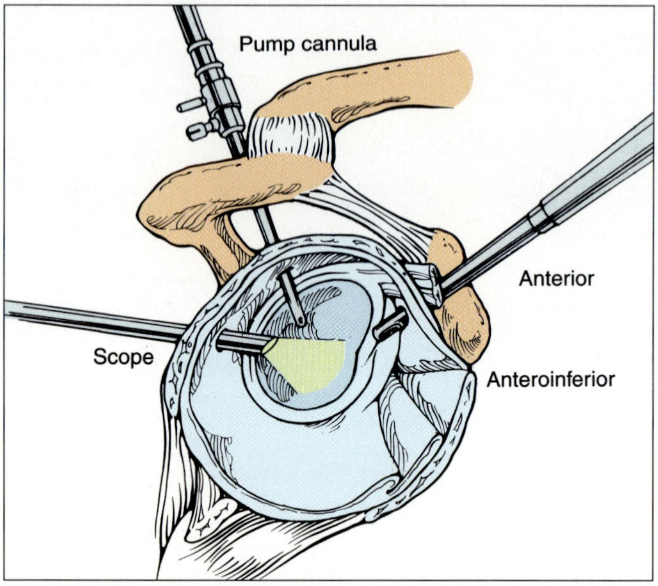

Figure 3-8. Pump cannula in the superior portal. The arthroscope is placed posteriorly; the shaver is placed anteriorly.

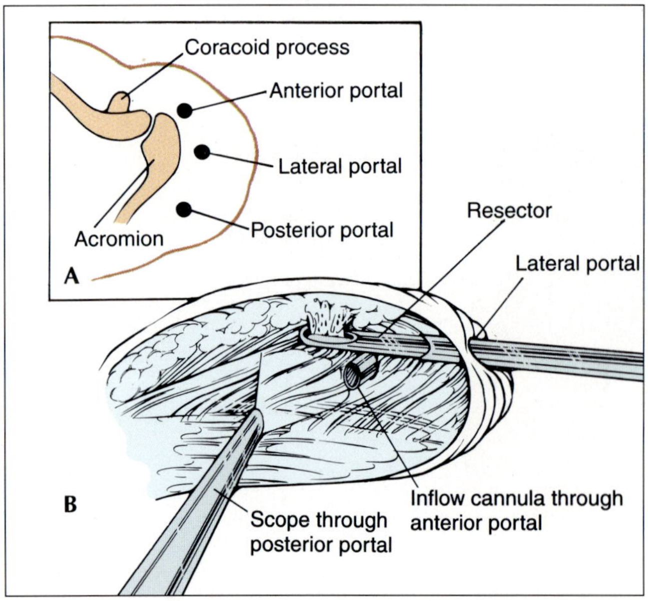

Figure 3-9. Subacromial decompression. **A**, Subacromial portals. **B**, Subacromial space with the arthroscope through the posterior portal, the shaver through the lateral portal, and the inflow cannula through the anterior portal.

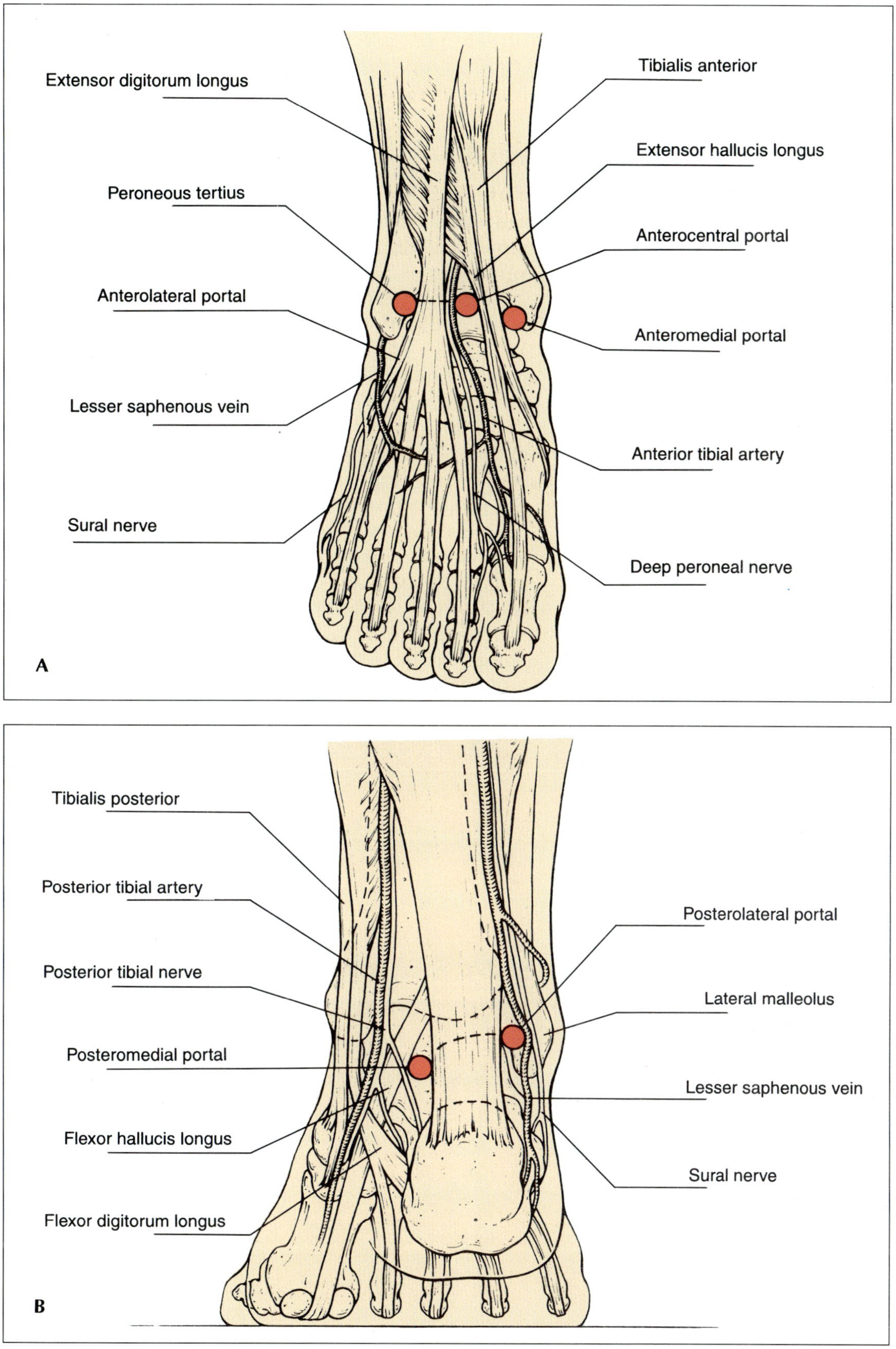

Figure 3-10. Ankle arthroplasty. **A**, Anterior portals for ankle arthroscopy. **B**, Posterior portals for ankle arthroscopy. The inflow cannula can be placed through the posterolateral portal.

Elbow

For elbow arthroscopy, the patient can be placed in any of the following three positions: supine, prone, or lateral decubitus. The two anterior portals can be used for scope and instrumentation, respectively. An accessory medial portal can be added for the insertion of the pressure sensor (Fig. 3-13). Two different lengths of cannulas are available: 2.5 cm and 5 cm. The teardrop configuration of the cannula head prevents it from slipping out of the joint.

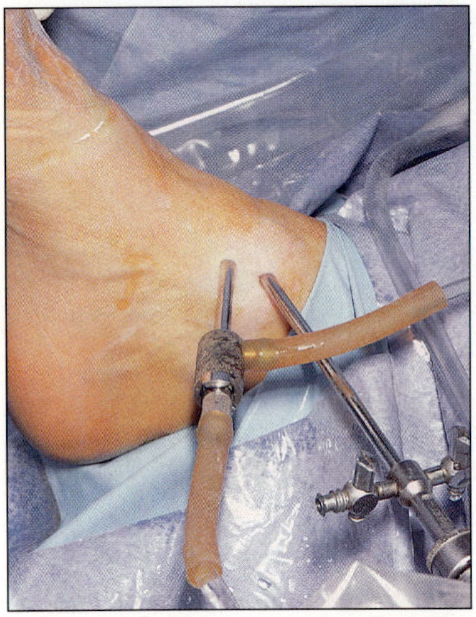

Figure 3-11. The pump cannula is placed through the accessory medial portal during ankle arthroscopy.

Wrist

Although the wrist is a small joint, infusion pumps can be used for arthroscopic surgical procedures. The same small cannulas previously described with lengths varying from 2.5 cm to 5 cm can be used.

The entry portal for the arthroscope is placed between the third and fourth compartments (Fig. 3-14). The 6-R portal, which is radial to the sixth compartment, is used for the insertion of the small-joint cannula [11]. The inflow tubing is attached to the stopcock of the arthroscopic sheath, while the outflow and pressure-sensing device are fitted to the small-joint cannula system. After distention of the joint with a pressure setting of 20 mm Hg, the flow can be adjusted accordingly. It is important to make sure that the cannula for the pump is free of any synovial debris and that fenestrations are inside the joint cavity [12]. The 4-5 portal can be used for instrumentation. During the procedure, exchange of portals can be performed when necessary.

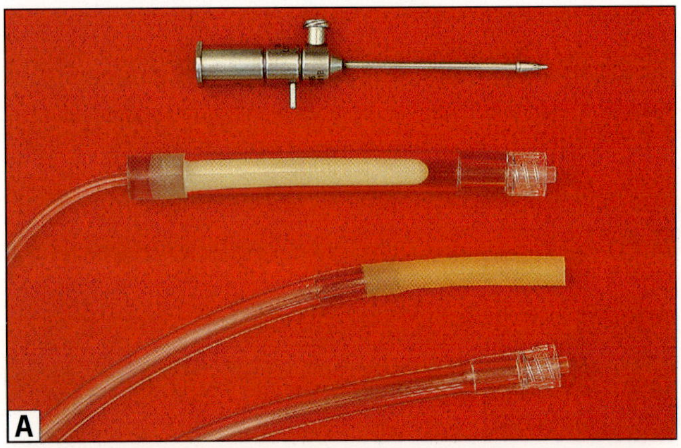

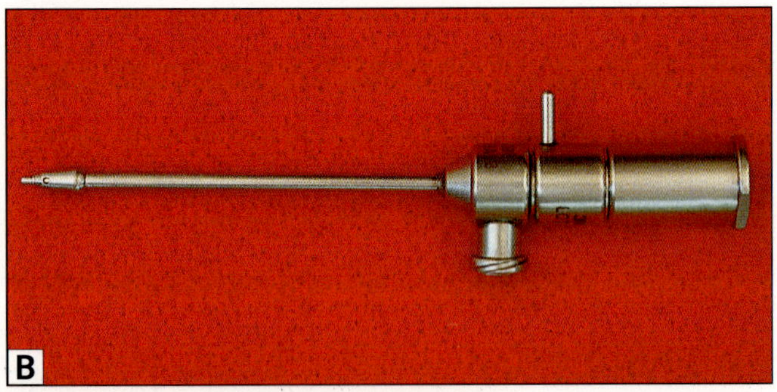

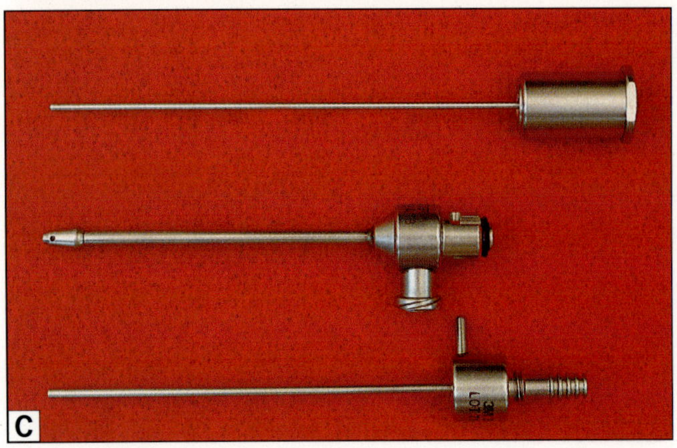

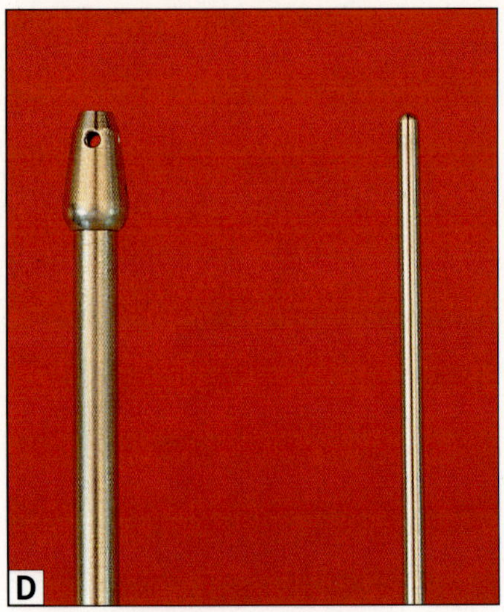

Figure 3-12. Small joint cannula fluid control system. **A**, Small tubing set for delivering fluids into a small joint. **B**, Small pump cannula. **C**, Pump cannula disassembled. **D**, Close-up of cannula showing teardrop configuration of the head.

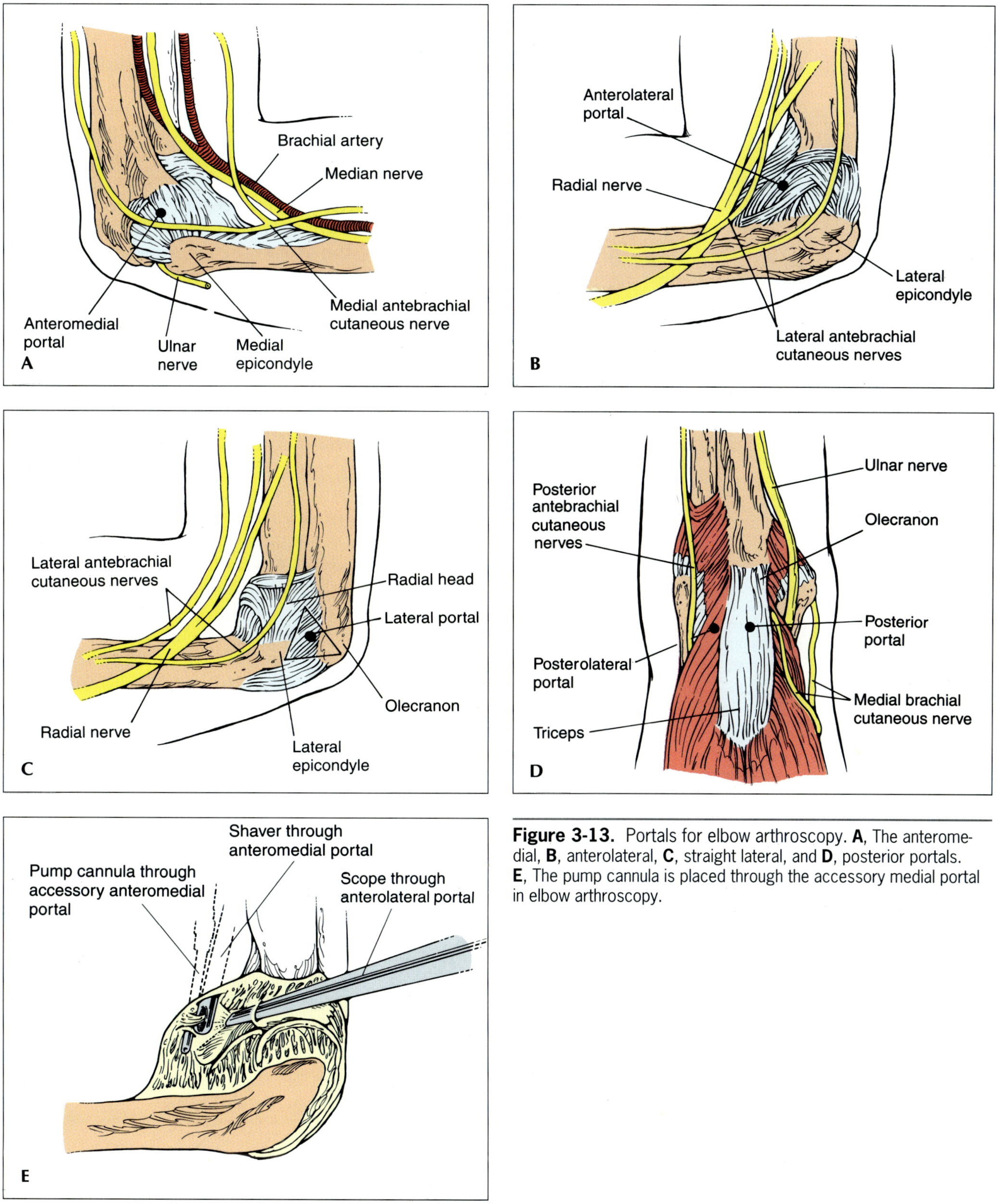

Figure 3-13. Portals for elbow arthroscopy. **A**, The anteromedial, **B**, anterolateral, **C**, straight lateral, and **D**, posterior portals. **E**, The pump cannula is placed through the accessory medial portal in elbow arthroscopy.

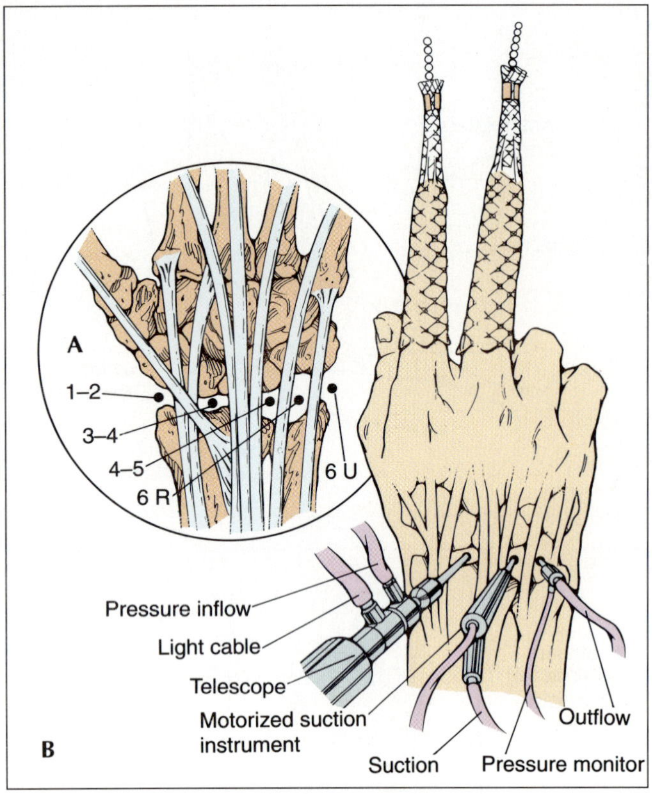

Figure 3-14. **A**, Portals for wrist arthroscopy. **B**, The scope with inflow is in the 3-4 portal, the motorized instrument is placed in the 4-5 portal, and the pump cannula with outflow is placed in the 6-R portal.

Hip

Hip arthroscopy can be performed with the patient supine or in the lateral decubitus position. When the infusion pump is used, the patient is usually placed laterally with the joint distracted using the Hip Distraktor (Arthronix, New City, New York). The three available portals, *ie*, the direct anterior and the anterolateral and posterolateral portals (placed anterior and posterior to the greater trochanter) can accommodate the scope, the cannula for the pump, and motorized instrumentation [13] (Fig. 3-15). An initial pressure of 20 mm Hg is sufficient to maintain joint distention with a low or medium flow. Again, care should be taken to minimize fluid extravasation.

Complications

Few reports on complications associated with the use of the infusion pump are available [14•,15]. Air extravasation and pneumoscrotum were reported during knee arthroscopy [14•] which were probably secondary to leaks of inflow tubing. Significant fluid extravasation has been reported by Noyes and Spievack [16] during arthroscopy with a foot-pedal–controlled fluid delivery system.

Compartment syndrome complications due to fluid extravasation during arthroscopic surgery have been reported with gravity flow as well as with the use of

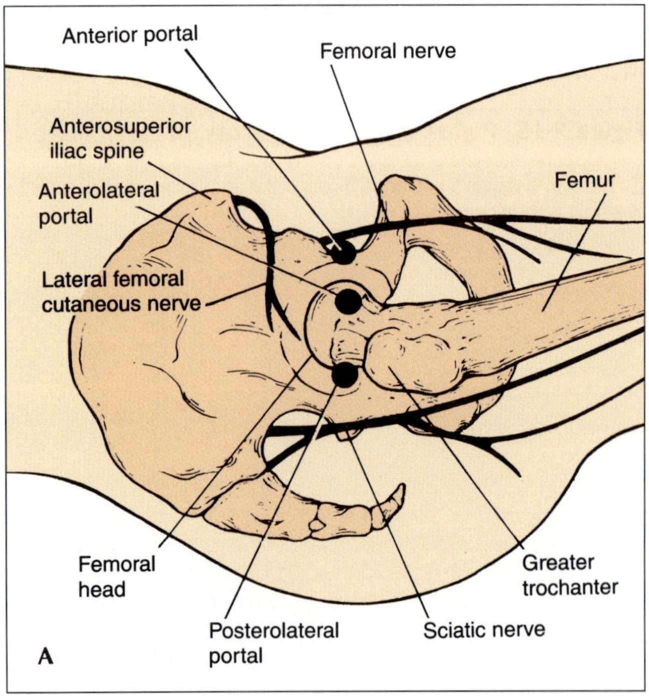

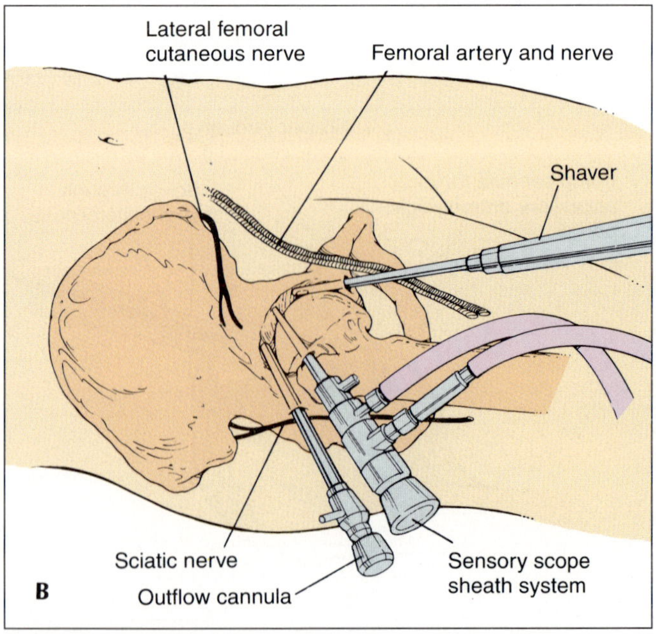

Figure 3-15. **A**, Portals for hip arthroscopy. **B**, With regard to the hip joint, the outflow cannula is placed in the posterior portal, the sensory scope sheath system is placed in the anterolateral portal, and the shaver is placed in the anterior portal.

the infusion pump [17,18]. Bomberg and coworkers [14•] reported a complication rate of 10% due to fluid extravasation after using the pump while performing knee arthroscopies on 283 patients. Two out of the four complications required fasciotomy for compartment syndrome.

Conclusions

Used properly, the infusion pump offers major benefits to the surgeon in terms of improving joint distention, controlling intra-articular pressure, and providing adequate flow while power instruments are used.

The main complication seems to be related to minor or serious cases of fluid extravasation. Familiarity with the device and early recognition are important in avoiding serious extravasation with possible vascular compromise.

It is important for the arthroscopic surgeon to keep the following in mind when using the infusion pump:

- The cannula tip and fenestrations must be intra capsular and free of any debris or excess synovium that can interfere with proper outflow.
- Snug portals should be developed during the procedure.
- The extremity being arthroscoped should be periodically inspected and palpated for fluid extravasation.
- Proper attention should be paid to the alarm while the inflow line is intra-articular; the cause of the malfunction should be identified and corrected before the procedure is resumed.

Extravasation of fluid into the soft tissue can be alarming at times, but fluid usually can be reabsorbed without untoward effects. Fluid extravasation–induced compartment syndrome—is extremely rare and can be managed successfully by fasciotomy [14•]. In my experience, having used the infusion pump in over 2000 arthroscopic procedures, I have not encountered such complications (Parisien, Unpublished data).

References and Recommended Reading

Recently published papers of particular interest have been highlighted as:
- • Of interest
- •• Of outstanding interest

1. Ericksson E, Seibik A: Arthroscopy and arthroscopic surgery in a gas versus a fluid medium. *Orthop Clin North Am* 1982, 13:293–298.

2. Reagan BF, McInerny VK, Treadwell BV, *et al.*: Irrigating solutions for arthroscopy. *J Bone Joint Surg* 1983, 65A:629–631.

3. Oretorp N, Elmersson S: Arthroscopy and irrigation control. *Arthroscopy* 1986, 2:46–50.

4. Morgan C: Fluid delivery systems for arthroscopy. *Arthroscopy* 1987, 3:288–291.

5. Johnson LL: *Arthroscopic Surgery: Principles and Practice.* edn 3. St. Louis: CV Mosby; 1986.

6. Gillquist J, Hagberg G, Oretorp N: Arthroscopy in acute injuries of the knee joint. *Acta Orthop Scand* 1977, 48:190.

7. Ewing JW, Noe DA, Kitaoka HB, *et al.*: Intraarticular pressures during arthroscopic knee surgery. *Arthroscopy* 1986, 2:264–269.

8. Dolk T, Augustini BG: Three irrigation systems for motorized arthroscopic surgery: a comparative experimental and clinical study. *Arthroscopy* 1989, 5:307–317.

9. Bergstrom R, Gillquist J: The use of an infusion pump in arthroscopy. *Arthroscopy* 1986, 2:41–45.

10. Wolf EM: A guide to arthroscopy of the shoulder using the 3M fluid control system. St. Paul:3M Health Care; 1993.

11.• Whipple TL: *Arthroscopic Surgery of the Wrist.* Philadelphia:JB Lippincott; 1992.

This is a comprehensive text on the use of arthroscopy in disorders of the wrist joint.

12. Poehling GG: A guide to arthroscopy of the wrist using the 3M joint cannula system. St. Paul:3M Health Care; 1993.

13.• Parisien JS: Portals and positioning in arthroscopic surgery: the shoulder, elbow, wrist, hip, and ankle. In *Current Techniques in Arthroscopy.* Edited by Parisien JS. Philadelphia: Current Medicine; 1994, 9–31.

The author makes a thorough review of the various portals and positions available in arthroscopic surgery.

14.• Bomberg BC, Hurley PE, Clark CA, *et al.*: Complications associated with the use of an infusion pump during knee arthroscopy. *Arthroscopy* 1992, 8:224–228.

Four complications were noted with the use of an automated infusion pump in 283 patients who underwent knee arthroscopy.

15. Henderson CE, Hopson CN: Pneumoscrotum as a complication in arthroscopy. *J Bone Joint Surg* [Am] 1982, 64:1238–1240.

16. Noyes FR, Spievack ES: Extraarticular fluid dissection in tissues during arthroscopy. A report of clinical cases and a study of intraarticular and thigh pressures in cadavers. *Am J Sports Med* 1982, 10:125–142.

17. Peek RD, Haynes DW: Compartment syndrome as a complication of arthroscopy. *Am J Sports Med* 1984, 12:464–468.

18. Fruensgaard S, Holm A: Compartment syndrome complicating arthroscopic surgery: Brief report. *J Bone Joint Surg* [Br] 1988, 70:146–147.

4

CHAPTER

The Use of Lasers in Arthroscopic Meniscal Surgery

STEPHEN P. ABELOW

Current orthopedic lasers are multipurpose tools that can cut, coagulate, vaporize, and shrink tissues. Just as a scalpel uses mechanical force to affect tissue, a laser uses a photon energy beam. When laser light energy is absorbed by a cell, photochemical and photobiologic reactions occur.

The surgical laser is a multipurpose tool that can simultaneously cut and coagulate. It obviates the need for a tourniquet or electrocautery, provides an effective soft-tissue release, and can ablate tissues by vaporizing them. Most importantly, surgical lasers allow easy access to tight spaces when used arthroscopically. After a very short learning period, laser surgery is technically easy.

Laser is an acronym for *L*ight *A*mplification by *S*timulated *E*mission of *R*adiation. Einstein postulated stimulated emission in 1917. Laser light is coherent, collimated, and monochromatic. When laser light is directed toward a material, the material can transmit, reflect, scatter, or absorb it. Laser light must be absorbed by a cell to provide energy for a photochemical or photobiologic reaction. If it is not absorbed, no reaction will occur. The specific optical properties of the material determine the effectiveness of the laser interaction.

What occurs when a laser beam strikes tissue depends on the wavelength, intensity, energy, and duration of the laser irradiation and the type, color, size, and composition of the tissue. The holmium:yttrium aluminum garnet (Ho:YAG) laser with its affinity for water may be used to selectively ablate chondromalacic cartilage tissue [1].

Current orthopedic lasers function in the infrared portion to the electromagnetic spectrum. Laser energy is absorbed by cellular water and is converted to heat. This essentially boils the cell and vaporizes tissue.

The first clinical studies using laser-assisted arthroscopic surgery were performed in the 1970s and 1980s using a carbon dioxide laser (Smith and Nance, paper presented at the Annual Meeting of the Arthroscopy Association of North America, Coronado, 1983) [2–5]. In the mid-1980s, Smith and coworkers [6] stimulated the curiosity of many orthopedic surgeons by publishing a large, successful study of arthroscopic surgeries using a pulsed CO_2 laser. In the late 1980s, Fanton and Dillingham [1] found less pain, swelling, and inflammation with holmium laser arthroscopic meniscectomies. In 1990, Sherk [7••] edited his text *Lasers in Orthopaedics* (Table 4-1).

THE HOLMIUM LASER

The Ho:YAG laser has a wavelength of 2.1 µm (Figs. 4-1A and 4-1B). The laser energy is created by stimulating a YAG crystal (yttrium, aluminum, and garnet crystal with small impurity concentrations of holmium, thulium, and chromium). The holmium

Table 4-1 Table of orthopedic lasers

Laser type	Wavelength hs, *µm*	Power, *W*	Depth of penetration, *µm*	Delivery system	Arthroscopic medium
Ho:YAG	2.1	0–80	200–400	Fiberoptic	Aqueous
1.44 Nd:YAG	1.44	0–60	200–400	Fiberoptic	Aqueous
1.06 Nd:YAG	1.064	0–100+	200–1000	Fiberoptic	Aqueous
KTP	0.532	0.05–40	500–2000	Fiberoptic	Aqueous
CO_2	10.64	0–120	50–200	Articulated arm with mirrors	Gas or ambient air
Excimer*	0.308	Up to 300 mJ	24	Fiberoptic	Aqueous
Erbium*	2.94	Up to 500 mJ	10–15	Zirconium fluoride fibers	Aqueous

*Experimental.
Ho:YAG—holmium:yttrium aluminum garnet; KTP—potassium titanyl phosphate; Nd—neodymium.

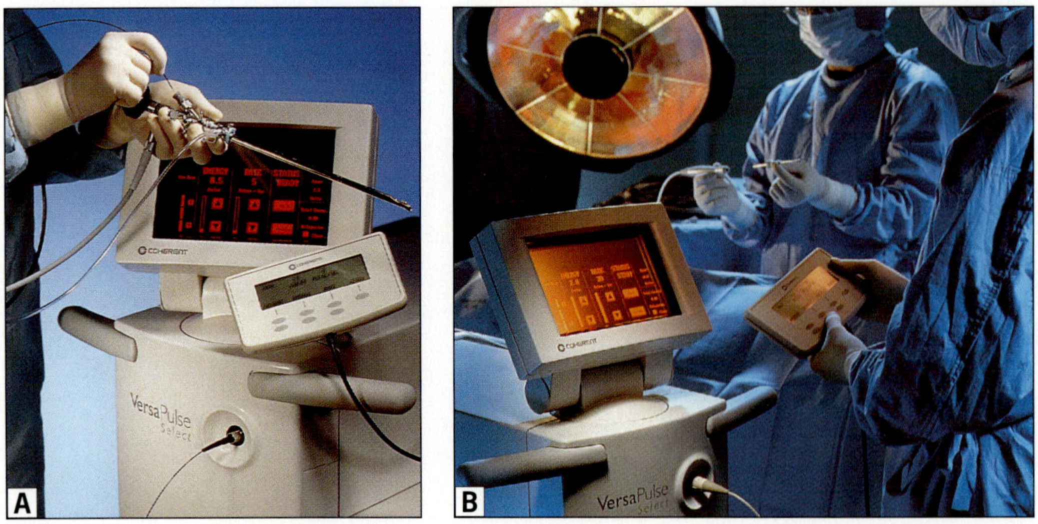

Figure 4-1. **A**, **B** Holmium 2.1µm laser. (Courtesy of Coherent Laser, Palo Alto, CA).

laser wavelength is strongly absorbed by the water component of tissues and allows for precise vaporization and cutting of tissues. The Ho:YAG laser can be effectively used in a saline medium and is able to vaporize water-laden tissue effectively [1,8]. It is transmitted via a 0.4-mm quartz fiberoptic fiber and has a low-profile handpiece 1.5 to 1.7 mm in diameter. The low-profile handpiece (Figs. 4-2A and 4-2B) operates in a near-contact–contact mode and is ideal for access to tight spaces such as the extreme posterior portions of the knee joint. Thermal necrosis averages 82 µm [9].

Trauner and coworkers [10•] reported thermal damage in bovine meniscus to be 400 µm laterally and 450 µm deep to the base of the crater. Thermal damage in bovine articular cartilage was less than 250 µm laterally and less than 500 µm deep to the base of the crater. Disruption of the lacunae extended 350 to 400 µm (Fig. 4-3).

The Ho:YAG laser is able to vaporize, cut, coagulate, shrink, smooth, and sculpt tissue. It is useful for joint debridement, meniscectomy, chondral ablation, soft-tissue release, and synovectomy. With practice, it allows an arthroscopist to smooth and contour a joint surface or meniscus with elegance.

Clinical indications for the Ho:YAG laser in the knee include debridement, meniscectomy, chondroplasty (photochondroplasty), synovectomy, plica excision, lateral release, chondral or osseous drilling, capsular shrinkage, and cauterization of bleeding vessels.

Meniscal tissue appears to be best cut or ablated by using 40 to 60 W of power at 10 to 15 pulses per second. At high-repetition rates and low-power settings, the holmium laser is able to feather, smooth, and contour meniscal tissue with great precision and is technically easier than any other arthroscopic tool currently available (Figs. 4-4A and 4-4B).

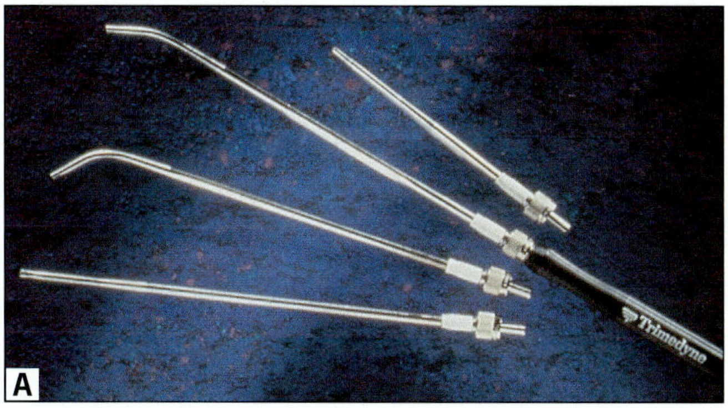

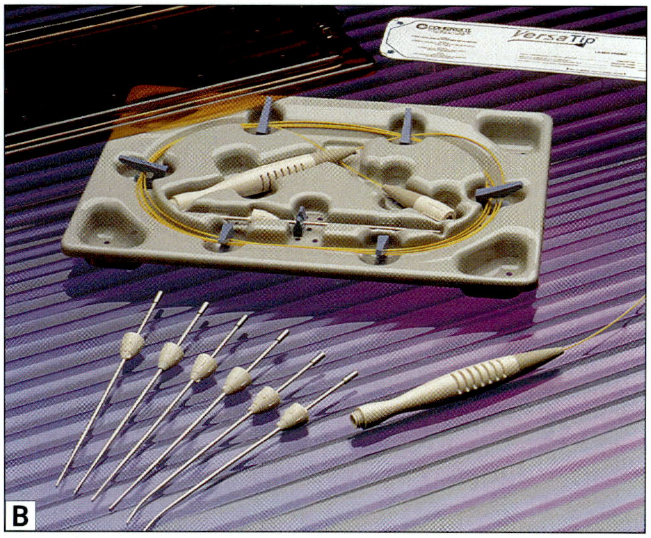

Figure 4-2. **A**, **B**, Low-profile switchable handpieces offer easy access to tight spaces, are reusable, and offer significant cost advantages. (Part A courtesy of Trimedyne, Irvine, CA; Part B courtesy of Coherent Laser, Palo Alto, CA).

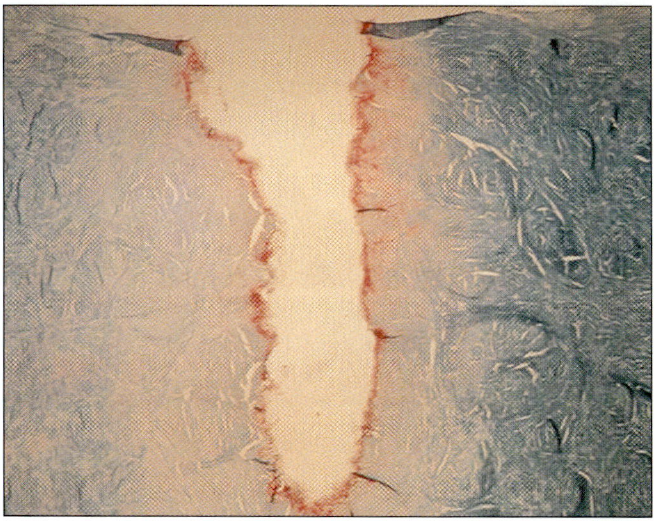

Figure 4-3. Trichrome stain of holmium:yttrium aluminum garnet (Ho:YAG) laser cut in meniscus. Thermal damage measures 400 µm laterally and 450 µm deep. Note the precise laser cut.

Fanton and Dillingham [1] reported less inflammation, pain, and swelling with Ho:YAG laser meniscectomy. They also reported that postoperative recovery with respect to pain, swelling, range of motion, and return to activity after lateral release has been significantly accelerated compared with mechanical or electrocautery techniques. Operative time was longer for lateral release.

Lane and Mooar reported 8 min less arthroscopy time for chondral and meniscus lesions. The Ho:YAG was felt to be safe and effective (Lane and Mooar, Paper presented at the 11th Annual Meeting of the American Society for Laser Medicine and Surgery, San Diego, 1991).

Waltenberger and Abelow [11] retrospectively analyzed 100 cases of debridement, chondroplasty, and meniscectomy using laser and conventional instrumentation. Laser-assisted arthroscopic surgical cases averaged 12.64 min longer compared with surgeries without laser. Laser-assisted arthroscopy cost $944.19 more than paired cases of conventional arthroscopy.

Newer lasers have a significantly less cost per Watt of power, and handpieces are now reusable. This has brought the cost of laser usage down to approximately $150 per case, which can come to approximate the cost of disposable shaver blades.

Complications of the Ho:YAG laser include tip breakage, fiber breakage, lasing the arthroscope, and inadvertent lasing of articular cartilage resulting in full-thickness cartilage defects.

A 1.7-mm diameter flexible holmium laser arthroscope is currently available. This allows arthroscopic visualization and simultaneous laser tissue ablation. As the resolution of this laser arthroscope improves, it will become a useful tool for minimally invasive arthroscopic laser surgery. Through a single small portal, laser ablative arthroscopic surgery may become a routine office procedure.

The future will bring lasers with increased powers. An 80-W, 7-J laser with the ability to function at more than 50 Hz will enable us to use the laser to ablate significant volumes of meniscal tissue and to bevel and contour the remaining meniscus with phenomenal accuracy.

The Ho:YAG laser offers the advantages of using fiberoptic delivery, standard instrumentation, standard portals, standard distension, minimal scuffing of chondral surfaces, easy access to difficult places, and good hemostasis. With minimal depth of penetration, minimal thermal damage, and excellent absorption by water, the 2.1 µm wavelength appears to be ideally suited for arthroscopic use.

THE 1.44 NEODYMIUM:YAG LASER

The 1.44-µm laser is a pulsed neodymium (Nd):YAG laser operating at 1.44 µm. It has nearly the same absorption by the water component of tissue as 2.1 µm laser energy. Thus, the 1.44-µm Nd:YAG laser has surgical precision and hemostasis very similar to that of holmium lasers.

The 1.44 Nd:YAG laser can be used in a saline medium. It is transmitted via a 0.6-mm quartz fiberoptic fiber and has a 1.7-mm low-profile handpiece. As with the holmium laser, the 1.44 Nd:YAG laser operates in a near-contact–contact mode and is ideal for access to tight spaces (Figs. 4-5 A–C). Thermal damage is 450 µm in meniscal fibrocartilage. The 1.44 Nd:YAG laser provides up to 60 W of power, 3.5 J per pulse, and up to 50 pulses per second.

The 1.44 Nd:YAG laser is able to vaporize, cut, coagulate, smooth, sculpt, and shrink tissue. It is

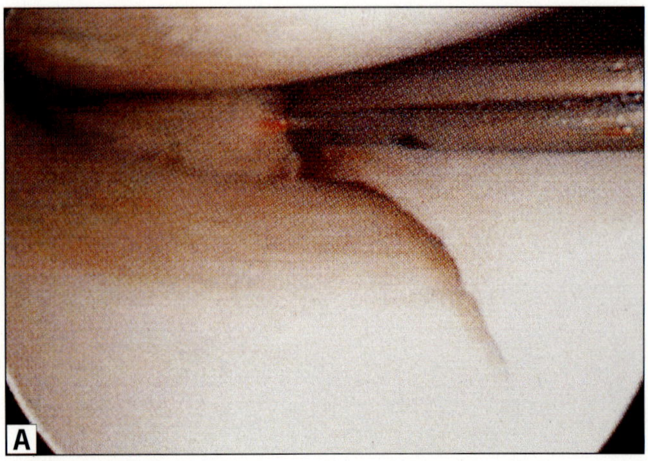

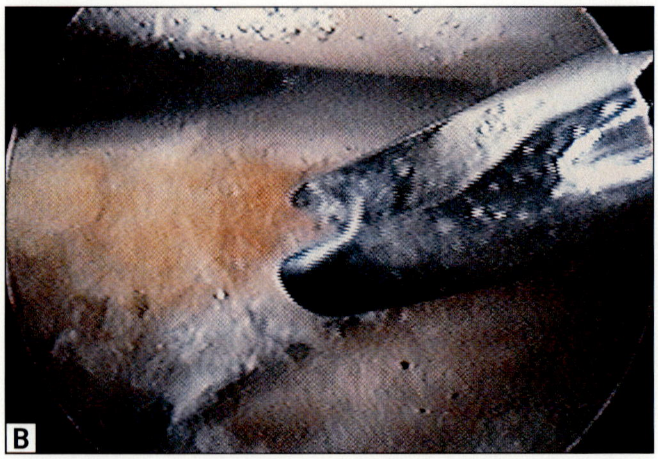

Figure 4-4. A, B, Holmium laser meniscectomy. Note the low-profile handpiece. No contact is made with the articular surface.

useful for joint debridement, meniscectomy, chondral ablation, soft-tissue release, and synovectomy.

The 1.06 Neodymium:YAG Laser

This Nd:YAG laser has a wavelength of 1.064 µm. The laser energy is created by stimulating a YAG crystal doped with a small quantity of neodymium-lasing medium. It is transmitted via fiberoptics and can be used in an aqueous medium. It is diffusely absorbed by tissue protein.

O'Brien and Miller [12] reported the contact Nd:YAG laser to be a safe and effective arthroscopic tool for performing meniscectomies. They felt it provided technical and biologic advantages over existing instrumentation.

Although the contact 1.06 Nd:YAG laser cuts hemostatically using standard arthroscopic portals and technique, the wavelength has not gained acceptance by laser arthroscopists.

Meniscal Repair

The 1.32-µm Nd:YAG laser has been used for tissue welding and meniscal repair. Dew and coworkers (Paper presented at the 17th Annual Meeting of the American Orthopedic Society for Sports Medicine, Orlando, 1991) [13] found that 1.32-µm Nd:YAG lasers were successful in welding scalpel-induced full-thickness meniscal cartilage wounds in a pig model. Thermal denaturation of tissue protein and resulting seal of tissue edges was achieved with the laser using powers of less than 2 W.

The wound edges were completely smooth and there was no evidence of wound dehiscence, infection, or unusual healing. Laser welding of cartilage was nontactile, did not require foreign material in the wound, *ie*, suture material, and did not result in any charring of the tissues.

Future of Lasers

The future will bring us more powerful and efficient lasers of lesser size and cost. As the optical properties of human tissues are analyzed and wavelength-specific lasers are developed, we will have a way to eliminate diseased tissue (with different optical properties) from healthy and normal tissues.

The potential for photoagglutination and tissue welding is exciting. The ability to repair torn meniscus by tissue welding with a "no touch" technique through

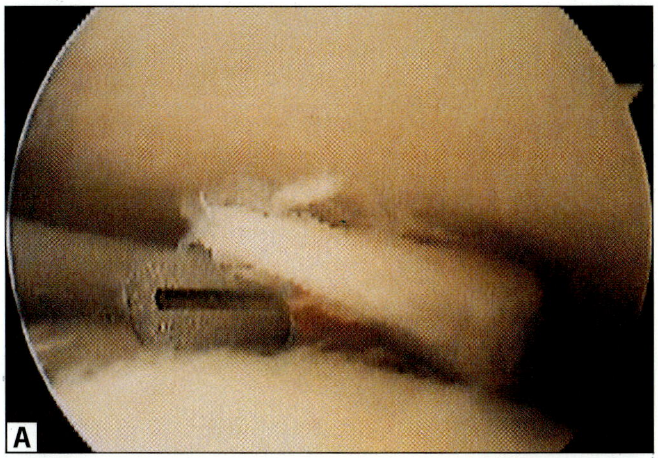

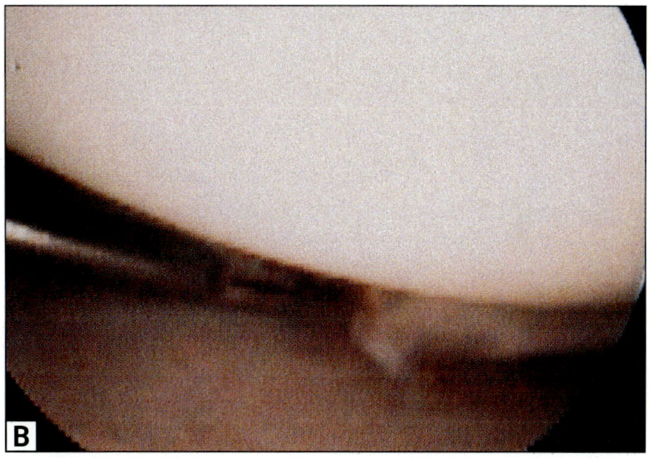

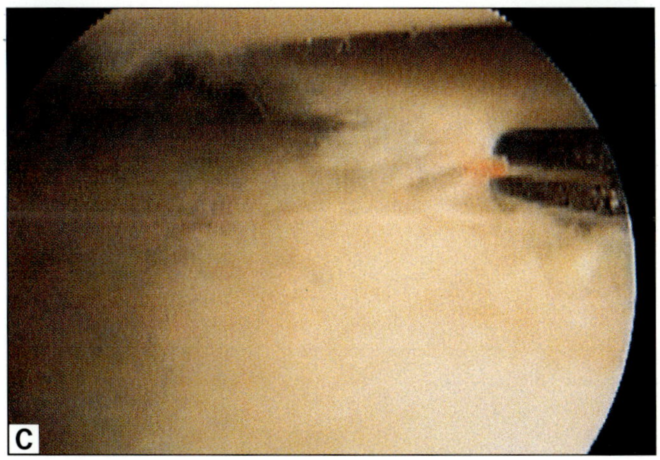

Figure 4-5. **A**, **B**, **C**, Meniscectomy performed with a 1.44 neodymium:yttrium-aluminum-garnet (Nd:YAG) laser. This laser provides easy access to tight spaces with no scuffing of the articular surface.

a small uniportal arthroscopy site is intriguing. New orthopedic wavelengths are being investigated.

The thulium laser (2.01 μm) is strongly absorbed by water. Because it is closer to the water absorption peak at 1.930 μm, thulium laser energy is absorbed even more strongly in most tissues, giving it the potential for great surgical precision.

The erbium (Er) lasers have a wavelength of 2.94 μm (Er:YAG) or 2.79 μm (Er:yttrium scandium gallium garnet [Er:YSGG]). This wavelength is very strongly absorbed by the water component of tissue. It can easily vaporize cartilage, fibrous tissue, and bone. It has a shallow depth of penetration and affords surgical precision better than that of the holmium laser. It has poor hemostatic qualities. The major drawback with the erbium laser is that it cannot be transmitted through standard quartz fiberoptics. There is no economical optical fiber that offers significant transmission and flexibility [14].

Photodynamic therapy is a new treatment modality that combines the use of a photosensitive drug, laser light, and fiberoptics to destroy cancer cells. With appropriate photopharmaceuticals and appropriate laser wavelengths, many synovial proliferative disorders can possibly be approached arthroscopically.

Combined instruments are currently being developed. Combining standard arthroscopic mechanical instruments with laser fibers allows for more efficient cutting, trimming, ablation, and sculpting of tissues.

The future will bring research in basic cellular mechanisms, laser interactions with tissues, function-specific wavelengths, dose thresholds, target organs and organelles, long-term effects of laser irradiation, and instrumentation.

Conclusion

The surgical laser is a new multipurpose tool that can cut, coagulate, and vaporize tissues. It utilizes a low-profile handpiece that allows easy access to tight places, such as the posteromedial or posterolateral corners of the knee joint. The holmium laser, at a 2.1 μm wavelength, is a useful arthroscopic tool and is gaining wide acceptance among orthopedic surgeons. It can cut, vaporize, and contour meniscal tissue easily and rapidly.

References and Recommended Reading

Papers of interest, published recently, have been highlighted as:

- • Of interest
- •• Of outstanding interest

1. Fanton GS, Dillingham MF: The use of the holmium laser in arthroscopic surgery. *Semin Orthop* 1992, 7:113.
2. Whipple TL, Caspari RB, Meyer JF: Arthroscopic laser meniscectomy in a gas medium. *Arthroscopy* 1985, 1:2–7.
3. Whipple TL, Caspari RB, Meyer JF: Laser subtotal meniscectomy in rabbits. *Laser Surg Med* 1984, 3:297–304.
4. Whipple TL, Caspari RB: Laser energy in arthroscopic meniscectomy. *Orthopedics* 1983, 6:1165–1169.
5. Philandrianos G: Carbon dioxide laser in arthroscopic surgery of the knee. *Presse Med* 1985, 14:2103–2104.
6. Smith CF, Johansen WE, Vangsness CT, *et al.*: The carbon dioxide laser, a potential tool for orthopedic surgery. *Clin Orthop* 1989, 242:43–50.
7. •• Sherk HH: *Lasers in Orthopaedics* Philadelphia:JB Lippincott; 1990.

First textbook on lasers in orthopedic surgery.

8. Fanton GS: Ho:YAG laser emerges as significant clinical tool for orthopedic and general surgery cases. *General Surgery News* 1990, XX:8.
9. Black J, Sherk HH, Meller M, *et al.*: Wavelength selection in laser arthroscopy. *Semin Orthop* 1992, 7:72.
10. • Trauner K, Nishioka N, Patel D: Pulsed holmium:yttrium-aluminum-garnet (Ho:YAG) laser ablation of fibrocartilage and articular cartilage. *Am J Sports Med* 1990, 18:316–320.

Excellent article defining the extent of Holmium laser effects on fibrocartilage and articular cartilage.

11. Waltenberger A, Abelow SP: Cost analysis of laser arthroscopy. *Arthroscopy* 1993, 9:341.
12. O'Brien S, Miller D: The contact neodymium: yttrium aluminum garnet laser: a new approach to arthroscopic surgery. *Clin Ortho* 1990, 252:95–100.
13. Dew DK, Supik L, Darrow CR, *et al.*: Tissue repair using lasers: a review. *Orthopedics* 1993, 16:581–587.
14. JGM Associates, Inc: Orthopedic surgery applications of advanced solid state laser. Burlington, MA: JGM Associates; 1991:5–32.

5

CHAPTER

Meniscal Allograft Reconstruction in Arthroscopic Surgical Technique

E. MARLOWE GOBLE

The knee menisci perform vital biomechanical functions that contribute to the maintenance of healthy articular cartilage and protect against degenerative joint disease. The functions of the menisci include load transmission across the tibiofemoral joint, shock absorption to protect the articular cartilage, secondary mechanical stability, and joint lubrication and nutrition. Damage to or removal of the meniscus will lead to cartilage degeneration and the development of osteoarthritis [1].

Total meniscectomy, which was once the standard treatment for all types of meniscus tears, is rarely indicated because of its many deleterious effects. As early as 1948, Fairbank [2] reported arthritic changes following complete meniscectomy including joint space narrowing as well as spurring and flattening of the femoral condyle on the operated side. Many researchers have demonstrated increased incidence of degenerative changes after partial and total meniscectomy [3–6]

Degenerative changes associated with total meniscectomy are owing to changes in the load distribution functions of the menisci. Removal of the medial meniscus causes a reduction in the contact area by 50% to 70%, and the pressure gradient is considerably more severe near the margins of the contact area [7]. The single most predictive factor in the development of degenerative arthritis is the time elapsed since meniscectomy [3].

Theoretically, restoration of the normal meniscal anatomy should be able to decelerate or prevent further degenerative changes. Currently, however, no long-term study has been able to demonstrate that meniscal allograft reconstruction has any impact on the inevitable joint degeneration. Short-term studies have demonstrated that patients who undergo meniscal allograft reconstruction experience relief of pain and improved functional activity levels (Noyes and Barber-Westin, paper presented at AAOS, Orlando, 1995) [8,9,10].

Medial Meniscus Allograft Technique

Arthroscopically assisted meniscal allograft reconstruction is performed as an elective outpatient procedure. Prior to the operation, a magnetic resonance image of the contralateral meniscus is obtained, and the donor meniscus is sized in the anterior-posterior and lateral planes to within 7% of the normal meniscus. Cost containment has prompted recent evaluation of plain radiographic techniques for sizing purposes.

The affected knee is placed in a leg holder applied at the level of the thigh tourniquet. This stabilization of the lower extremity will allow full extension and approximately 120° of knee flexion.

Arthroscopic portals are placed adjacent to the proximal patellar tendon, both medial and lateral. When the patient is anterior cruciate ligament (ACL) deficient (as well as medial meniscus deficient), and it is necessary to harvest the central one third of the patellar ligament, I prefer not to place portals through the harvest defect. Portals medial and lateral to the patellar ligament provide better angles of approach to the corners of knee compartments.

The arthroscope and arthroscopic instruments are freely exchanged between portals as the need dictates. The peripheral rim of the medial meniscus is debrided to the junction of capsule and meniscus. Do not injure the capsule or its expansions.

An assistant should apply constant valgus force (proximal to the ankle) with the knee flexed but not rotated at 20°. Continuous valgus pressure will gradually open the medial joint because the medial viscoelastic passive restraints lengthen as a function of time within their elastic limit. By the time the meniscal rim resection is complete, medial rim opening will be remarkably increased.

The medial compartment can be tightly controlled by a firm medial collateral ligament (MCL) and posterior oblique ligament (POL). Occasionally, it will be needful to increase the space between the medial femoral condyle and the tibia. It is better to provide for this opening than to struggle and perhaps iatrogenically injure remaining articular cartilage.

A 3-cm incision is made between the inferior border of the vastus medialis oblique and the medial epicondyle of the femur. The exposure is completed by dissecting directly down to bone, exposing the proximal portion of the epicondyle. A curved 0.5-in osteotome is inserted at the proximal base of the medial epicondyle. Osteotomize the epicondyle, with its attached origins of the deep MCL and POL, but the distal cortex of the epicondyle should be left intact (Fig. 5-1). Valgus stress should be applied to the leg until tension in the MCL and POL distract the osteotomized epicondyle, causing a green stick fracture at its distal base (Fig. 5-1).

A full-radius soft-tissue resector blade is used to carefully remove synovium at the interval between the posterior cruciate ligament and the medial tibial eminence. When the peaked ridge of the medial tibial eminence is fully visible, the proximal one third of this eminence is removed with a 0.25-in osteotomy introduced through the medial portal (Fig. 5-2). This I describe as the Mt. Saint Helen's maneuver.

After the Mt. Saint Helen's maneuver, a 30° arthroscope can easily pass through the interval provided, allowing full view of the insertion of the posterior horn of the medial meniscus. The posterior horn insertion provides a footprint, once debrided, similar to that of the ACL on the tibia. In a similar guided fashion to tibial drilling of the ACL, a tibial drill guide is inserted through the medial portal; its target point is passed over the resected medial tibial eminence and placed within the footprint of the posterior horn on the back slope of the medial tibial eminence. Verification and observation of this target can be easily accomplished by inserting the 30° arthroscope through a posteromedial portal. The reason this is so easy is because the medial meniscus is absent.

The tibial guide is positioned within a 2-cm incision at the anterolateral tibia, 3 cm distal to the tibial tuberosity. A guidewire is drilled from distal to proximal, entering the knee joint at the guide target, *ie*, the footprint of the posterior horn. The guidepin is overdrilled with a cannulated 6-mm drill. A small curved curette is passed through this 6-mm tunnel, and the proximal opening of the tunnel is expanded to 8 mm (Fig. 5-3). Further expansion of this proximal opening to the tunnel can be achieved by introducing the curved curette through a posteromedial portal.

A looped pull suture is passed up the tunnel and retrieved back through the medial portal (Fig. 5-4) (*point A*). Two additional pull sutures are placed within the medial compartment. The first is introduced through a 16-gauge spinal needle inserted at the posteromedial corner of the knee, advanced deep to the posterior capsule, and finally enters the joint posteriorly within 2 cm of the posterior horn of the medial meniscus (Fig. 5-4) (*point B*). A monofilament suture is urged through the spinal needle from outside-in. A grasper is inserted through the medial portal to retrieve the suture and pull it out through the medial portal.

A second pull suture is similarly passed. However, it enters into the knee joint from the posteromedial corner at the junction of the central and posterior thirds of the medial meniscus (Fig. 5-4) (*point C*).

The meniscal allograft is prepared on the back table by an assistant. A centrally cannulated bone block is left attached at both anterior and posterior horns of the allograft. The anterior bone block measures 9 x 9 mm; the posterior horn plug measures 8 x 9 mm (9 mm deep). A braided #2 polyethylene suture is sewn to the base of the meniscal horn, and then both arms of the suture are passed through the 1.5-mm drill hole (cannulation) in the bone blocks. These sutures will be used as transosseous sutures to secure both ante-

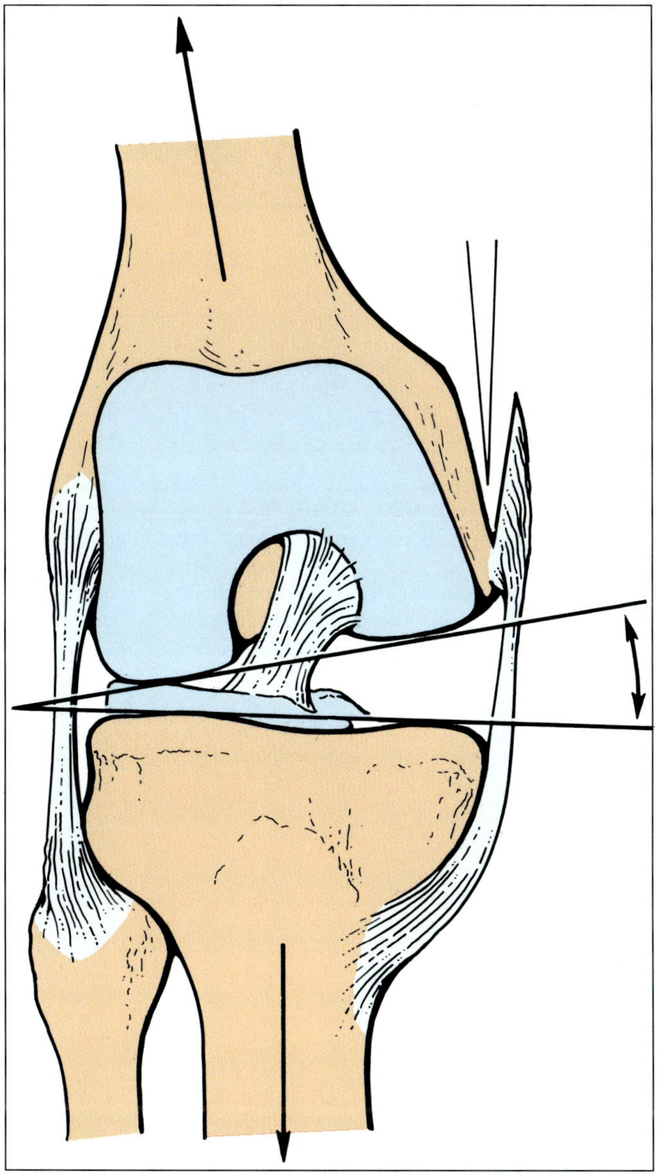

Figure 5-1. If an additional medial compartment opening is required, an incomplete osteotomy of the medial epicondyle can be performed through a 3-cm subvastus medialis oblique incision.

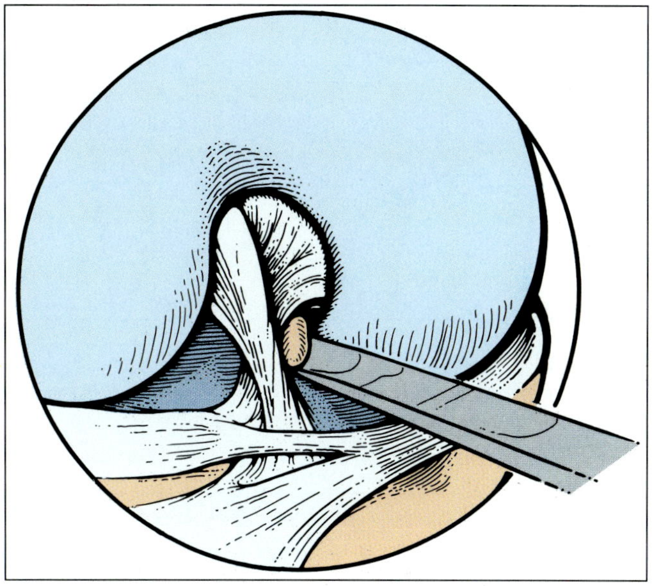

Figure 5-2. Mt. Saint Helen's maneuver. The top of the medial tibial eminence is removed with a 0.25-in osteotome. This maneuver 1) permits thorough visualization of the posterior horn region of the medial meniscus and 2) permits passage of the medial meniscal allograft between the eminence and the medial femoral condyle.

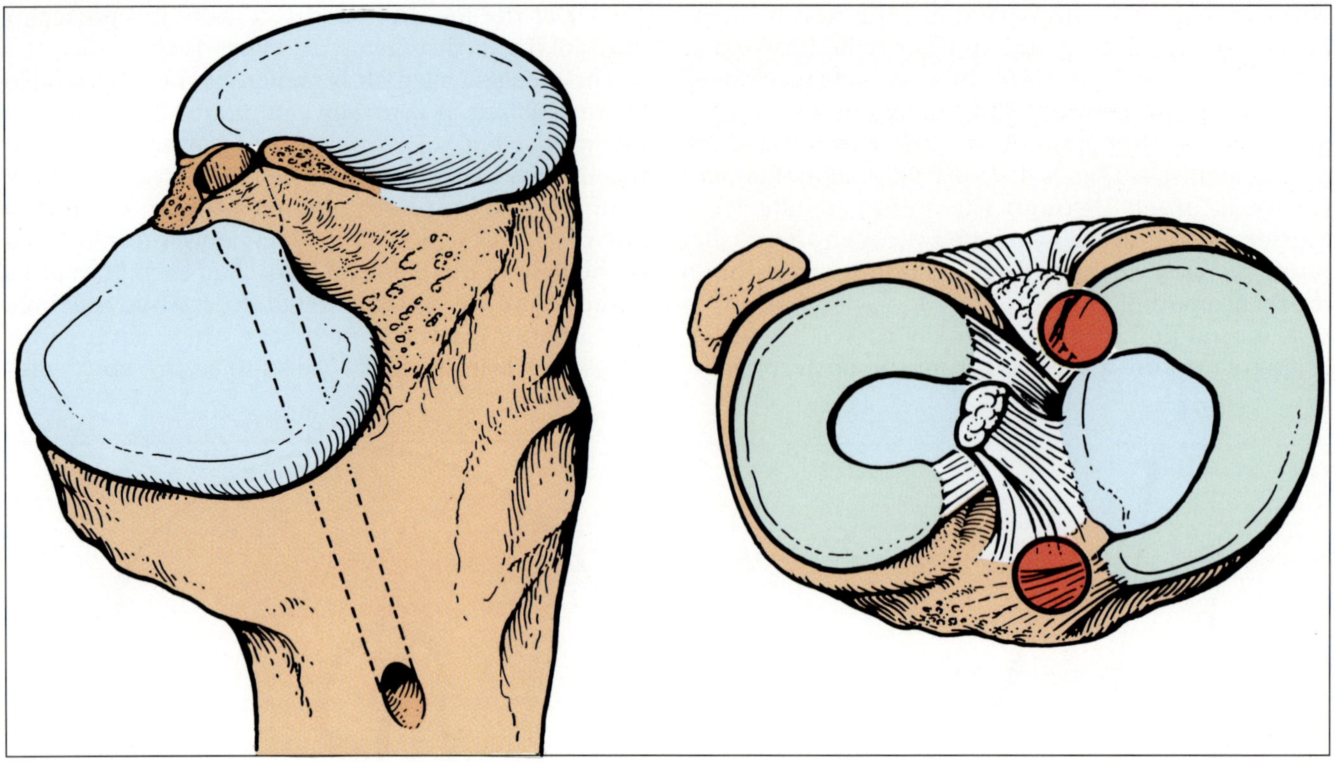

Figure 5-3. Using a tibial guide (anterior cruciate ligament type), a 6-mm tunnel is drilled proximally from the anterolateral tibia to the insertion of the posterior horn of the medial meniscus. The proximal opening of the tunnel is expanded (with a curette) to an 8-mm diameter.

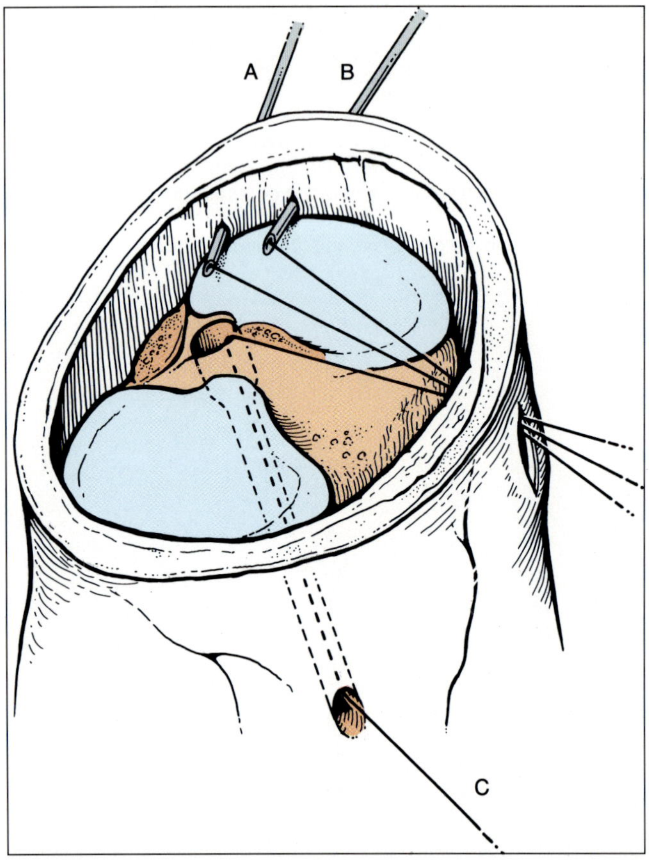

Figure 5-4. It is important to insert three strategic pull sutures: the first through the posterior capsule, *point A*, the second through the posteromedial capsule, *point B*, both of which are introduced through 16-gauge spinal needles. The third pull suture is introduced through the tibial tunnel, *point C*. The free intra-articular ends of all three sutures are advanced to the outside of the knee by pulling them out through the medial portal.

rior and posterior horns of the allograft within their respective tunnels (Fig. 5-5) (*point A*).

Three absorbable sutures are placed within the outer rim of the allograft. The first suture is placed at the posterior horn, 2 cm from the bone block (Fig. 5-5) (*point B*). The second suture is placed at the junction of the central and posterior thirds of the allograft (Fig. 5-5) (*point C*). Both of these sutures correspond to the pull sutures introduced with spinal needles described previously.

A third suture is placed at the anterior horn about 1 cm from the bony anterior horn (Fig. 5-5) (*point D*).

All three of the preplaced sutures, in addition to the two sutures placed within the bone blocks of the anterior and posterior horns of the allograft, are used to maneuver the allograft into position within the medial compartment (Fig. 5-6).

The medial portal is extended distally to the level of the tibial plateau. Care must be taken not to cut the existing pull sutures. The edges of the incision are retracted, exposing the anterior margin of the tibial plateau. Here is found the bony anchor of the anterior horn of the medial meniscus, hidden (from the arthroscopic view) by the intermeniscal ligament and the fat pad. This bony bed can be directly prepared nonarthroscopically through the expanded medial portal. The anterior horn attachment should be removed with a 0.25-in osteotome, or a 10-mm drill, deepening the bed to 10 mm. A transosseous hole is

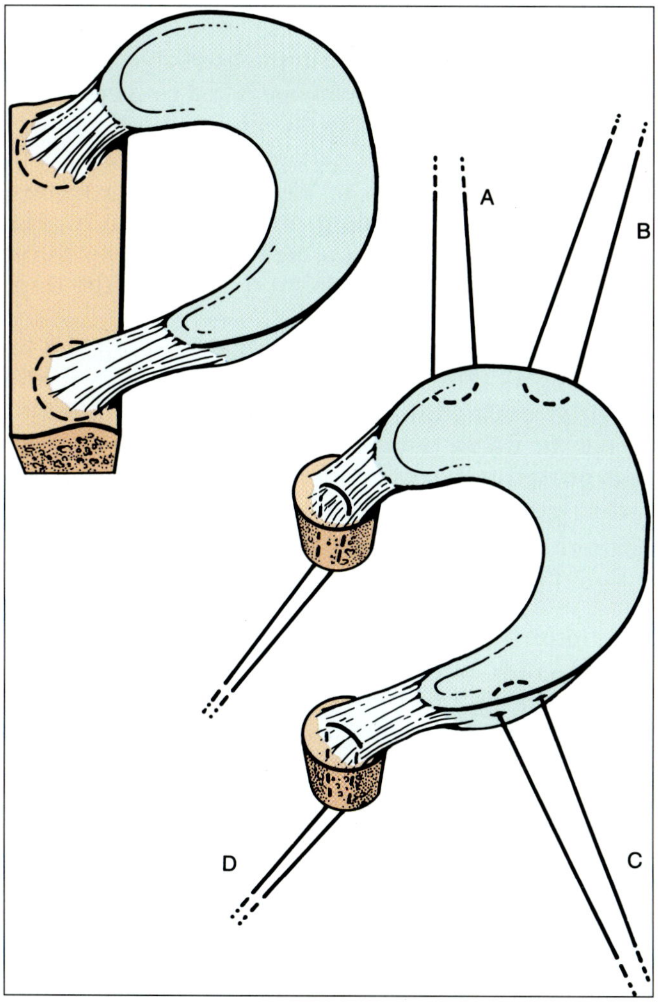

Figure 5-5. Three pairs of sutures are sewn to the edge of the medial meniscal allograft, *point A*, *point B*, and *point C*. These sutures will spread the allograft into proper position within the joint. They also supply suture-to-capsule attachment where arthroscopic suturing techniques would be difficult. Two additional preplaced sutures are placed in the bone plugs to be used as transosseous sutures within their respective tibial tunnels, *point D*.

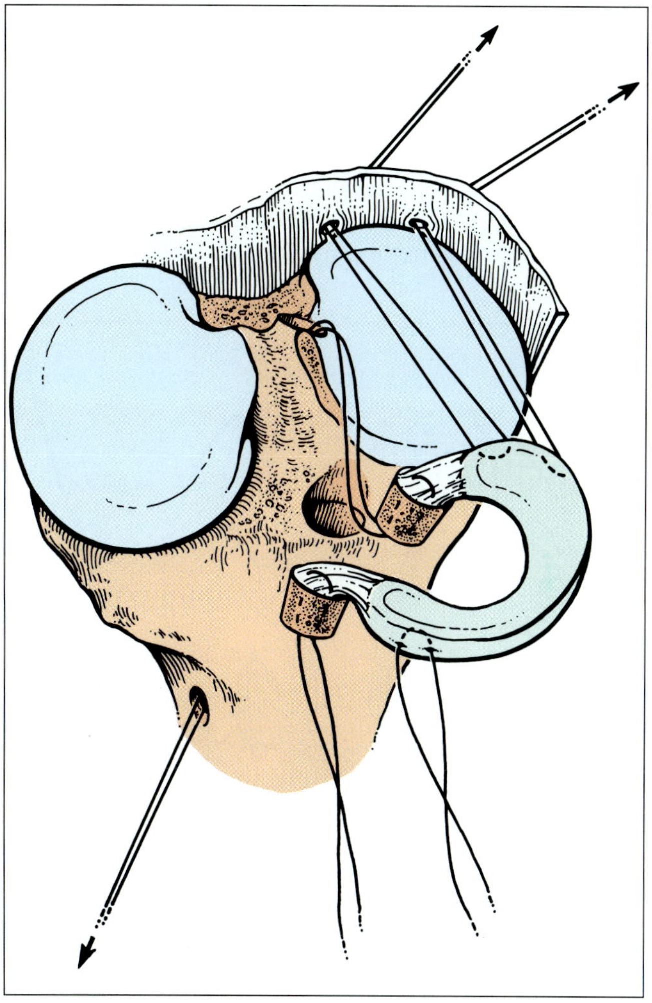

Figure 5-6. Each of the three pull sutures is tied to its corresponding medial meniscal allograft suture. These paired sutures are drawn into the joint (through the medial portal), exiting the joint through the posterior capsule, posteromedial capsule, and posterior (horn) tibial tunnel. The medial meniscal allograft is now ready to be pulled into the knee joint.

passed from the anteromedial tibia to the center of the bony bed of the anterior horn.

The enlarged medial portal should allow easy passage of an index finger. Each allograft suture is connected with its corresponding pull suture exiting the enlarged medial portal. Each of the five sutures is then pulled into its respective hole. While an assistant sequentially applies tension to each suture, the allograft is urged through the medial portal, leading with the posterior horn (Fig. 5-7). The knee should be bent to 60° while valgus stress is applied. This maneuver will permit the posterior third of the allograft to pass through the interval between the medial tibial eminence and the medial femoral condyle. Once this bottleneck is passed, each of the peripheral sutures is tightened to expand the allograft into anatomic position.

The bony block at the posterior horn must be teased into proper orientation with a curved probe to drop into its tunnel. The anterior bone block is press-fit into its bony bed using a blunt-ended tamper. This is done with direct visualization through the expanded medial portal.

With the medial meniscus allograft (MMA) in anatomic position, the periphery is sewn in a technique similar to repairing a full bucket-handle tear (Fig. 5-8). I prefer an inside-out series of sutures, beginning posteriorly and advancing to the anterior aspect of the joint. Approximately eight additional sutures will be sufficient. The preplaced anterior horn meniscal suture (*see* Fig. 5-5, *point D*) is loaded on a free-curved Davis needle and passed through the anterior capsule (Fig. 5-9) (inside-out type technique).

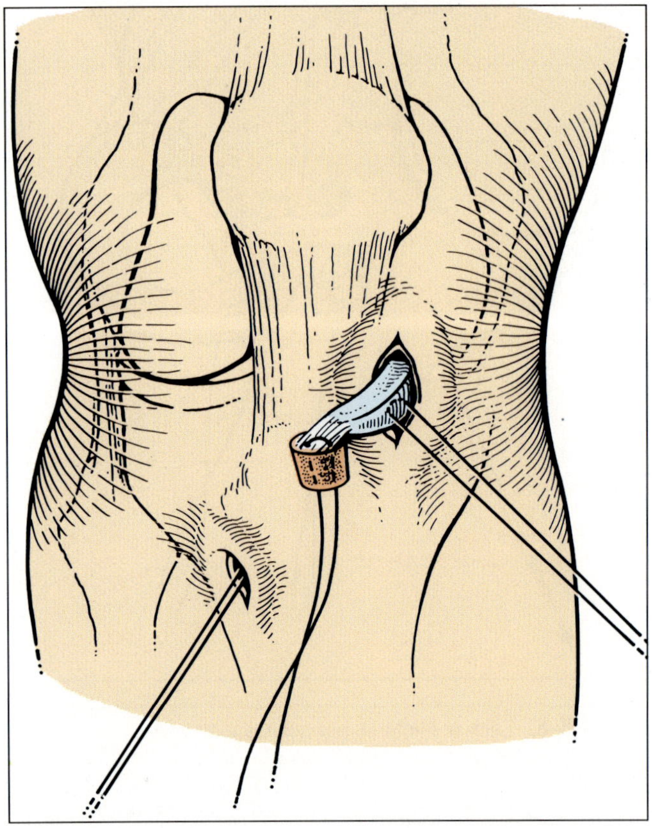

Figure 5-7. The medial meniscal allograft is pulled (*sutures*) and pushed (*index finger*) into the enlarged medial portal.

Lateral Meniscal Allograft Technique

Arthroscopic portals used for lateral meniscal allograft technique (LMA) are the same as described for the medial meniscus. Because the anterior and posterior horns of the lateral meniscus are located only 13 mm apart, the LMA is implanted in the lateral compartment of the recipient knee with a bone island connecting the two horns (Fig. 5-10). This island of donor bone will measure approximately 9 mm in diameter by 22 mm in length. Guy wire sutures are placed in the same relative position on the LMA as described for the MMA (*see* Fig. 5-5). This includes a suture near the posterior horn, another in the posterior lateral corner, and the third adjacent to the anterior horn (Fig. 5-10).

The recipient lateral compartment is prepared by removing all of the remnants of the meniscus to the capsular expansion. A trough is now prepared to accept the donor bone island containing the anterior and posterior horns of the lateral meniscus. The arthroscope is placed in the medial portal and the instruments are introduced through the lateral portal. A 0.25-in osteotome is introduced through the lateral portal and a 10-mm section of bone is removed beginning immediately adjacent to the lateral edge of the ACL. A cut is made from anterior to posterior beginning anteriorly adjacent to the most anterior fibers of the ACL. The cut is then extended posteriorly for a distance of 22 mm remaining alongside the lateral border of the ACL. A second parallel cut is made beginning 10 mm lateral to the first cut and extended for 20 mm from anterior to posterior. Bone in-between these two cuts is removed to a depth of 10 mm. The trough thus formed will remove half of the girth of the lateral tibial eminence. The remaining lateral border to the trough is made up of the elevation of the lateral tibial eminence and will serve as a restraining buttress, preventing the allograft bone from escaping into the lateral compartment (Fig. 5-11).

A flexible silicone template that matches the allograft bone island in size is fitted within the prepared trough to determine appropriate size. Additional bone is removed until this template fits comfortably within the trough without excessive elevation. The template is removed in preparation for installation of the allograft. The lateral portal is enlarged, extending distally to the articular edge of the lateral tibial plateau. It should be large enough to allow passage of the surgeon's index finger into the joint.

The allograft that has been prepared on the back table is now ready for implantation.

In a similar manner to that described for the MMA, two pull sutures are placed in the posterior aspect of the lateral compartment (Fig. 5-12). The first suture is introduced through a 16-gauge spinal needle from an exterior point at the head of the fibula (with the knee at 90° flexion) as the spinal needle is extended along the posterior capsule of the lateral compartment and enters this compartment posteriorly in line with the lateral border of the prepared bony trough.

The second spinal needle and suture are directed to the posterior lateral corner at the junction of the central and posterior thirds of the compartment. Each of these two sutures is pulled forward through the lateral portal. The two sutures sewn through the posterior aspect of the meniscal allograft are placed through the loops in these pull sutures. The pull sutures are then pulled out, thus delivering the allograft sutures into their respective positions in the posterior aspect of this compartment (Fig. 5-12). The meniscus is then urged through the enlarged lateral portal; tugging on the guy wires will pull this allograft into anatomic position. A small tamper is used to advance the donor bone island into its trough, and at the same time, with the knee in varus and 60° flexion, the posterior third

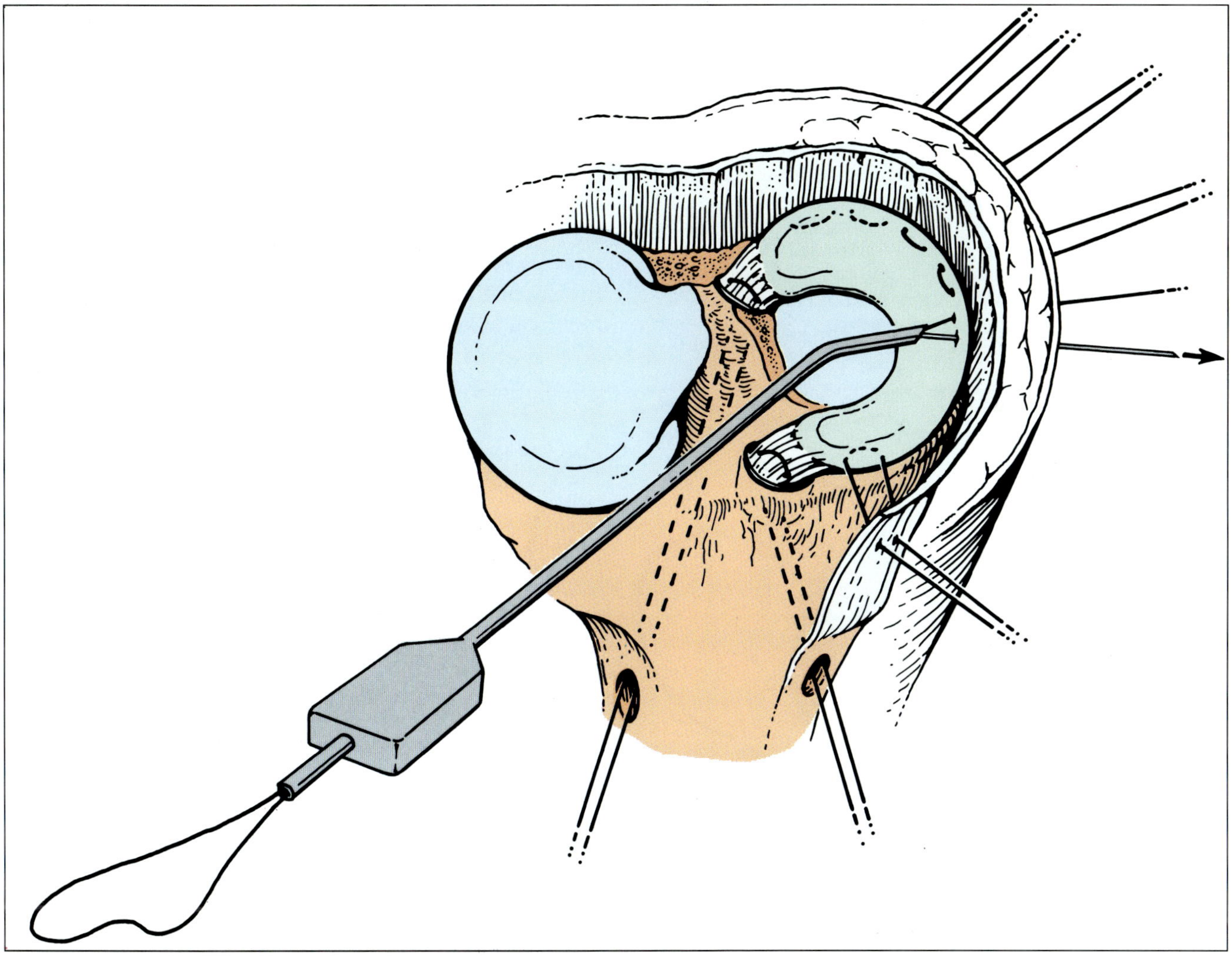

Figure 5-8. The peripheral edge of the body of the transplant is secured to the capsular margin with a series of horizontal mattress sutures using an inside-out suture technique. The author prefers the use of absorbable sutures (size 0 or #1).

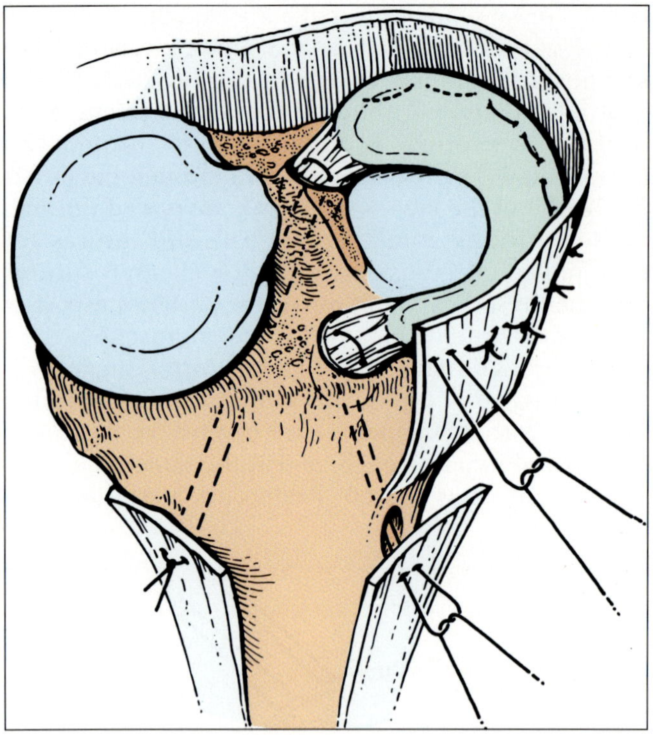

Figure 5-9. The anterior horn suture is preplaced within the edge of the transplant. A sharp free needle is loaded with each of the free ends of the sutures. The capsule is now penetrated on either side of the medial portal, thus closing this arthroscopic portal. The transosseous sutures securing the anterior and posterior horns of the meniscus are tied over deep fascia or a button.

of the allograft is pushed through the interval bordered by the lateral femoral condyle and the lateral tibial eminence. The bony trough measures 10 mm in diameter and the donor bone island measures 9 mm, thus allowing the allograft 1 mm of tolerance within the trough. This tolerance is necessary to permit passage.

The anatomically installed bone island is then carefully tamped into its trough, thus providing a press-fit. The meniscus should be in anatomic position at this time. An optional 3.5-mm cortical screw (30 mm in length) can be added on the back table. This screw is directed from proximal and anterior to distal and posterior through the bone island of the LMA (*see* Figs. 5-10 and 5-13). If the allograft is properly positioned, there will be no draping of meniscal tissue over either the anterior or posterior ridges of the lateral tibial eminence.

The periphery of the lateral meniscus is sewn beginning in the posterior compartment, using outside-in sutures as described by Morgan [10]. The knee is flexed to 90° and the head of the fibula and the biceps tendon are marked on the skin. Outside-in sutures are then placed anterior to the fibular head and biceps tendon, thus preventing injury to the peroneal nerve. After two sutures are placed in the posterior third of the meniscal allograft, the technique should be changed to an inside-out technique, using zone-specific cannulas to complete the suturing of the middle and anterior thirds of the meniscal allograft (Fig. 5-13).

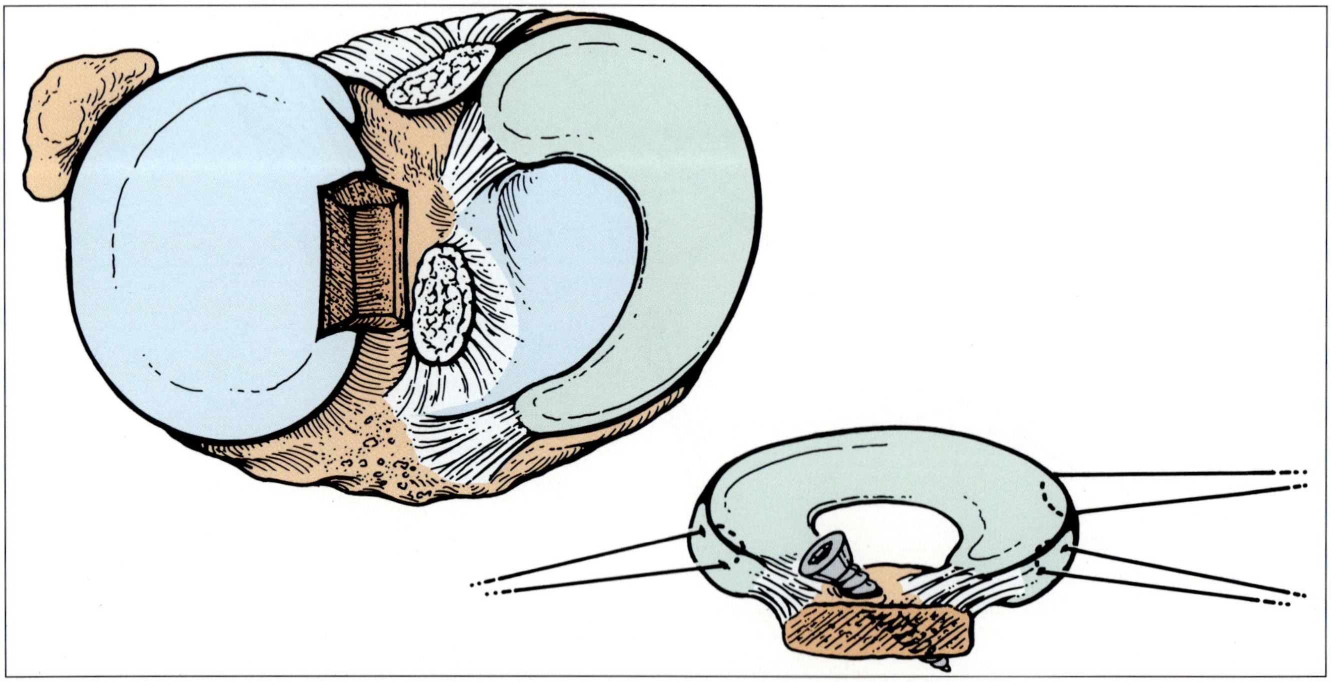

Figure 5-10. Sutures are preplaced in the posterior horn region, the posterolateral corner, and the anterior horn region. This procedure is similar to the medial meniscal allograft preparation.

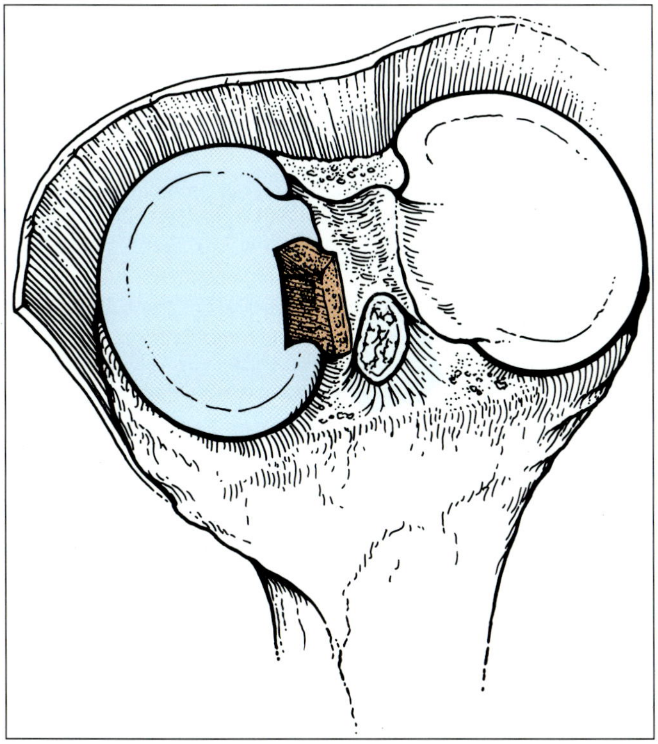

Figure 5-11. A trough (10 x 10 x 20 mm) is prepared lateral to the anterior cruciate ligament.

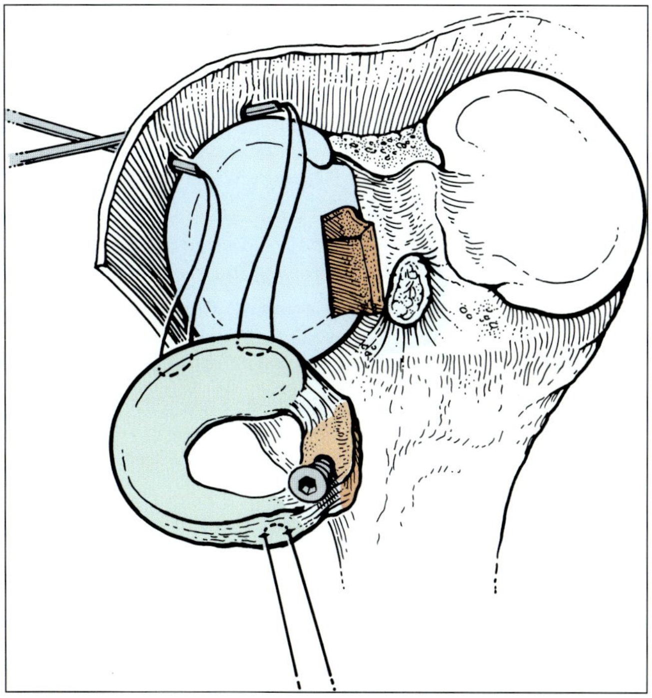

Figure 5-12. The lateral portal is enlarged enough to permit passage of the lateral meniscal allograft. The horns are left attached by a bony bridge.

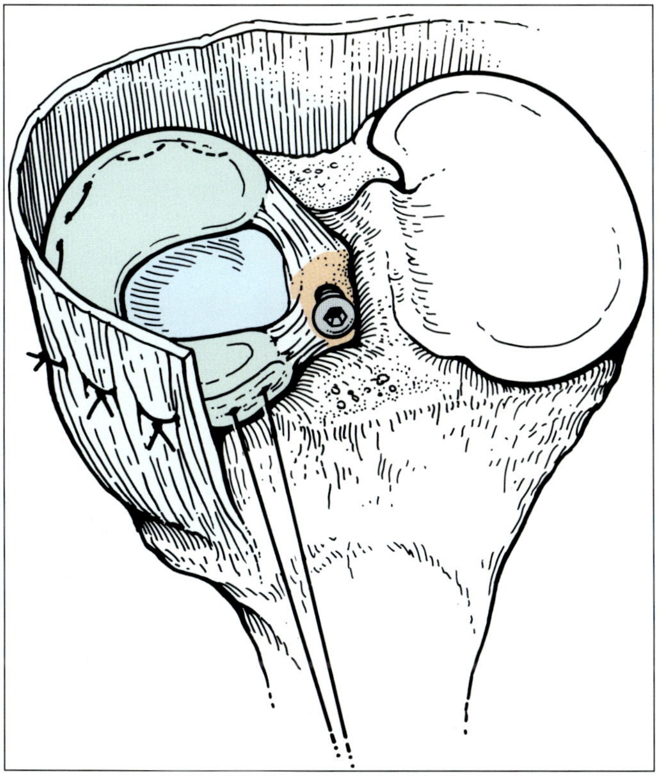

Figure 5-13. The bony bridge is tamped into a press-fit within the trough. A preplaced screw is advanced into the cancellous bone in the path of the bony trough.

REFERENCES

1. Mow VC, Ratcliffe A, Chern KY, *et al.*: Structure and function relationships of the menisci of the knee. In *Knee Meniscus Basic and Clinical Foundations* edn 1. Edited by Mow VC, Arnoczky SP, Jackson DW. New York: Raven Press, 1992, 37–57.
2. Fairbank TJ: Knee joint changes after meniscectomy. *J Bone Joint Surg* 1948, 30B:664–670.
3. O'Brien WR: Degenerative arthritis of the knee following anterior cruciate ligament injury: Role of the meniscus. *Sport Med Arthroscopy Review* 1993, 1:114–118.
4. Lynch MA, Henning CE, Glick KR: Knee joint surface changes: Long-term follow-up meniscus tear treatment in stable anterior cruciate ligament reconstructions. *Clin Orthop* 1983, 172:148–153.
5. Lynch MA, Henning CE: Osteoarthritis in the ACL-deficient knee. In *The Cruciate Ligaments* edn 1. Edited by Feagin JA JR New York: Churchill Livingstone, 1988, 385–391.
6. Johnson RJ, Kettlekamp DB, Clark W, *et al.*: Factors affecting late results after meniscectomy. *J Bone Joint Surg* 1974, 56A:719–729.
7. Ahmed AM: The load bearing role of the knee menisci. I n *Knee Meniscus Basic and Clinical Foundations* edn 1. Edited by Mow VC, Arnoczky SP, Jackson DW. New York: Raven Press, 1992, 59–73.
8. Zukor DJ, Cameron JC, Brooks PJ, *et al.*: The fate of human meniscal allografts. In *Articular Cartilage and Knee Joint Function: Basic Science and Arthroscopy.* Edited by Ewing JW. New York: Raven Press, 1990, 147.
9. Garrett JC: Meniscal transplantation: a review of 43 cases with 2–7 year follow-up. *Sports Med Am Arth Rev* 1993, 1:164–167.
10. Morgan CD: The arthroscopic outside to inside meniscus repair technique. *Techniques in Orthopedics* 1993, 82:99–104.

6

CHAPTER

Arthroscopically Assisted Proximal Extensor Mechanism Realignment of the Knee

NEAL C. SMALL
ALEXANDER I. GLOGAU

The treatment of recurrent lateral patellofemoral instability has been a difficult problem for the orthopedist for many decades. There are numerous surgical procedures that have been developed for the treatment of this condition (Friedman, exhibit at the AAOS, Atlanta, GA, 1991) [1–9]. In 1983, the senior author developed a procedure that addressed this problem using an arthroscopically assisted proximal extensor mechanism realignment. During the past 10 years, 67 procedures have been performed. Twenty-seven knees in 24 patients were studied in detail and followed postoperatively for a minimum of 18 months. The results were published in 1993 [10]. Eighteen of the 24 patients in the original series have been followed for a minimum of 40 months. The data on these patients are currently being compiled.

CASE I

A 27-year-old man sustained a right patellar dislocation defending a pass during a flag football game. The patellar dislocation was reduced by the patient with lateral pressure. He was placed in a knee immobilizer by the athletic trainer and referred for orthopedic evaluation.

Physical examination revealed a moderately effused right knee with a positive apprehension sign and diffuse tenderness. The knee was ligamentously stable to testing. Radiograph results demonstrated evidence of a patellar fracture dislocation with intra-articular fragments noted on the Merchants 45° axial view (Fig. 6-1). The radiographs also demonstrated a mild patellar tilt and lateral subluxation.

Surgical intervention was recommended. The patient underwent an arthroscopic evaluation. Osteochondral fragments were excised and arthroscopically assisted proximal extensor mechanism realignment was performed. There was noted to be a large defect in the medial patellar facet. Four loose fragments were removed. The medial retinaculum was noted to be torn at the time of surgery.

Three months after surgery, the patient was noted to have a stable patellofemoral joint and was returned to unrestricted athletic activity. His follow-up visit 54 months postoperatively demonstrated a full active range of motion, no effusion, and no significant patellofemoral pain.

Isokinetic testing demonstrated symmetrical extensor strength at 60° and 300° per second. Radiographs demonstrated a concentrically positioned patella on the Merchant's 45° axial view (Fig. 6-2). The patient has remained at full activity without limitations.

CASE II

A 15-year-old girl with a history of recurrent left patellar subluxation while running hurdles during high school track sustained an acute subluxation playing basketball. The patient felt and heard a "pop" with jumping.

The initial examination demonstrated significant medial retinacular tenderness and discoloration. Her apprehension test was markedly positive with an easily dislocatable patella. A large effusion was noted. The remainder of the examination was unremarkable.

Radiographs obtained (Merchant's 45° axial view) demonstrated a lateral subluxation and tilt (Fig. 6-3). The congruence angle and sulcus angle were +17° and 132°, respectively. The patellofemoral index was 2.5 with a lateral tilt noted.

The patient and parents elected to undergo operative intervention. At surgery, the patella was easily dislocatable during the examination under anesthesia. The medial retinaculum was disrupted. The patient underwent an arthroscopically assisted extensor mechanism realignment. The patella was reduced, thus correcting the tilt and lateral subluxation (Fig. 6-4).

The patient experienced a local suture reaction postoperatively that required suture removal 3 months later and slowed her initial recovery. She regained 90° of motion by the third postoperative month. She began jogging by the fourth postoperative month. At the 76th month postoperatively, she was noted to have a stable patellofemoral joint and continued to play basketball. Her radiographs demonstrated a stable patellofemoral joint with a congruence angle of -5° and no lateral tilt.

SURGICAL PROCEDURE

Under general anesthesia, the patella is often easily subluxed or completely dislocated with laterally directed passive pressure during the examination with the knee in 30° of flexion. An arthroscopic assessment of patellofemoral tracking is then performed. This examination includes attention to lateral patellar overhang at varying degrees of knee flexion and

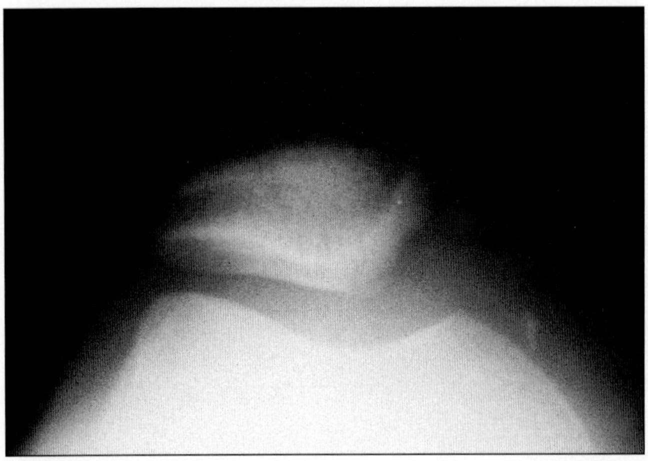

Figure 6-1. Merchant's 45° axial view of the patellofemoral joint demonstrating patellar tilt and lateral subluxation with osteochondral fragments.

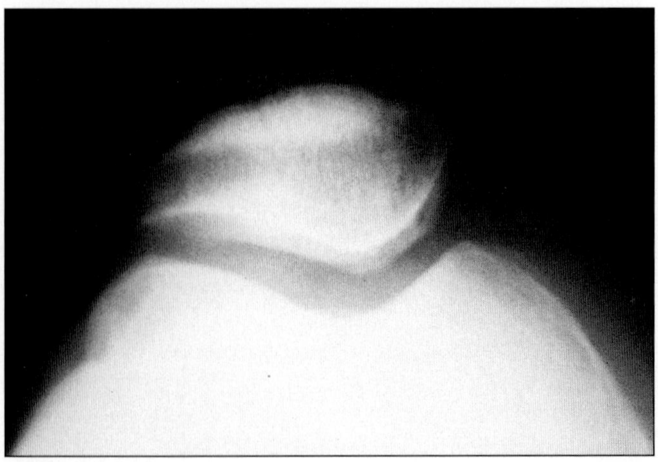

Figure 6-2. Merchant's 45° axial view of the patellofemoral joint, 54 months postarthroscopically assisted proximal extensor mechanism realignment.

incongruity of tracking in the intertrochlear sulcus. Areas of contact and articular surface wear are noted. The patellofemoral articulation is viewed from both the superior lateral and inferior lateral portals. Recently, viewing from the superior medial portal has been found to be useful. In acute cases, the medial retinacular defect is visible. This is usually immediately adjacent to the medial border of the patella. Osteochondral fragments from the medial patellar border or lateral femoral condylar margin are easily visible. The fragments are removed arthroscopically if they are loose or extensively detached from the soft tissues. The extent of the tear is examined and probed. If required, the defect is extended proximally to expose 2 to 3 cm of the vastus medialis muscle fibers or distally to the medial border of the patellar tendon. This extension is performed using an endoscopic scalpel blade.

Multiple #2 polydioxanone sutures are then passed percutaneously under direct arthroscopic visualization (Figs. 6-5 and 6-6). A large half-round trocar cutting needle is used for the percutaneous insertion of this

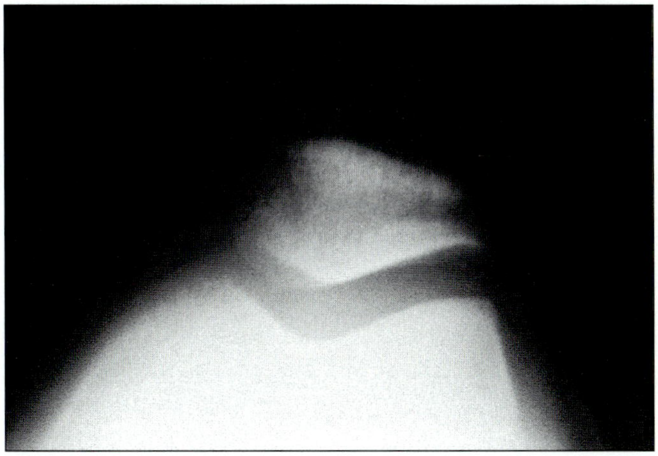

Figure 6-3. A 45° axial view of the patellofemoral joint demonstrating lateral subluxation and tilt.

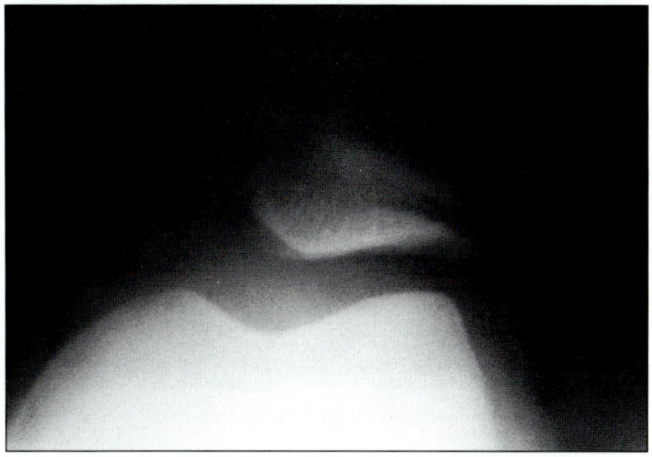

Figure 6-4. Merchant's 45° axial view of the patellofemoral joint 76 months following arthroscopically assisted extensor mechanism realignment showing no significant subluxation or lateral tilt.

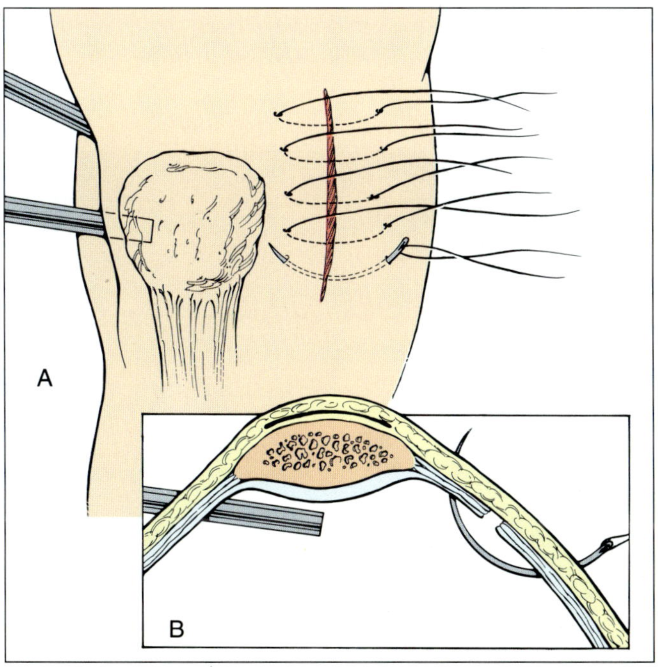

Figure 6-5. Under arthroscopic control, #2 polydioxanone sutures are passed percutaneously through the posterior and anterior margins of the medial retinacular defect. **A**, External perspective. **B**, Arthroscopic perspective.

suture. The needle enters the medial retinaculum, approximately 1 cm posterior to the edge of the retinacular defect. The needle is then passed under arthroscopic control across the retinacular defect to exit 1 cm anterior to the edge of the tear. The anterior exit point is often adjacent to the medial border of the patella. The needle is then brought out through the skin anteriorly. Four to six sutures are usually required to close and plicate the defect in the medial retinaculum.

A 2-cm skin incision is then fashioned medially between the two ends of the sutures. Blunt subcutaneous dissection is used to retrieve the sutures into the single small medial incision (Figs. 6-7 and 6-8). A lateral retinacular release is then performed using either an endoscopic or subcutaneous technique under arthroscopic control (Fig. 6-9). With a medially directed force on the patella and with the knee in full extension, the sutures are then tied individually

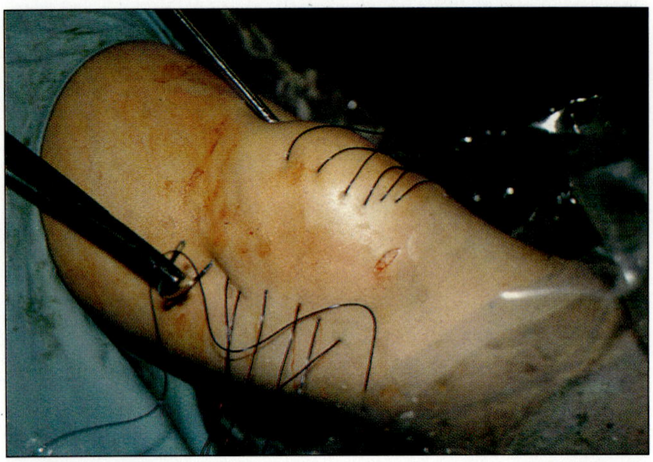

Figure 6-6. A #2 polydioxanone suture placed percutaneously under arthroscopic control.

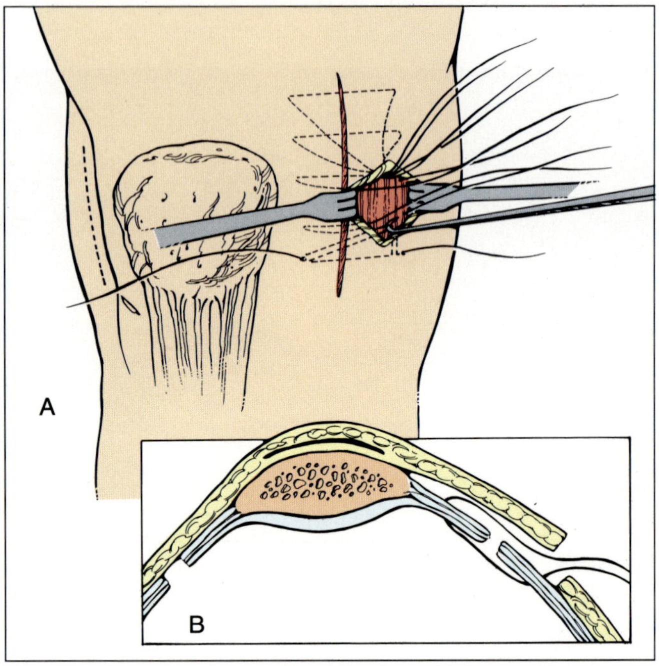

Figure 6-7. Retinacular plicating sutures being passed into the 2-cm medial incision. **A**, External perspective. **B**, Arthroscopic perspective.

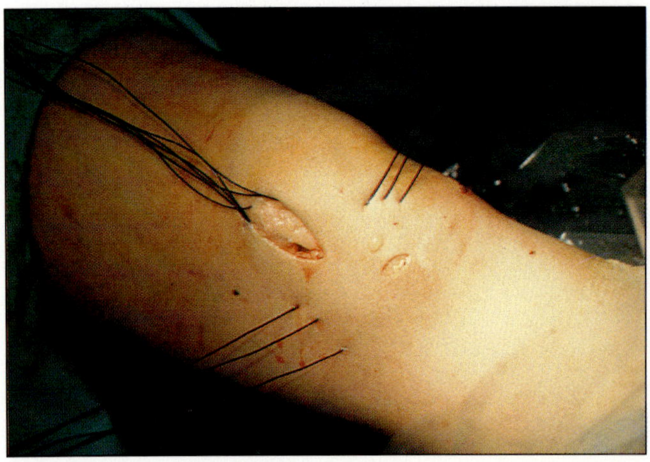

Figure 6-8. Sutures passed into small medial incision (2 cm).

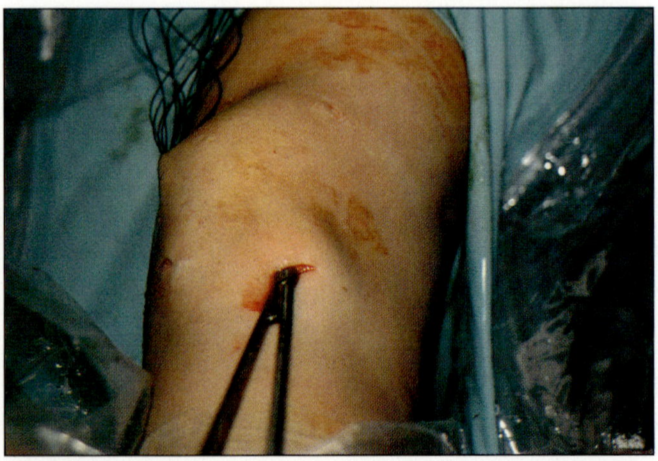

Figure 6-9. Subcutaneous lateral retinacular release performed.

(Fig. 6-10). This substantially plicates the medial retinaculum and the distal fibers of the vastus medialis (Figs. 6-11 and 6-12). The patella is then checked for stability through a range of motion from full extension to 90° of flexion. Patellar tracking is observed arthroscopically. The sutures are usually not visible at this point because of the significant plication and overlap of the medial retinaculum. The small medial wound is then closed with one or two sutures. The knee is then placed in a knee immobilizer splint in full extension. Postoperative weight bearing is allowed as tolerated. Range of motion is allowed postoperatively at 2 weeks. Usually a continuous passive motion (CPM) machine is utilized. The knee immobilizer is used during ambulation until 4 weeks following surgery.

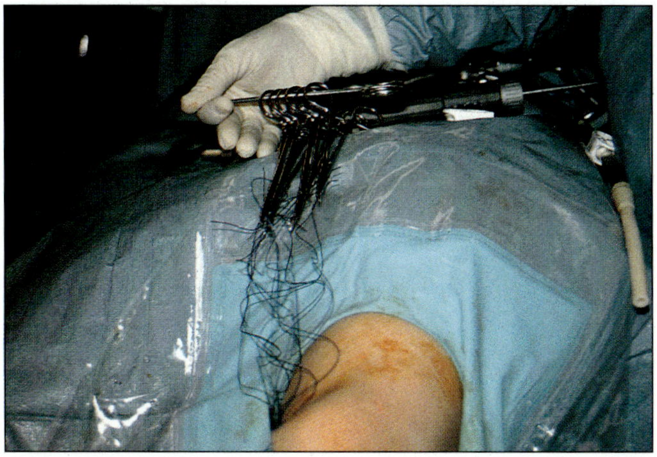

Figure 6-10. Sutures kept in order for individual tying after lateral retinacular release.

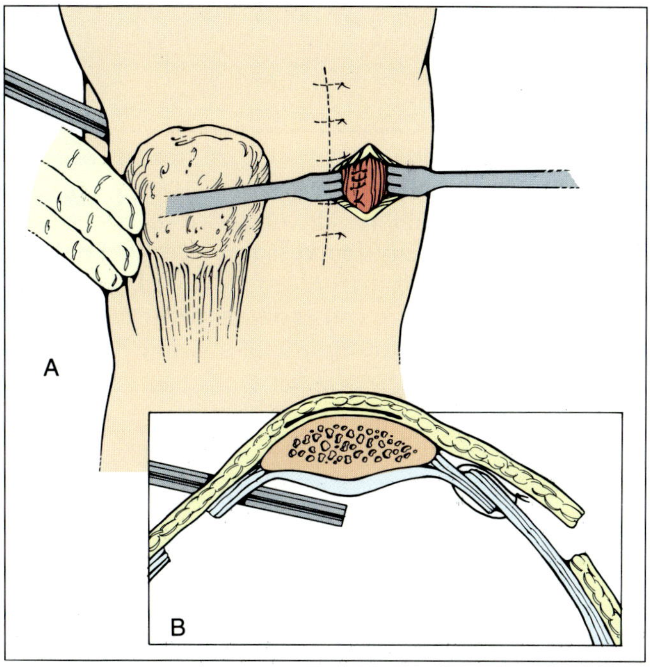

Figure 6-11. Medially directed pressure is applied to the lateral margin of the patella as the sutures are being tied individually. This allows maximum plication of the medial retinaculum. **A**, External perspective. **B**, Arthroscopic perspective.

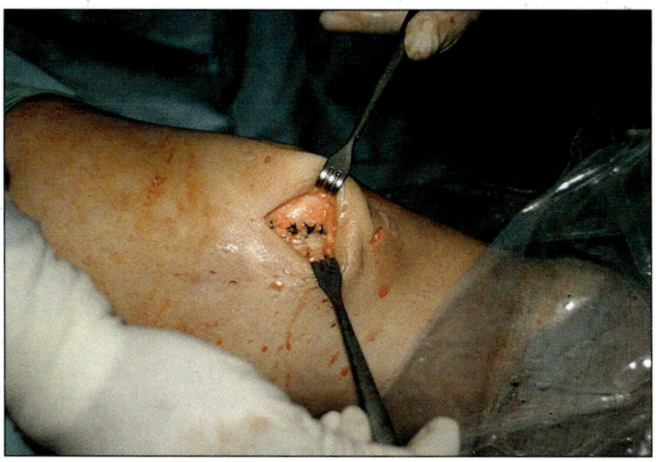

Figure 6-12. Sutures plicating medial patellar retinaculum.

Postoperative Care

Twenty-seven knees in 24 patients were followed for a minimum of 18 months postoperatively. The patients were asked to complete a detailed questionnaire. They were also brought back for a detailed physical examination by one of the junior authors.

The objective success rate of the procedure is 96% (one recurrent episode of instability). The patients subjectively rated the procedure a success in 93% of the knees.

Discussion

This minimally invasive procedure has been quite helpful in the treatment of patients with recurrent patellofemoral instability. The objective success rate of 96% and the subjective success rate of 93% are both impressive. If indeed the procedure does fail, a distal realignment procedure can easily be performed. Clinical indications for this minimally invasive procedure include recurrent dislocation of the patella, a first-time dislocation with an osteochondral fragment, a first-time dislocation in a highly competitive athlete, and recurrent major subluxation of the patellofemoral joint.

This procedure has now been performed by the senior author for over 10 years. The procedure has recently been modified to allow immediate weight bearing in full extension and early range of motion beginning at approximately 2 weeks using a CPM machine. This has minimized the amount of postoperative stiffness. This procedure is simple, effective, and does not preclude the use of distal realignment should there be a clinical failure following the arthroscopically assisted procedure. The return to active competition following the procedure is quite rapid, averaging about 3 months for return to full sports participation.

In summary, the procedure is simple, predictable, and allows a rapid return to full function. Patient satisfaction with the procedure is quite high. The recurrent rate among the initial 27 procedures performed is 4% at a minimum 18-month follow-up.

References

1. Betz RR, Magill JT III, Lonergan RP: The percutaneous lateral retinacular release. *Am J Sports Med* 1987, 15:477–482.
2. Dainer RD, Barrack RL, Buckley SL, *et al.*: Arthroscopic treatment of acute patellar dislocations. *Arthroscopy* 1988, 4:267–271.
3. Henry JH, Goletz TH, Williamson B: Lateral retinacular release in patellofemoral subluxation. *Am J Sports Med* 1986, 14:121–129.
4. Metcalf RW: An arthroscopic method for lateral release of the subluxing or dislocating patella. *Clin Orthop* 1982, 167:9–18.
5. Scuderi G, Cuomo F, Scott WN: Lateral release and proximal realignment for patellar subluxation and dislocation. *J Bone Joint Surg* [Am] 1988, 70:856–861.
6. Schonholtz GJ, Zahn MG, Magee CM: Lateral retinacular release of the patella. *Arthroscopy* 1987, 3:269–272.
7. Yamamoto RK: Arthroscopic repair of the medial retinaculum and capsule in acute patellar dislocations. *Arthroscopy* 1986, 2:125–131.
8. Hawkins RJ, Bell RH, Anisette G: Acute patellar dislocations. *Am J Sports Med* 1986, 14:117–120.
9. Sherman OH, Fox JM, Sperling H, *et al.*: Patellar instability: treatment by arthroscopic electrosurgical lateral release. *Arthroscopy* 1987, 3:152–160.
10. Small NC: Arthroscopically assisted proximal extensor mechanism realignment of the knee. *Arthroscopy* 1993, 9:63–67.

7

CHAPTER

The Use of Hamstring Tendons in Anterior Cruciate Ligament Surgery

ROGER V. LARSÓN

The use of semitendinosus and gracilis tendon autografts for reconstruction of the anterior cruciate ligament (ACL) has been well established [1–3]. They may in fact offer several advantages over other commonly used autografts such as the patellar tendon. The potential advantages of these grafts include increased strength, stiffness characteristics similar to the normal ACL, a large surface area for revascularization, ease of tensioning, and adaptability to precise positioning.

When the semitendinosus and gracilis tendons are both doubled and used as an anterior cruciate graft, they provide a large diameter, strong ACL substitute. Noyes and coworkers [4] have shown that a 14-mm wide patellar tendon graft is approximately 175% as strong in tension as a normal ACL. These data are commonly used to argue that the patellar tendon autograft is the strongest ACL autogenous substitute. In actuality, it is much more common to use a patellar tendon graft of 10-mm width, which by extrapolation would provide a graft approximately 125% the strength of a normal ACL. This same study on graft strength shows that a semitendinosus tendon is approximately 75% the strength of a normal ACL and that the gracilis tendon is approximately 50% of the strength of a normal ACL. If these two tendons are doubled and then combined we can obtain a graft with actual strength in excess of 200% than that of the normal ACL. Another way to view this would be to consider the cross-sectional area of collagen that is being used to replace the normal ACL. The cross-sectional area of the average patellar tendon graft is 10 mm x 3 mm or approximately 30 mm^2. The cross-sectional area of an 8-mm tunnel is 50 mm^2. A double loop of semitendinosus and gracilis tendons normally fills an 8 mm tunnel tightly, therefore providing a cross-sectional area of collagen approximately 1.7 times that provided by a patellar tendon graft.

The ability to place a hamstring tendon graft precisely is enhanced over that of a patellar tendon graft. Figure 7-1 demonstrates that if a bone tunnel is placed in the desired region for ACL attachment and is filled with a soft-tissue graft, the precise location of the collagen is known. When a bone–block-tendon composite graft is placed into a tunnel, the exact position of the collagen portion is less well controlled because of the dependence on the final position of the bone block and perhaps the fixation device. The ability for a multistranded graft to obtain nutrition either by diffusion or by vascular ingrowth is enhanced over that of a solid graft due to the increased surface area and smaller depth of penetration needed for either revascularization or nutrient diffusion (Fig. 7-2).

Another potential advantage of using hamstring tendons for ACL reconstruction is that this procedure produces a graft that is similar in stiffness to the normal ACL compared with the patellar tendon autograft, which is significantly more stiff than the normal ACL [5]. The use of a graft with the stiffness characteristics of hamstring tendons also allows more leeway when tensioning the reconstruction, thus making over constraint of the joint less likely. Recent studies by Steiner and coworkers [6] have also demonstrated that when hamstring tendon grafts are fixed by the method to be described, the initial fixation strength is greater than that of bone blocks fixed with interference-fit screws. The recently published study of Rodeo and coworkers [7] has documented the process of tendon healing in bone tunnels and has demonstrated that biological fixation in this situation occurs relatively early.

Probably the most compelling reason to consider hamstring tendon autografts for ACL reconstruction is the decreased surgical morbidity associated with this procedure. In our experience, problems with motion or with patellofemoral arthrosis are extremely rare. Several recent studies comparing hamstring tendon ACL reconstruction with patellar tendon ACL reconstructions did not show a significant difference in success rates between the two grafts but have shown increased morbidity with the use of patellar tendon autografts. The increased morbidity includes decreased quadriceps strength, decreased range of motion, and increased patellofemoral pain complaints (Callaway and coworkers, Paper presented at the 61st Annual Meeting American Academy of Orthopaedic Surgeons, New Orleans, 1994) (Friedman and coworkers, paper presented at the Combined Congress of the International Arthroscopy Association and the International Society of the Knee, Copenhagen, 1993) [8,9•]. It has been demonstrated by Lipscomb [10] that there is no significant loss of knee flexion strength after sacrificing both the semitendinosus and gracilis tendons if appropriate rehabilitation is undertaken.

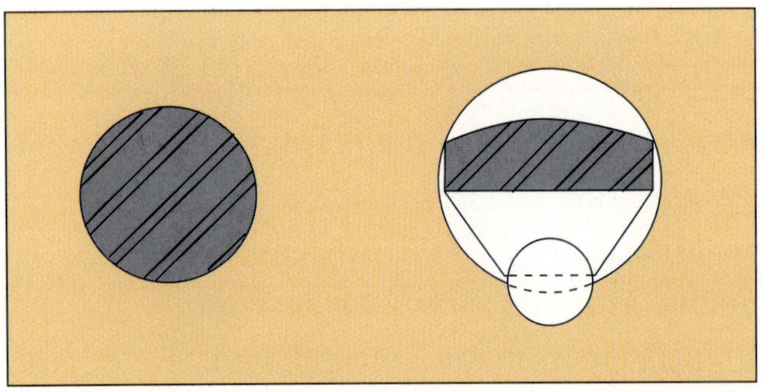

Figure 7-1. The location of the collagen portion of a graft (*cross hatched*) is better controlled when a tunnel is completely filled with a soft-tissue graft (*left*) than when a bone block and fixation device also are near the tunnel opening (*right*).

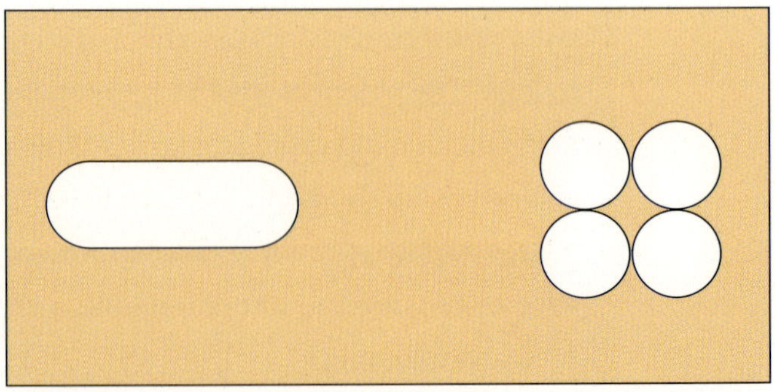

Figure 7-2. A multistranded graft (*right*) has more surface area for vascularization and less depth of penetration needed for nutrition than a solid piece of collagen (*left*).

Technique for Reconstruction With Double Loops of Semitendinosus and Gracilis Tendons

Set-up

The set-up for this procedure includes a tourniquet placed as proximal as possible on the thigh. A thigh holder is used that is very low profile (Fig. 7-3). It is important to avoid a bulky thigh holder that would interfere with the ability to obtain the proper drilling angle for the femoral tunnel. It is our current practice to exsanguinate the limb and inflate the tourniquet at the beginning of the case, however, diagnostic arthroscopy and any meniscal work could be accomplished prior to inflation of the tourniquet if desired. There needs to be a break in the table at the level of the knee joint so that the knee can be flexed to 90°.

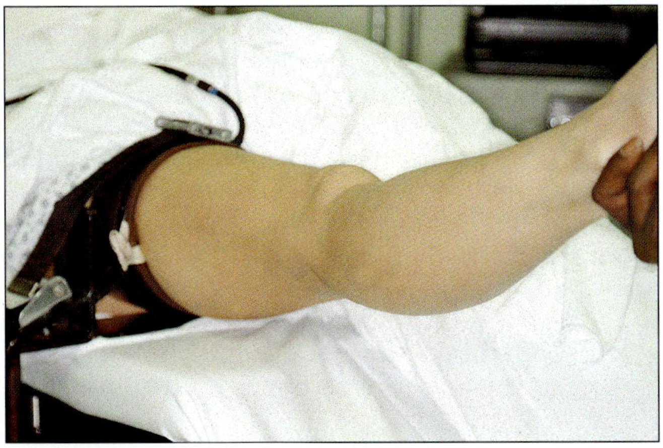

Figure 7-3. Proper set-up requires a proximal tourniquet, low bulk thigh holder, and a table that bends at the knee level to allow flexion to 90°.

Diagnostic Arthroscopy

At the beginning of the case, a diagnostic arthroscopy is carried out. Any meniscal work or joint debridement is done. It is important to make the anteromedial and anterolateral portals as close as possible to the patellar tendon to allow easier access to the intercondylar notch (Fig. 7-4). One point that is worth emphasizing is that if a medial meniscus repair is going to be accomplished, the semitendinosus and gracilis grafts should be obtained prior to the meniscal repair. Harvesting the hamstring tendons after the meniscal repair has been completed puts the meniscus repair sutures at risk for disruption.

Notchplasty

Proper visualization of the intercondylar notch usually requires at least a minimal notchplasty. In the case of chronic ACL insufficiency with intercondylar notch narrowing, it may be necessary to perform a much greater notchplasty. To begin the notch debridement, a motorized shaver with a full-radius resector is used to debride a portion of the fat pad anteriorly, anterolaterally, and anteromedially. This allows for the arthroscope to be "backed up" to provide a better perspective of the anterior portion of the intercondylar notch.

The notchplasty is performed by using a 0.25-in curved osteotome on the lateral aspect of the notch

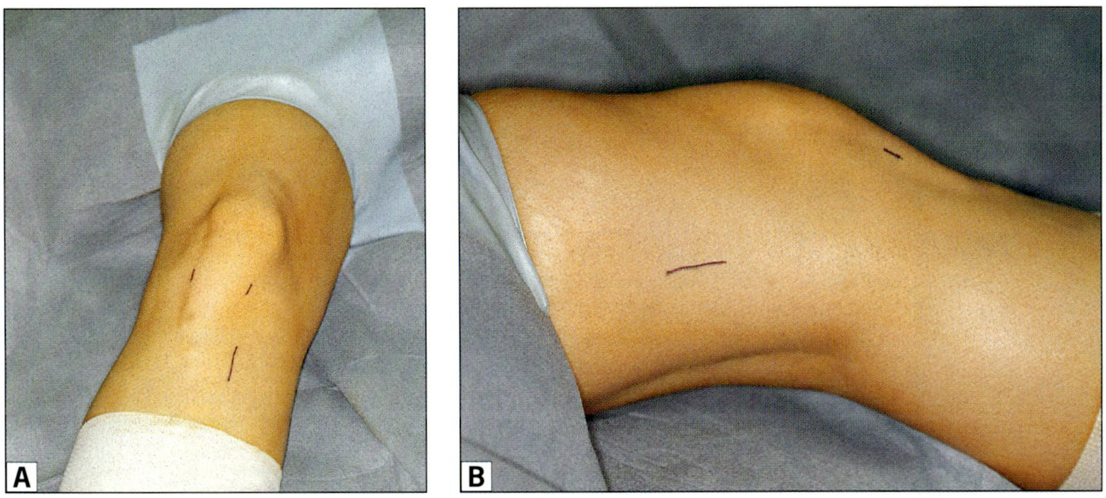

Figure 7-4. A, B, Incisions include anterolateral and anteromedial portals both adjacent to the patellar tendon. The tibial incision begins approximately 1 in distal to the anteromedial portal and extends 1 to 1.5 in. The lateral incision is centered over the iliotibial band and extends distally to the level of the superior pole of the patella.

with the knee flexed near 90° (Figs. 7-5A and 7-4B). The initial notchplasty can then be carried superiorly and also deep within the notch using a curette (Fig. 7-5B). In most knees, the notchplasty can be completed with a curette and smoothed with a rasp (Fig. 7-5C). In some knees where the bone is particularly hard a motorized burr can be used. Care should be taken to remove all bone fragments from the joint as they are created. Removal of soft tissue should include synovium from the lateral border of the posterior cruciate ligament (PCL) so that the lateral border can be clearly identified. There should be approximately 1 cm of clearance between the lateral margin of the PCL and the lateral wall of the intercondylar notch (Fig. 7-5D). Enlargement of the intercondylar notch should be carried posteriorly to the posterior capsule so that the "over the top" area can be clearly defined. Care should be taken not to misinterpret a ridge in front of the "over the top" area as the "over the top" area because this may lead to an inappropriate placement of the femoral tunnel.

Tibial Stump

In most cases, there is a tibial stump of the ACL present. Depending on the condition of the stump, it can be either debrided or sutured and pulled out of the way. If it is debrided, which is the usual case, only enough stump is removed to allow visualization of the bony landmarks for placement of the tibial and femoral tunnels. When the graft is placed, if it can pass through the residual tibial stump, this may provide vascularized tissue that may help revascularize the grafts. If it is elected to pass sutures through the stump, these sutures can be pulled through the femoral tunnel after the graft has been placed.

Harvest of Grafts

For graft harvest, a skin incision is made vertically over the insertion of the semitendinosus and gracilis tendons. This same incision is used as an exit point for the tibial tunnel. The incision starts approximately 1 in distal to the anteromedial portal and need extend distally approximately 1 to 1.5 in only (Fig. 7-4A and 7-4B). Once the semitendinosus and gracilis tendons have been identified, they are isolated with a clamp (Fig. 7-6A) then freed from their tibial attachments. They are harvested with a closed-end tendon stripper (Figs. 7-6B and 7-6C). It is very important to identify any extraneous bands or insertions to make sure there is a clear pathway for the tendon stripper to pass proximally to the muscle belly [11]. If this precaution is not taken, it is possible for the tendon stripper to follow an aberrant pathway and sever the tendon far short of the muscle belly. To best avoid this, it is advisable to clamp the free end of each tendon with a clamp and apply tension while carefully dissecting

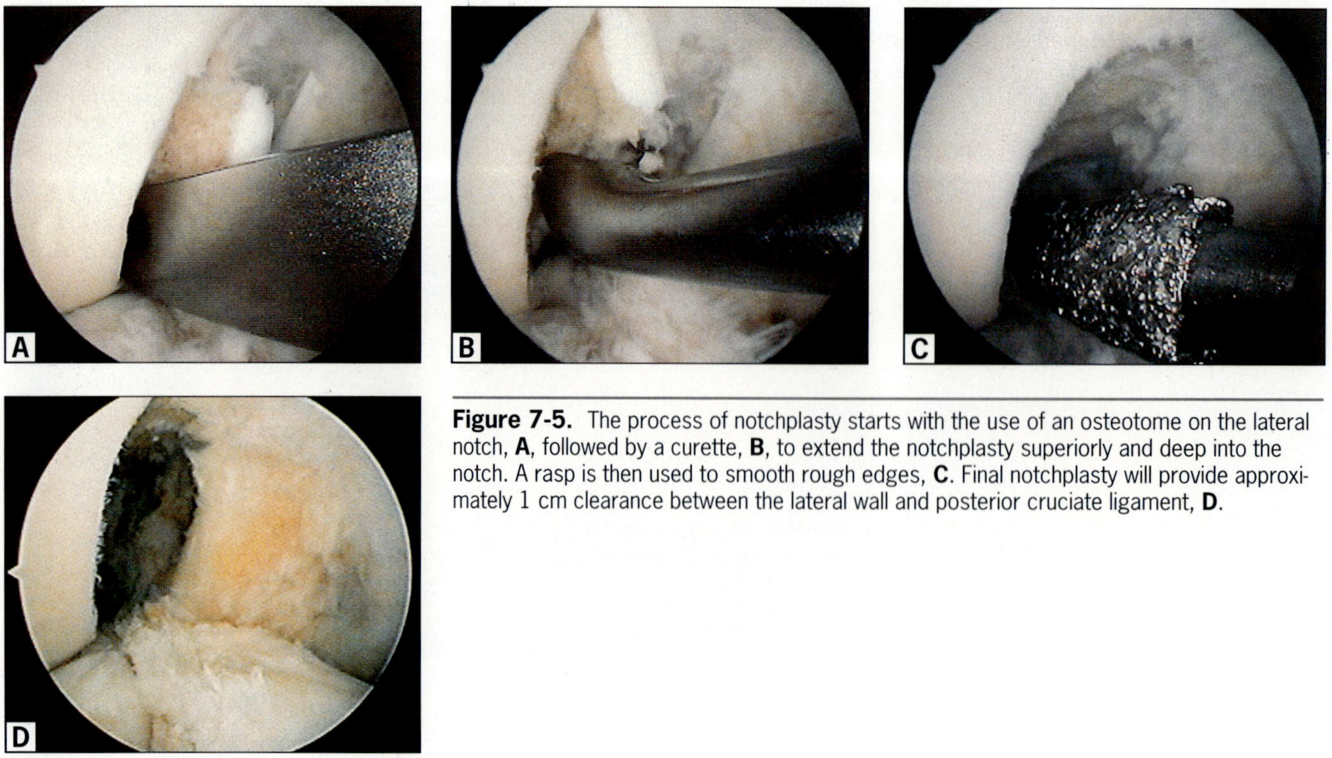

Figure 7-5. The process of notchplasty starts with the use of an osteotome on the lateral notch, **A**, followed by a curette, **B**, to extend the notchplasty superiorly and deep into the notch. A rasp is then used to smooth rough edges, **C**. Final notchplasty will provide approximately 1 cm clearance between the lateral wall and posterior cruciate ligament, **D**.

each tendon with scissors until the tendon is clearly free. If there is difficulty in identifying or separating the two tendons, it is best to identify the upper border of the gracilis tendon, then release all attachments distal from the tibia. The combined insertion can then be inverted and from the underside it is usually very easy to identify and separate the two tendons. Usually approximately 28 to 30 cm of tendon length can be obtained, and most often the two tendons are of nearly equal length. There are occasions when the gracilis graft is somewhat shorter than the semitendinosus, and a means for dealing with this will be discussed in the graft fixation section.

Graft Preparation

Once the tendons have been harvested, a sharp scalpel or curette is used to scrape the retained muscle belly from the tendon. Each end of each graft is then sutured for approximately 4 cm using a Bunnel stitch of #2 nonabsorbable sutures as demonstrated in Figure 7-7A. The suturing of each end of the graft is a very important step that allows the fixation at the terminal ends to extend up to the major body of the tendons. The prepared grafts are demonstrated in Figure 7-7B. The grafts are then sized by passing them through sizing tubes as demonstrated in Figure 7-7C. The smallest tunnel that will allow graft passage will be created in the tibia and femur.

Preparation of Tibial Tunnel

After the grafts have been harvested, a point is selected for exit of the tibial tunnel proximal to the insertion of the pes anserinus at the junction of the diaphysis and metaphysis of the anteromedial tibia. This region can be easily palpated. A tibial drill guide with a narrow angle of approximately 30° to 35° is then used to place a guidepin from this point to an intra-articular point corresponding to a central tibial attachment site. The goal is to provide a central tibial attachment or an attachment site that approximates the center of the anatomic ACL. This is a site that allows for complimentary graft attachment to the femur in an area that provides minimal strain to the ACL substitute [12]. The central tibial attachment site also avoids impingement with the roof of the intercondylar notch. If the graft is positioned so that superior notch impingement occurs, the result will be compromised due to possible extension block, broken anterior graft fibers, and delayed graft healing [13].

The appropriate tibial attachment site can be accomplished by placing the tip of the tibial aiming guide intra-articularly just lateral to the midportion of the medial tibial spine (Fig. 7-8A). Usually there is enough of a tibial stump present to aid in the selection of this point. When the initial guidepin has been placed, it is imperative that it be passed approximately 1 in into the intercondylar notch region and then

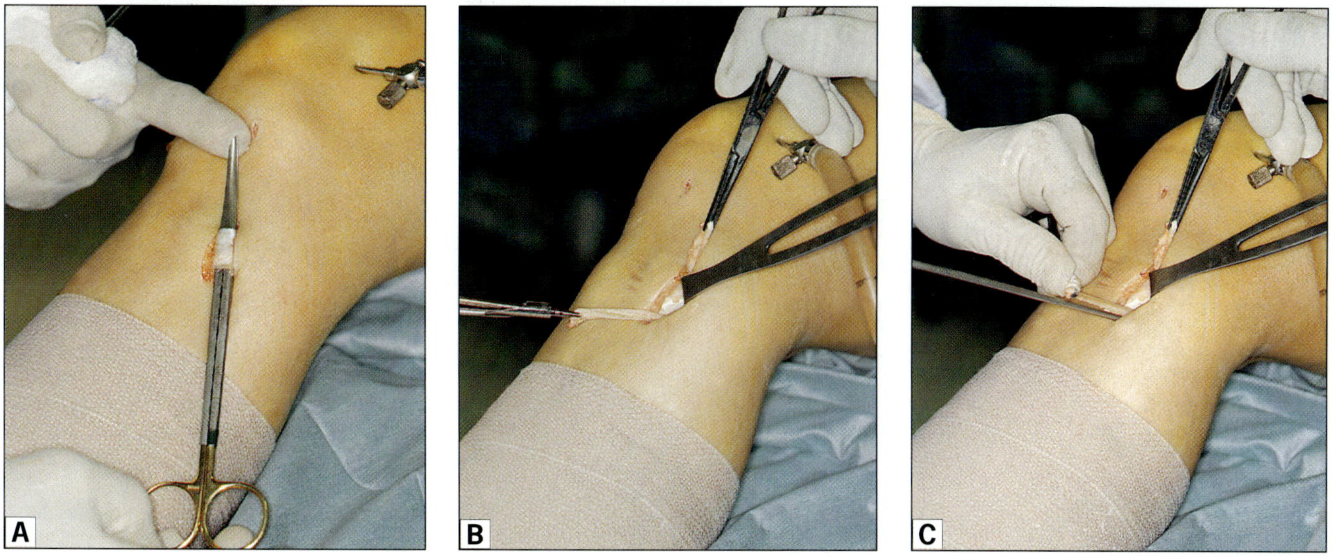

Figure 7-6. Harvest of the semitendinosus and gracilis tendons begins by isolating the two tendons, **A**, then releasing them from the tibia, **B**. They are then inverted and separated and harvested with a tendon stripper, **C**.

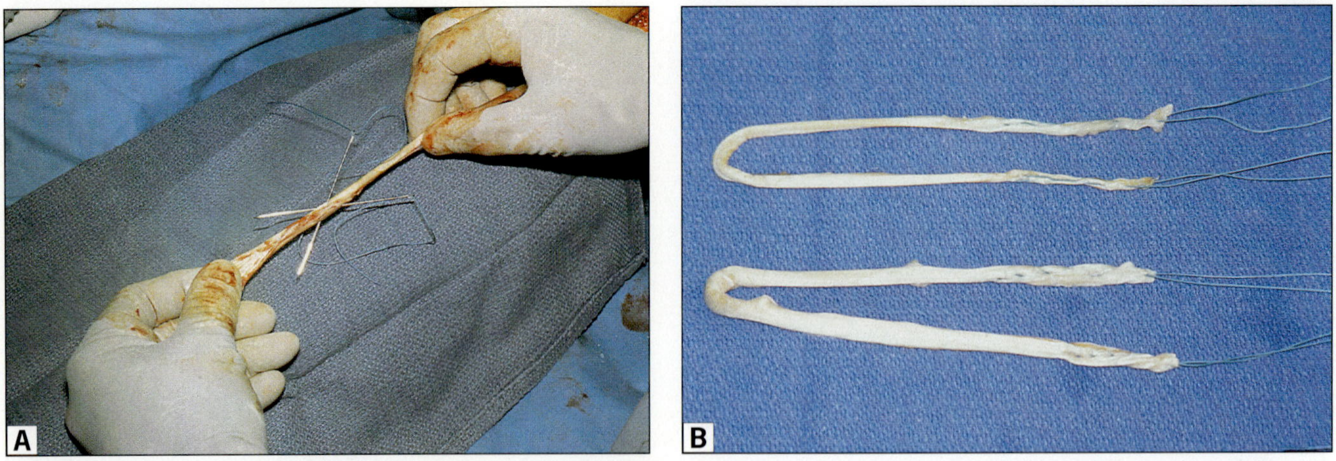

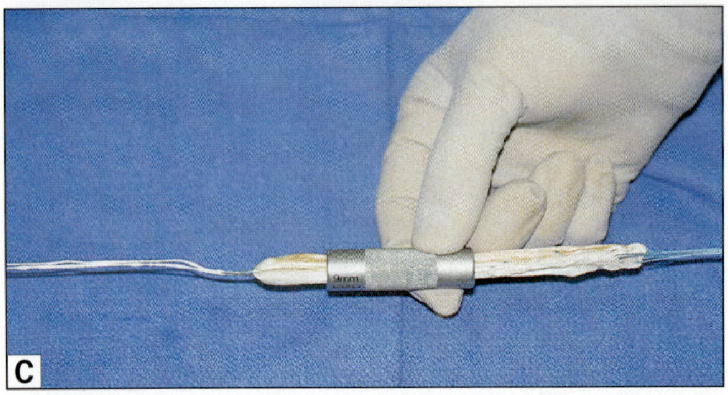

Figure 7-7. The hamstring tendons are prepared by tagging each end of each tendon with a nonabsorbable suture, **A, B**. The doubled tendons are then sized by passing them through a sizing tube, **C**. The smallest tunnels that will allow passage of the grafts will be drilled.

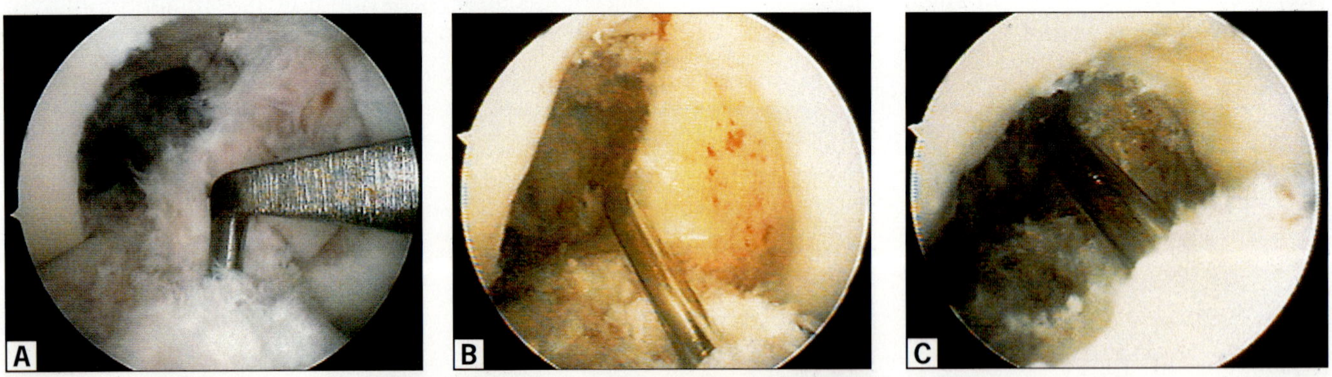

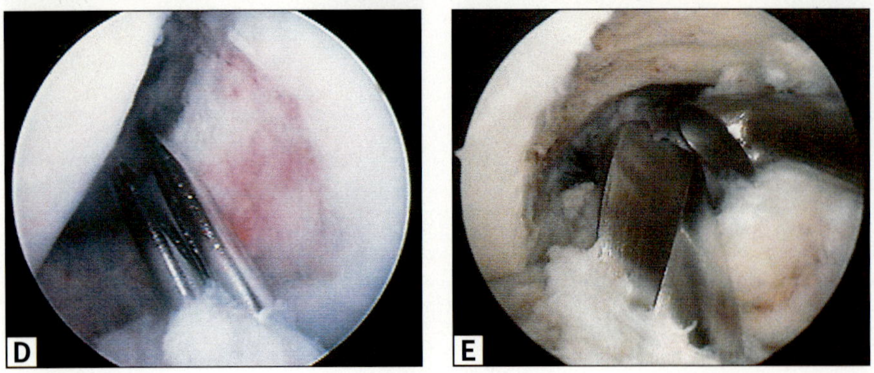

Figure 7-8. The central tibial tunnel is created by first placing a guidepin with a drill guide, **A**. The position of the guidepin should be adjacent to the posterior cruciate ligament, **B**, and as the knee is extended the pin should move directly toward the apex of the notch. At terminal extension clearance should exist between the pin and the notch roof equivalent to the radius of the tunnel to be drilled, **C**. If the position is not ideal a parallel drill guide can be used to "fine tune" the position, **D**. When the optimal position is achieved the pin is over-drilled with the appropriate cannulated drill, **E**.

observed as the knee is passed through a range of motion. The guidepin should pass directly adjacent to the PCL (Fig. 7-8B), and as the knee is brought into full extension the guidepin should move directly toward the apex of the notch, and at terminal extension there should be a clearance between the guidepin and the superior notch equal to the desired radius of the tibial tunnel (Fig. 7-8C). If the position is not perfect, it can be fine tuned by placing a parallel guidepin with the desired correction (Fig. 7-8D). The placement of parallel guidepins can be facilitated by commercially available parallel drill guides. As the guidepin is observed with knee motion, a careful evaluation of the notchplasty can also be made and any additional modifications carried out.

When the position of the guidepin has been optimized, it is overdrilled with a cannulated drill (Fig. 7-8E). The size of the drill is selected based on the size of the graft. The smallest tunnel that will allow passage of the graft is created.

Preparation of Femoral Tunnel

A second skin incision is made in the distal lateral thigh. The incision is centered over and parallel to the midportion of the iliotibial band. The incision is 1 to 1.5 in long with the distal end extending to the level of the superior pole of the patella (Fig. 7-4B). The incision is then carried down to the iliotibial tract, which is incised just anterior to the intermuscular septum. The vastus lateralis is elevated from the intermuscular septum and the lateral femur. Z-retractors are used to hold the vastus lateralis anteriorly. A point is selected for exit of the femoral tunnel approximately 1 cm anterior to the "over the top" area. The "over the top" area can be palpated by releasing a small portion of the intermuscular septum to allow passage of a fingertip into this region. Care should be taken while making this exposure to identify and cauterize circumflex vessels. The desired exit point for the femoral tunnel is selected and marked with a bovee.

Arthroscopy is next resumed and a point for the femoral tunnel entrance into the joint is selected. This point is very high and to the extreme back of the intercondylar notch as described by Sidles and Larson [12]. This position is complimentary to the previously selected central tibial attachment site. If the tunnel edge is properly placed, the medialmost edge of it will be at approximately 12 o'clock high. There will be almost no bone in the back of the tunnel, and if the back of the tunnel is "blown out" while drilling, thus creating a trough, it is acceptable if not desirable. Thus, the point for centering the drill guide is at either the 11-o'clock or 1-o'clock position and extends to within 3 to 5 mm of the extreme back edge of the notch (Fig. 7-9A). This point is marked with a small right angle curette that serves as a receptacle for the tip of the femoral drill guide.

A posterior entry drill guide is now pulled into the knee joint. The tip is placed in the previously created pilot hole. The opposite end of the drill guide is placed at the previously selected point on the distal lateral femur. Once the guidepin has been placed and its position verified, it is overdrilled with the appropriate sized cannulated drill (Fig. 7-9B). The anterior edge of the now created femoral tunnel is chamfered to relieve stresses at this crucial area. The final femoral tunnel position is shown in Figure 7-9C.

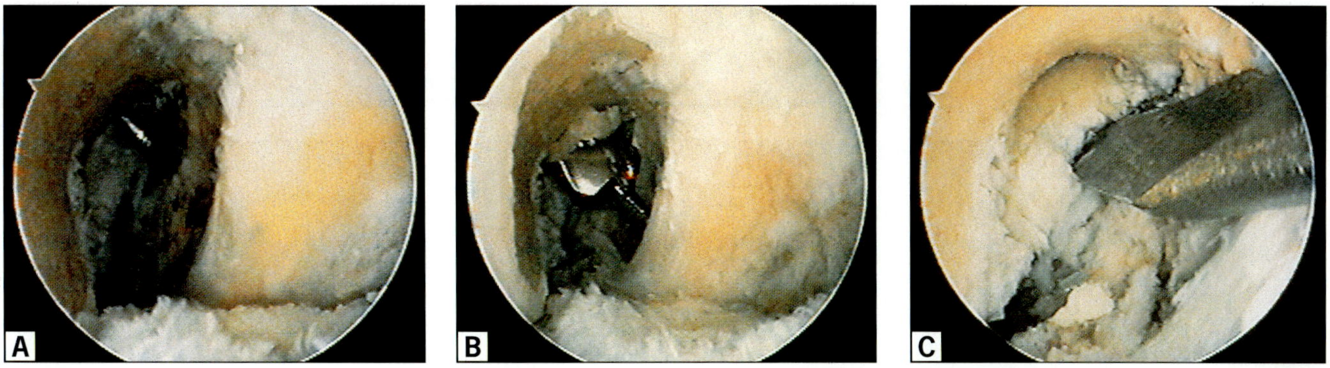

Figure 7-9. Proper femoral tunnel position is achieved by placing the tip of a drill guide at the 11-o'clock or 1-o'clock position and approximately 3 to 5 mm from the extreme back of the notch, **A**. The guidepin is then overdrilled with the appropriate cannulated drill, **B**, creating a tunnel with a medial edge extending to 12 o'clock high and the back edge extending to or into the "over the top" area, **C**.

Use of an Isometer

An isometer is not usually needed to locate the ideal position for placement of the femoral tunnel. If an isometer is used, care must be taken when interpreting the information that it provides, and it will optimally lead to the area of minimal strain for a single fiber. To assume that this is the ideal location for centering a graft of 8 to 10 mm in diameter would, however, be incorrect. The goal is to place the finite-sized graft so that no fibers overstrain, and centering on the fiber of least strain will not accomplish that goal. If the point of minimal strain is used as the center of a 1-cm diameter tunnel, the tunnel created will be too far forward in the notch. It will become even more forward if proper chamfering of the tunnel edge is accomplished. It is more appropriate to be certain that no part of the femoral tunnel extends more forward in the notch than the point that the isometer indicates as the ideal location for a single fiber. This would allow the bulk of a finite-sized graft to be located within an area that provides acceptable strain. If the femoral tunnel is placed so the medial edge is at 12-o'clock and the back edge extends to or into the "over the top" area, then it will almost always be correctly placed. Bony landmarks are adequate for defining this position.

Graft Passage

When performing a two-incision technique, graft passage is accomplished by passing a wire loop through the femoral tunnel into the joint (Fig. 7-10A). This loop is then retrieved by a grabber passed through the tibial tunnel, thus delivering the tip of the wire loop out of the tibial tunnel (Fig. 7-10B). The grafts are then passed through the loops so that the midportion of each of the two grafts can then be pulled through the tibial tunnel across the joint and out the femoral tunnel, leaving all four free ends near the tibial exit site (Figs. 7-10C–E).

Graft Fixation and Tensioning

The grafts are fixed to the femur by placing a screw and washer through the looped midportion of each tendon that has been pulled through the femoral tunnel. This fixation can take place at the point where the grafts exit the femoral tunnel, thus preserving length. Titanium screws with low-profile washers work particularly well for fixation at this location, because the minimal prominence seldom causes any problems with irritation of the iliotibial band. Care should be taken to equalize the length of the two

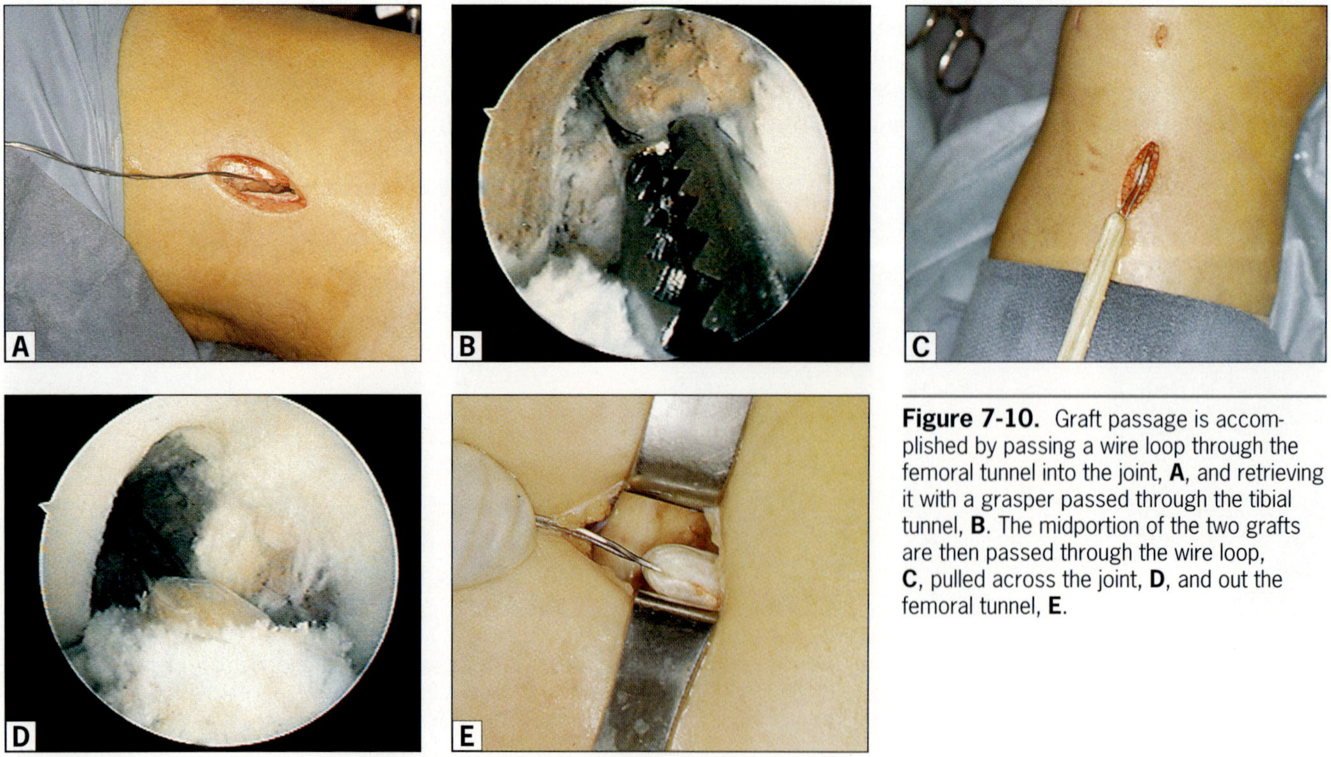

Figure 7-10. Graft passage is accomplished by passing a wire loop through the femoral tunnel into the joint, **A**, and retrieving it with a grasper passed through the tibial tunnel, **B**. The midportion of the two grafts are then passed through the wire loop, **C**, pulled across the joint, **D**, and out the femoral tunnel, **E**.

arms of each tendon prior to advancing the femoral screw (Figs. 7-11A–C).

Tibial fixation is accomplished by tensioning and tying each of the two grafts separately around a titanium screw and low-profile washer on the anteromedial tibia. The screw should be placed near the distal end of the most distal graft so that the sutures can be tied tightly around the post. After the sutures have been tied, the knee is flexed to 20° and the grafts are pulled with approximately 10 to 20 lbs of force while the screw and washer are advanced to directly fix the grafts (Fig. 7-12). The tibial fixation is usually bicor-

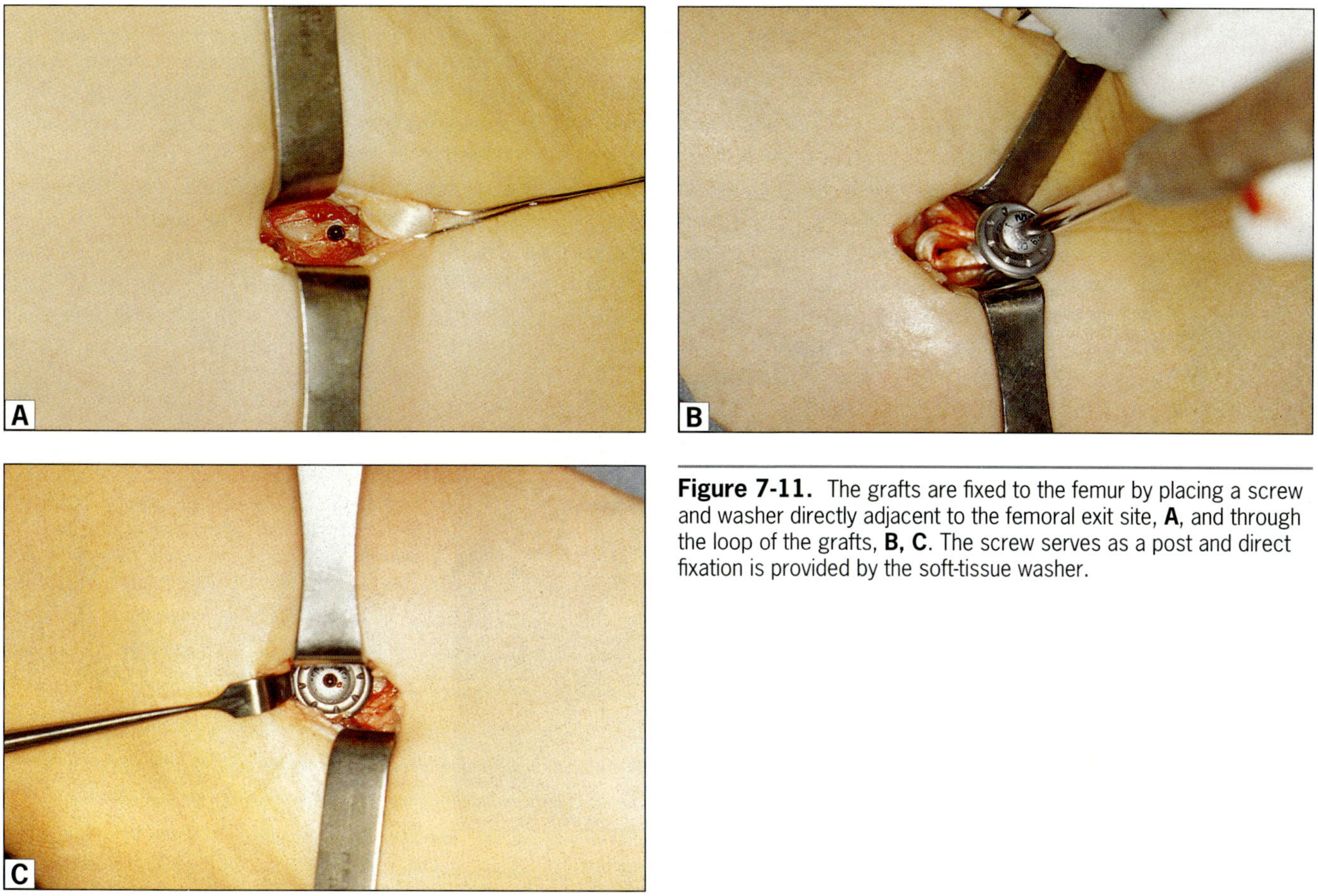

Figure 7-11. The grafts are fixed to the femur by placing a screw and washer directly adjacent to the femoral exit site, **A**, and through the loop of the grafts, **B, C**. The screw serves as a post and direct fixation is provided by the soft-tissue washer.

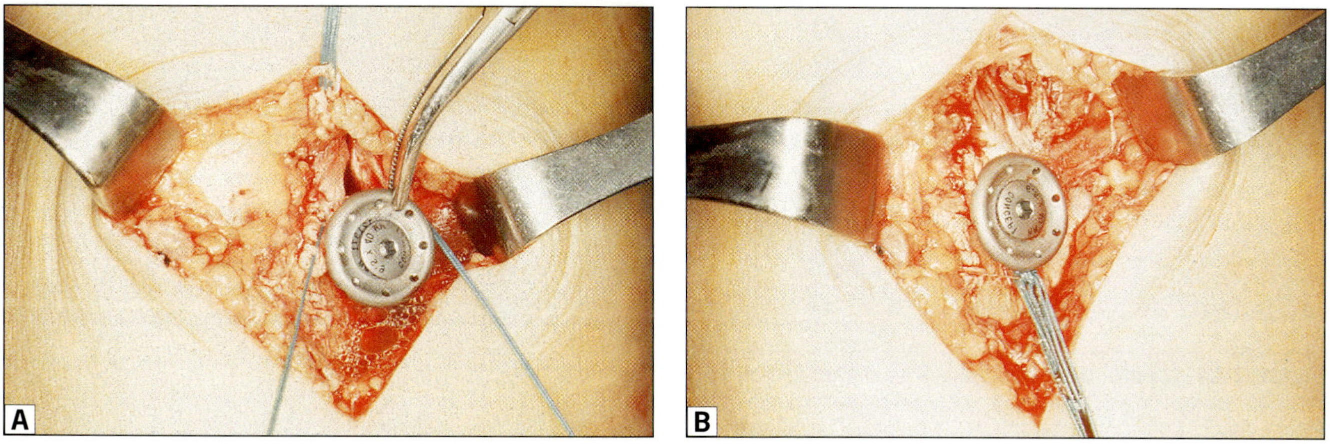

Figure 7-12. Tibial fixation is accomplished by placing a screw at the distal ends of the grafts, **A**. The graft sutures are then tied to this post and the grafts are directly fixed by the soft-tissue washer, **B**.

tical. It is unnecessary to wrap the grafts around the post, but is instead preferable to end the grafts at the level of the screws so that the sutures can be secured tightly. Once the graft has been fixed, it should be carefully observed arthroscopically. The graft should be adjacent to and in contact with the PCL. It should have good clearance from the lateral wall of the intercondylar notch and the graft should merely touch the superior roof at terminal extension (Fig. 7-13).

Short Grafts

Most often, the semitendinosus and gracilis tendons are of sufficient length to allow double loop passage and fixation. There are occasions, however, when either one or both of the grafts are too short to allow fixation by the method previously described. In this instance, a ligament extender is used to add length to one or both of the grafts. This is accomplished by taking a Mercilene (Ethicon Inc., Somerville, NJ) or Dacron (Dupont Co., Wilmington, DE) tape and tying it into a double loop. The midportion of the short graft can then be passed through this loop (Fig. 7-14) and the loop fixed to the femur with the screw and washer. This allows for the grafts so fixed to recess slightly into the femoral tunnel, providing adequate length on the tibia for fixation.

Closure and Bracing

Following graft fixation, the tourniquet is deflated and hemostasis is secured. Usually the procedure discussed can be completed in about 60 to 80 minutes of tourniquet time. Closure is accomplished using interrupted absorbable sutures in the iliotibial band, subcutaneous sutures, and a running subcuticular suture followed by steristrips. A drain is not normally used. Intravenous antibiotics are started before the tourniquet is inflated. A second dose is given following deflation of the tourniquet. No further antibiotics are used. Following dressing application, the patient is placed in a hinged knee brace.

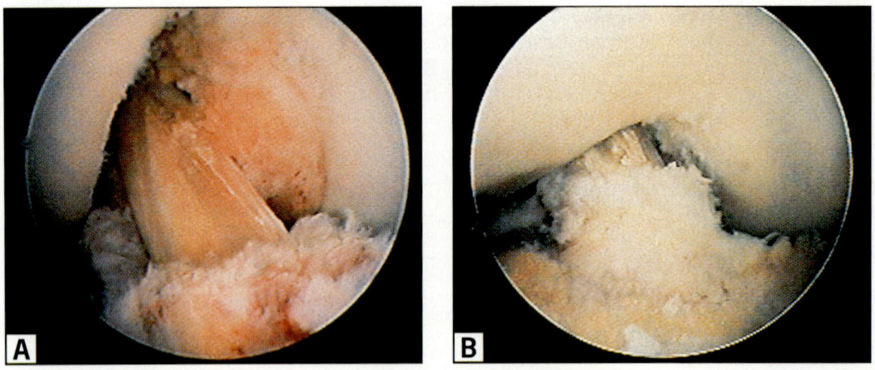

Figure 7-13. Final graft position showing direct contact with the posterior cruciate ligament and good lateral wall clearance, **A**. The graft barely touches the superior notch at terminal extension, **B**.

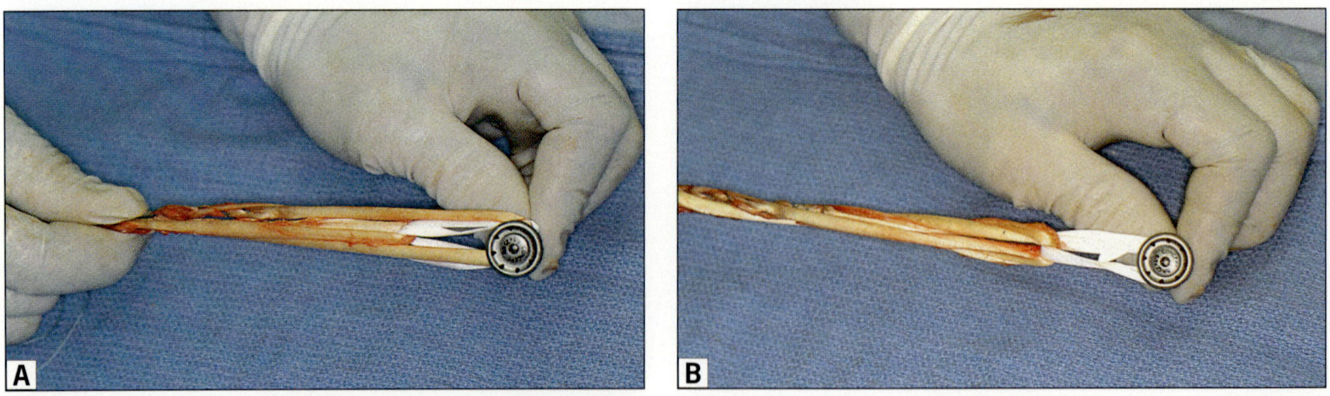

Figure 7-14. It either one or both grafts are too short to allow doubling and fixation as described, they can be lengthened with a ligament extender as shown for the gracilis, **A**, or for both tendons, **B**.

REHABILITATION

Most patients are treated as outpatients or discharged the morning following surgery. Their knee brace is set from 15° to unlimited flexion. They are started on quad sets and leg raises and active motion in the brace. The brace is removed several times daily for full passive extension. Crutches are used initially with weight bearing as tolerated. Formal physical therapy is started approximately 1 week following surgery with a phased program. (Tables 7-1 to 7-4).

DISCUSSION

The previously described technique has been used at the University of Washington Medical Center in over 500 cases of ACL reconstruction. It has proved highly effective in restoring normal anterior laxity in ACL insufficient knees in both acute and chronic situations. It has also been extremely effective in avoiding complications, particularly motion problems and patellofemoral pain complaints. Figure 7-15 shows the appearance of a double loop semitendinosus and gracilis graft approximately 1 year postimplantation. The graft is well synovialized and both the tibial and femoral attachments have a "splayed" appearance similar to the normal ACL. This procedure is also cosmetically acceptable particularly because it avoids an incision on the anterior aspect of the knee where the skin needs to adapt to considerable motion. The incision location below the joint line on the tibia and on the distal lateral thigh are in regions where there is very little skin motion, thus incisions do not normally tend to spread. Figure 7-16 is an example of these incisions in a young woman approximately 1 year following surgery.

The importance of adhering to technical detail in performing this or any other procedure for ACL reconstruction cannot be overemphasized. Attention to graft preparation, tunnel placement, avoidance of notch impingement, fixation, and rehabilitation are much more important factors to the success of ACL reconstruction than is the origin of the autogenous graft. Although the described technique is applicable in almost all situations of ACL insufficiency, it is particularly applicable to those patients in whom a patellar tendon ACL reconstruction has failed, or those with preexisting patellofemoral disease, or any other situation where avoidance of the extensor mechanism is desirable. The procedure is also appropriate when cosmesis is of more than a casual concern.

Table 7-1 Phase I-A: Physical therapy following arthroscopic anterior cruciate ligament surgery (0–6 weeks)

Therapy	Goals
Range-of-motion–limiting brace 15° to unlimited flexion	Demonstrated independent home exercise program
Weight bearing as tolerated with crutches and brace, discontinue crutches as tolerated	Passive range of motion between 0° and 5° of extension and between 115° and 125° of flexion.
Physical therapy will work for full passive range of motion and patellar mobility	Normal gait at 6 weeks without a brace on level ground
Daily stretching out of brace for full passive extension	Stationary bike at 80 rpm for 20 minutes
Electrical muscle stimulator used as needed	
Daily low-resistance stationary biking when range of motion allows (out of brace); resistance as tolerated	
Exercises performed in brace include quad sets, straight leg raises, hamstrings, abductors, adductors, and gluteals; add weights as tolerated with the exception of no weights on straight leg raises	
Stretching of hamstrings and heel cords	

Table 7-2 Phase I-B: Physical therapy following arthroscopic anterior cruciate ligament surgery (6–12 weeks)

Therapy	Goals
Off crutches	At 8 weeks bike with resistance for 20 minutes
Brace worn when away from home	At 12 weeks, 0 lbs straight leg raise without a quad lag
Range of motion in brace 10° to unlimited flexion	Able to walk 15 to 20 minutes without a limp
Full active extension out of brace, no resistance	Stairmaster 20 minutes
Full active flexion with resistance	Normal gait without a brace
Stationary biking with increasing resistance as tolerated	Upstairs step-over-step two flights
Swimming kicking from the hip only, no wall push-offs	Sit-to-stand transfer normal
Physical therapy continued at least on a limited basis	Full passive range of motion
Gym weights equipment or ankle weights used for strengthening exercises. Precaution: straight leg raise must be limited to 5 lbs and resisted knee extension range from 90°–45° only	
Stairmaster and closed kinetic chain exercises	
Sport cord	

Table 7-3 Phase II: Physical therapy following arthroscopic anterior cruciate ligament surgery (12–24 weeks)

Therapy	Goals
No brace or crutches	At 16 weeks, 5 lbs straight leg raise without a quad lag
Full passive and active range of motion	At 16 weeks, stairs step-over-step for two flights ascending and descending
More aggressive strengthening via cycling, stairs, closed kinetic chain activities as tolerated	Unlimited walking without a limp
Patient monitors pain and swelling and reports this to physical therapist	At 24 weeks, or 6 months, 10 lbs straight leg raise without a quad lag
Progressive resistive exercises continued, straight leg raise weights increased to 10 lbs	Stair climbing for exercise
No resisted knee extension through full range of motion until 6 months postoperatively	At 24 weeks, balance on one leg for 2 minutes
Being proprioception-balance training	

Table 7-4	Phase III: Physical therapy following arthroscopic anterior cruciate ligament surgery (6 months–1 year)
Therapy	**Goals**
Aggressive strengthening exercises and return-activity exercises (straight line running) are initiated Aggressive contact, pivoting, and quick acceleration-deceleration movements avoided until 9 months following surgery If deemed appropriate, patient is measured for a derotation brace before starting jumping or pivoting	Able to run without a limp Quads and hamstrings at 90% of uninvolved leg on a Cybex test with quad-to-hamstring ratio at a minimum of 3 to 2 Full muscle mass for brace fitting Return to unrestricted activity including sports Derotation bracing as indicated

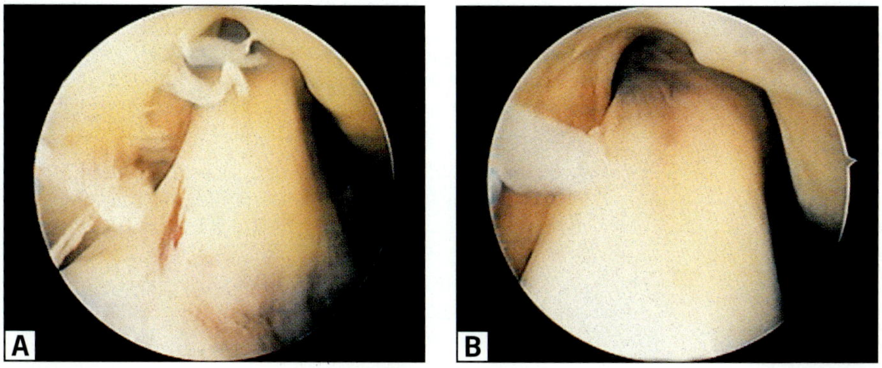

Figure 7-15. Semitendinosus and gracilis grafts 1 year postimplantation. The grafts are well synovialized. The attachment sites on the tibia, **A**, and femur, **B**, have a normal "splayed" appearance.

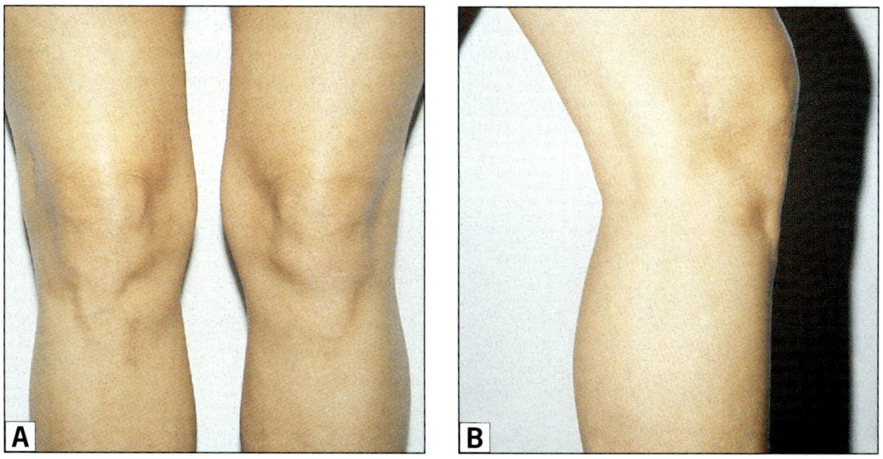

Figure 7-16. Leg and thigh incisions 1 year following anterior cruciate ligament reconstruction by the described technique, **A, B**. Because both incisions are in areas of minimal skin motion, a good cosmetic result is usually obtained.

REFERENCES AND RECOMMENDED READING

Papers of interest, published recently, have been highlighted as:

- Of special interest
- •• Of outstanding interest

1. Cho KO: Reconstruction of the anterior cruciate ligament by semitendinosus tenodesis. *J Bone Joint Surg* 1975, 57A:608–612.

2. Mott HW: Semitendinosus anatomic reconstruction for cruciate ligament insufficiency. *Clin Orthop* 1983, 172:90–92.

3. Gomes JLE, Marczyk LRS: Anterior cruciate ligament reconstruction with a loop or double thickness of semitendinous tendon. *Am J Sports Med* 1984, 12:199–203.

4. Noyes FR, Butler DL, Paulos LE, *et al.*: intra-articular cruciate reconstruction. Perspectives on graft strength, vascularization, and immediate motion after replacement. *Clin Orthop* 1983, 172:71–77.

5. Noyes FR, Butler DL, Grood ES, *et al.*: Biomechanical analysis of human ligament grafts used in knee ligament repairs and reconstructions. *J Bone Joint Surg* 1984, 66A:344–352.

6.•• Steiner ME, Hecker AT, Brown CH, *et al.*: Anterior cruciate ligament graft fixation: Comparison of hamstring and patellar tendon grafts. *Am J Sports Med* 1994, 22:240–247.

This article compares initial fixation strengths of anterior cruciate ligament grafts fixed by different methods. It demonstrates that a double loop semitendinosus and gracilis graft fixed as described in this paper has greater initial fixation strength than patellar tendon grafts fixed with interference fit screws.

7.•• Rodeo SA, Arnoczky SP, Torzilli PA, *et al.*: Tendon-healing in a bone tunnel: A biomechanical and histological study in the dog. *J Bone Joint Surg* 1993, 75A:1795–1803.

This article studies tendon healing in a bone tunnel and demonstrates that biologic fixation occurs with the formation of Sharpey-like fibers.

8. Rosenberg TD, Franklin JL, Baldwin GN, *et al.*: Extensor mechanism function after patellar tendon graft harvest for anterior cruciate ligament reconstruction. *Am J Sports Med* 1992, 20:519–525.

9.• Aglietti P, Buzzi R, Zaccherotti G, *et al.*: Patellar tendon versus doubled semitendinosus and gracilis tendons for anterior cruciate ligament reconstruction. *Am J Sports Med* 1994, 22:211–218.

This paper compares groups of patients reconstructed with semitendinosus and gracilis tendon grafts and patellar tendon grafts. The patients demonstrated no statistically significant differences in the results.

10. Lipscomb AB, Johnston RK, Snyder RB, *et al.*: Evaluation of hamstring strength following use of semitendinosus and gracilis tendons to reconstruct the anterior cruciate ligament. *Am J Sports Med* 1982, 10:340–342.

11.•• Pagnani MJ, Warner JJP, O'Brien SJ, *et al*: Anatomic considerations in harvesting the semitendinosus and gracilis tendons and a technique for harvest. *Am J Sports Med* 1993, 21:565–571.

This paper reviews important anatomy relative to the insertion of the semitendinosus and gracilis tendons and outlines a technique of successfully harvesting these tendons.

12. Sidles JA, Larson RV, Garbini JL, *et al.*: Ligament length relationships in the moving knee. *J Orthop Research* 1988, 6:593–610.

13. Howell SM, Taylor MA: Failure of reconstruction of the anterior cruciate ligament due to impingement by the intercondylar roof. *J Bone Joint Surg* [AM] 1993, 75:1044–1055.

8

CHAPTER

Two-Incision Arthroscopy-Assisted ACL Reconstruction Using Patellar Tendon Substitution

CHERIE A. HOLMES AND BERNARD R. BACH, JR.

Treatment of anterior cruciate ligament (ACL) injuries during the past two decades has dramatically evolved. In the 1970s, Jones [1] recommended open arthrotomy using a central third strip of patellar tendon to reconstruct the ACL. Subsequently, Noyes [2] biomechanically demonstrated that a 14-mm patellar tendon graft was 158% stronger than a normal ACL. Other authors [3–5] popularized the use of vascularized medial and lateral one third patellar tendon grafts for ACL reconstruction. In light of these clinical and biomechanical studies, midthird bone–patellar-tendon–bone constructs gained popularity. Their appeal flourished with the further observations that these high-strength constructs allowed bone-to-bone union, early motion, minimal surgical morbidity, and consistent stability when properly anatomically placed and secured.

Further advances evolved with the use of arthroscopy to perform bone-tendon-bone reconstructions. Arthroscopically assisted techniques have been described using autogenous tissues [6–8,9•,10•,11], allograft tissues (Noyes, Paper presented at the American Orthopedic Society for Sports Medicine Annual Meeting, Orlando, 1987) [11–13], and synthetic ligaments [14–18]. The advantages of this technique over conventional open techniques are multiple: better joint visualization facilitating exact anatomic (isometric) attachment sites, prevention of articular cartilage desiccation, shortened hospitalization, and lack of an arthrotomy leading to less postoperative pain and theoretically less patellar pain from capsular mechanoreceptors not being violated. In reference to the last issue of postoperative patellar pain, studies that have indicated 19% to 37% incidence of patello-femoral pain [19–22] also revealed similar symptoms with hamstring reconstructions and advocated aggressive rehabilitation programs to decrease this complication.

Preliminary Technique

The patient is placed in the supine position. A lateral post or leg holder is used. Knee flexion is maintained between 45° and 60° during most of the procedure. A preoperative prophylactic cephalosporin (1 g) is administered intravenously 30 min prior to skin incision. Prior to diagnostic arthroscopy, a meticulous examination is performed under anesthesia and the results are recorded in the operative report. The Lachman test is performed and the presence or absence of an endpoint is compared with the opposite knee. The pivot shift test is performed and graded (grade I, slip; grade II, jump; grade III, transient lock). Varus and valgus laxity is assessed at 0° and 30°. Posterior cruciate ligament (PCL) and posterolateral findings are assessed with the posterior sag, recurvatum, and posterior and posterolateral drawer tests. A KT-1000 evaluation is performed preoperatively in the office. A padded tourniquet is placed high on the operative thigh and set at 300 mm Hg. However, much of this procedure is performed without tourniquet usage.

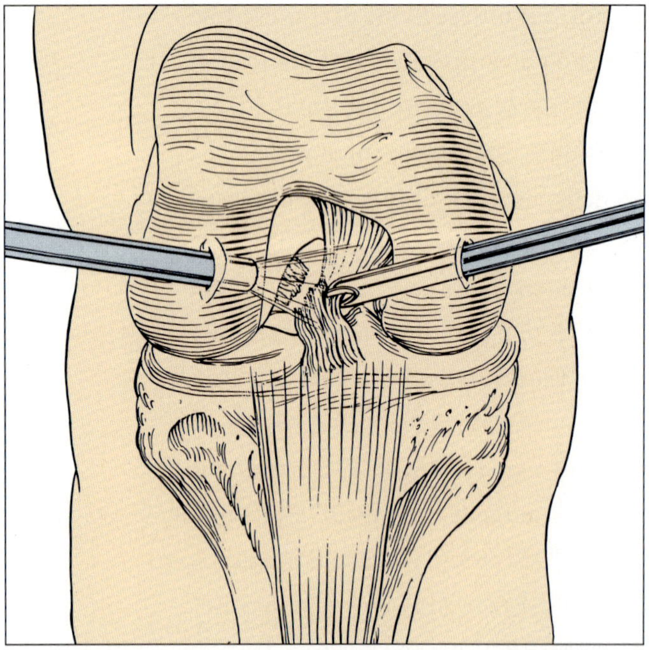

Figure 8-1. Residual anterior cruciate ligament (ACL) tissue is debrided using an arthroscopic shaver. The tissue is debrided along the femoral intercondylar notch wall and the insertion site of the former ACL. This is performed with the arthroscope in the inferolateral portal and a shaver is placed through the inferomedial portal. (*From* Hardin, *et al* [32]; with permission.)

Diagnostic Arthroscopy

The diagnostic arthroscopy is performed without tourniquet inflation to minimize potentially prolonged tourniquet time during ACL reconstruction or meniscal repair. A superomedial portal is used for pump or gravity inflow, along with inferolateral and inferomedial portals. Dilute epinephrine (1:300,000 solution) is injected intra-articularly and at each of the portal sites and contributes to reduced tourniquet usage.

Careful attention is paid to partial-thickness posterior-horn meniscal tears and bucket-handle tears. Vascular zones of the tear are assessed and attempts are made to salvage and repair bucket-handle tears by employing an inside-out technique [23,24]. Concomitant meniscal repair and ligament reconstruction are performed versus a staged operation because fibrin and platelet-derived growth factors from the hemarthrosis are important components of meniscal healing. Articular surface injuries, orientation of the remaining ACL fibers, the *empty wall* sign [25], and the lateral notch sign on the lateral femoral condyle are evaluated.

Intercondylar Notch Preparation

Intercondylar notch preparation is performed after diagnostic arthroscopy and meniscal resection or repair. Evaluation of notch architecture, stenosis, and osteophytes is performed. Although the anatomy of the intercondylar notch varies, a normal reference width of 22 mm [26–28] is applied. Initial removal of the ligamentum mucosum from the notch apex facilitates visualization throughout the procedure.

Aggressive debridement of remaining ACL tissue is performed (Fig. 8-1). A motorized 5.5-mm full-radius resector is used to debride the tibial eminence and lateral wall of the intercondylar notch. Overaggressive debridement of the tibial eminence may injure the intermeniscal ligament. Care is taken to prevent injury to the PCL by directing the shaver toward the lateral wall. Small amounts of synovial tissue encapsulating the PCL can be carefully removed to facilitate better visualization into the posterior notch. An arthroscopic osteotome or curette is used to remove remaining tissue from the lateral wall, roof, and posterolateral notch outlet. This allows better definition of the "over-the-top" position.

Notchplasty

Notchplasty aids in arthroscopic visualization, and it protects the graft from abrasion and impingement in full extension. Care should be taken not to misinterpret a vertical ridge two thirds of the way posteriorly as the true outlet. Using an aggressive shaver or 5.5-mm motorized burr, the surgeon carefully performs the notchplasty from anterior to posterior and from apex to inferior, allowing eventual ease of access to the "over-the-top" position (Fig. 8-2). Minimal bone is debrided at the femoral anatomic attachment site to prevent lateralizing the isometric point. A probe can be hooked over the "over-the-top" position to confirm thorough preparation of the notch.

Graft Harvest

The tourniquet remains deflated during this part of the procedure. The skin just medial to the patellar tendon is infiltrated with a 1:300,000 solution of epinephrine in saline. An 8-cm longitudinal incision located just medial to the midline and extending from the inferior pole of the patellar to 2 cm distal to the tibial tubercle is made (Fig. 8-3). Although mini-incisions can be used and are aesthetically pleasing, precise graft harvesting requires adequate visualization.

After exposure of the medial and lateral edges of the tendon and measurement of its width, the central aspect of the tendon is marked at both the distal patellar pole and the tibial tubercle. A 10-mm wide

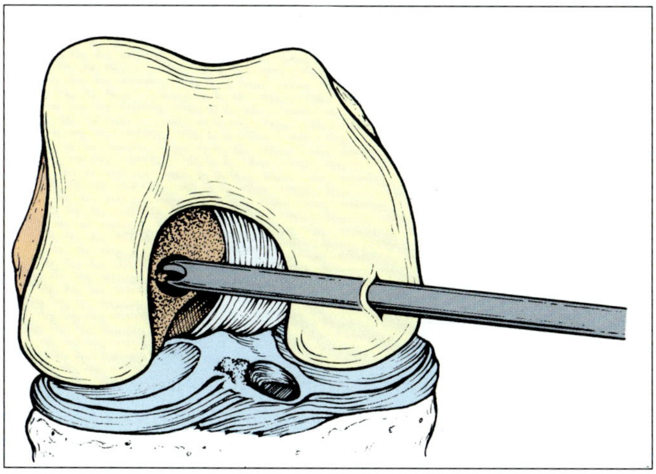

Figure 8-2. Notchplasty being performed with a 5.5 spherical burr. The lateral wall is expanded from anterior to posterior and from inferior to superior. Osteophytes are debrided in more chronic situations. (*From* Hardin, *et al* [32]; with permission.)

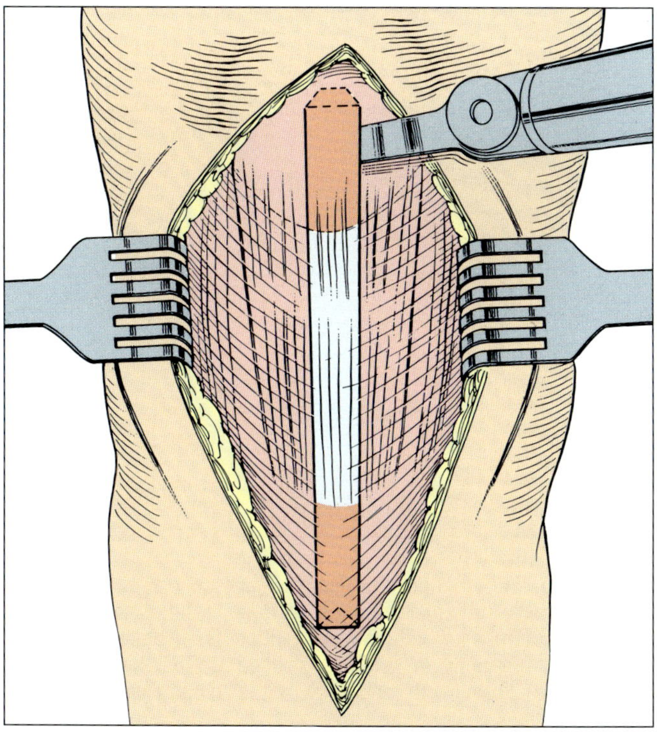

Figure 8-3. A 3.5-in incision is used for exposure to the patellar tendon. Graft edges are exposed and measured. A middle third graft is harvested, generally the 10-mm width that is currently being used. A #238 oscillating saw blade is employed to harvest the bone plugs from the patella and tibia. A trapezoidal-shaped profile patellar plug is obtained in contrast to a triangular profile tibial bone plug (*From* Bach [8]; with permission.)

patellar tendon graft is obtained. The surgeon should be careful to include 25-mm long bone blocks at each end and leave a 20-mm width of remaining tendon distally [29] (Figs. 8-3 and 8-4). Using an oscillating saw, the surgeon takes the tibial and patellar bone blocks with the saw blade directed 45° to the sagittal and coronal planes, creating a triangular-shaped tibial plug and trapezoidal-profiled patellar plug. A triangular tibial bone plug is harvested to maximize the remaining bone at the tibial tubercle region (Fig. 8-5). A trapezoidal patellar plug is taken to reduce the possibility of intra-articular violation. Each bone plug should be 5 to 6 mm thick. Curved osteotomes (0.25 and 0.5 in) are gently used to lift the grafts from their bone beds. Incorrectly using the osteotome as a lever may fracture the graft or result in a longitudinal patellar fracture. Residual fat pad and synovial tissue are dissected free of the graft by using a pair of Metzenbaum scissors. The graft is harvested and dissected from distal to proximal.

The graft is trimmed and contoured on a separate table by an assistant. Sharp edges and excess bone are removed from the graft to facilitate easy passage through an appropriate sizing tube (Fig. 8-6). A 0.062-mm K-wire is used to drill two or three holes transverse and parallel to the cortex in each bone plug at the corticocancellous junction. Ticron sutures (#5) are passed using a suture passer through the drill holes. Transverse—as opposed to perpendicular—drill holes are used to reduce the risk of suture laceration when using Kurosaka interference screw fixation. The orientation is less important if the grafts are stapled into place or tied over screw posts.

Supracondylar Femur Preparation

A 4-cm incision in the lateral supracondylar area is created. The iliotibial band is identified and divided parallel to its fibers for a similar length in its thicker middle third. The vastus lateralis is bluntly dissected from the intermuscular septum and retracted anteriorly by using a Chandler retractor placed over the anterior femur. If the intermuscular septum is not easily identified, the surgeon may be posterior to the septum. The lateral superior geniculate vessels are identified and cauterized. A longitudinal periosteal dissection "over-the-top" of the femoral condyle and posterior to the femoral metaphysis is performed with a 0.75-in Cobb elevator. Adequate dissection facilitates easy passage of a finger subperiosteally around the "over-the-top" position and palpation of the posterior intercondylar notch. This step is necessary for safe passage of the right or left rear-entry femoral guides.

Femoral Drill Hole Placement

The goal of femoral tunnel placement is to achieve a thin, intact (1- to 2-mm) posterior cortex that is oriented at the 11-o'clock to 11:15 position on a right knee or a 12:45 to 1-o'clock position on a left knee. The J-shaped retrieval guide is placed through the

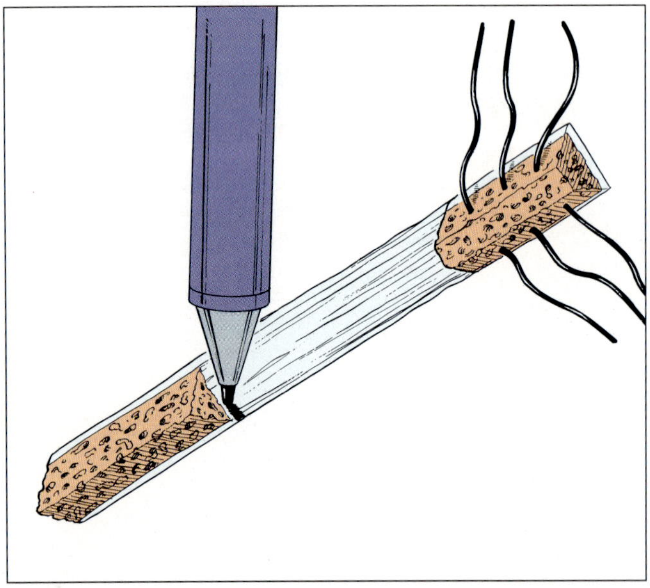

Figure 8-4. The graft is prepared by placing 0.062 K-wire drill holes parallel to the cortex. Two or three sutures of #5 Ticron (American Cyanamid Co., Danbury, CT) are placed through these holes. Passage is facilitated with a suture passer (Acufex Microsurgicals, Mansfield, MA). The tendo-osseus junction may be marked with a sterile marking pen. (*From* Bach [8]; with permission.)

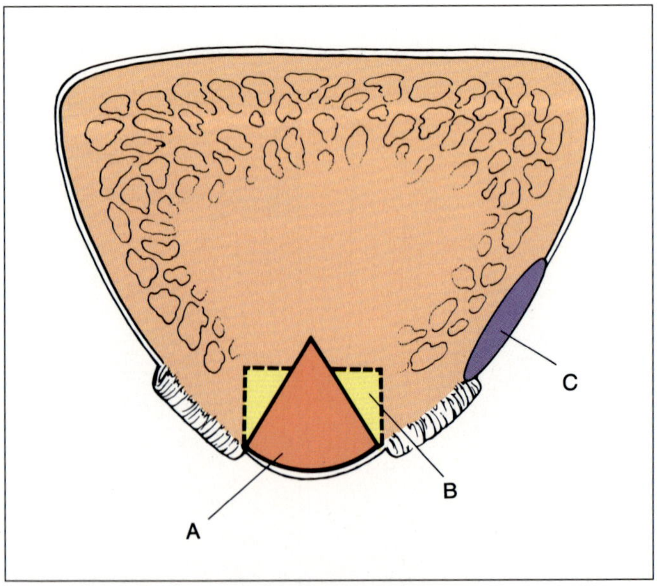

Figure 8-5. **A**, A triangular profile tibial tubercle plug is fashioned, thus maximizing the remaining bone left deep to the remaining medial and lateral third of the patellar tendon, **B**, which would be minimal if a rectangular graft is fashioned. **C**, The tibial tunnel entrance site. (*From* Hardin and Bach [33]; with permission.)

midpatellar rent and is passed to the "over-the-top" position under arthroscopic visualization. The rear-entry guide is subsequently introduced and positioned arthroscopically approximately 5 mm anterior to the "over-the-top" position (1-o'clock for the left knee and 11-o'clock for the right knee) (Fig. 8-7). A probe is used to confirm the entry position relative to the "over-the-top" position. Once confirmed, the guidepin is drilled from outside-in, with the pin entrance site located 4 cm proximal to the lateral epicondyle and slightly posterior to the midline of the femoral metaphysis. Intra-articular pin placement is visualized arthroscopically and confirmed with a probe (Fig. 8-8). If isometry testing is used, then the pin remains in place until after preparation of the tibial tunnel. Because we no longer perform isometry testing, the femoral guidepin is overreamed at this point. An arthroscopic curette is introduced through the anteromedial portal to protect the PCL. The outer femoral cortex is initially reamed with a small 7- to 8-mm cannulated reamer and then completed with the appropriately sized cannulated reamer, usually 10 mm (Fig. 8-9). After passage intra-articularly, the drill is removed and the tunnel edges are chamfered using a motorized synovial resector and arthroscopic rasp. Particular attention should be directed toward the most superior and lateral aspects of this hole because this is where graft impingement usually occurs.

Tibial Hole Placement

Through the central incision, the medial metaphysis of the proximal tibia is exposed. Electrocautery and a Cobb elevator are used to create a 1.5-cm × 2-cm osteoperiosteal medially based flap. The edges of the flap are bordered by the patellar tendon laterally, the medial edge of the patellar, and the distal aspect of the pes anserinus inferiorly and should be protected.

The arthroscope is replaced through the inferolateral portal to visualize the tibial eminence. Currently, our landmarks are to place the tibial pin in the middle third region of the former ACL insertion site. A general reference point is midway between the posterior edge of the anterior horn of the lateral meniscus and the anterior edge of the PCL. The original ACL insertion is rather broad based—2.5 cm to 3 cm on the intercondylar eminence.

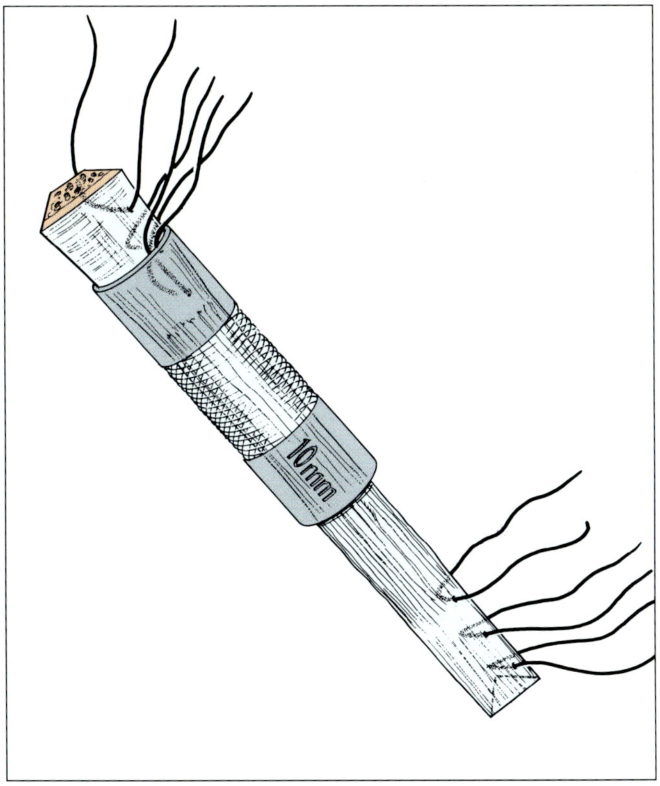

Figure 8-6. The graft is sized. In the late 1980s, our tendency was to use a slightly larger graft, sometimes using 11- and 12-mm grafts. Currently, our goal is to use a 10-mm width patellar tendon graft. Placement of slightly oblique drill holes that catch the cortical edge of the bone plugs is demonstrated. If drill holes are placed perpendicular to the cortex, they may be lacerated at the time of interference screw placement. Some authors prefer a press-fit on one of the bone plugs. (*From* Hardin, *et al* [32]; with permission.)

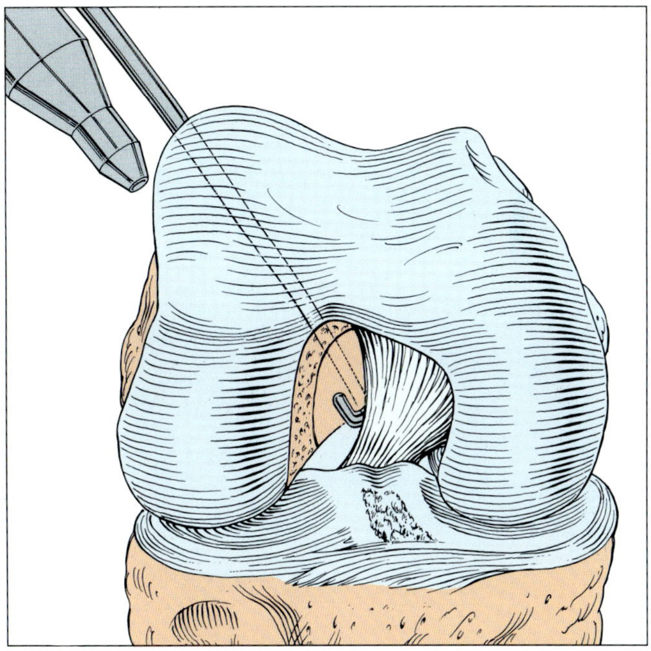

Figure 8-7. Visual placement of the stylet of the rear-entry guide. The stylet is positioned approximately 5 mm anterior to the "over-the-top" position. The subsequent goal of pin placement and over-reaming will create a thin posterior cortex of approximately 1 to 2 mm. The stylet is positioned at the 11-o'clock to 11:15 position on a right knee and the 12:45 to 1-o'clock position on a left knee. (*From* Hardin, *et al* [32]; with permission.)

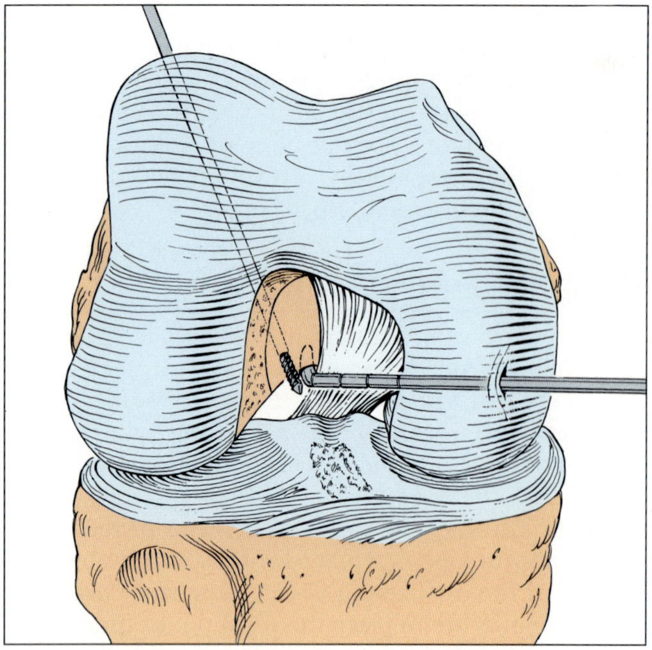

Figure 8-8. Once the femoral pin has been positioned, an arthroscopic probe may be placed in the "over-the-top" position to confirm its relative placement. (*From* Hardin, *et al* [32]; with permission.)

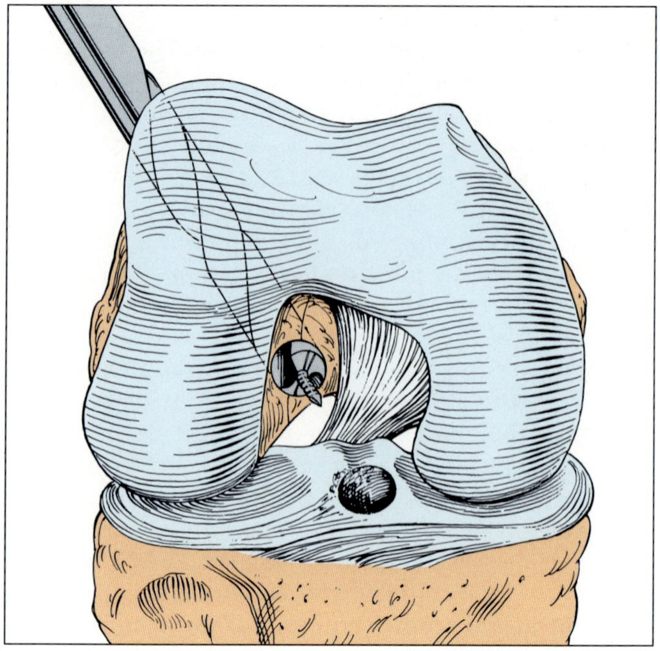

Figure 8-9. Intra-articular view of femoral tunnel reaming. Note that a small portion of posterior cortex remains. (*From* Hardin, *et al* [32]; with permission.)

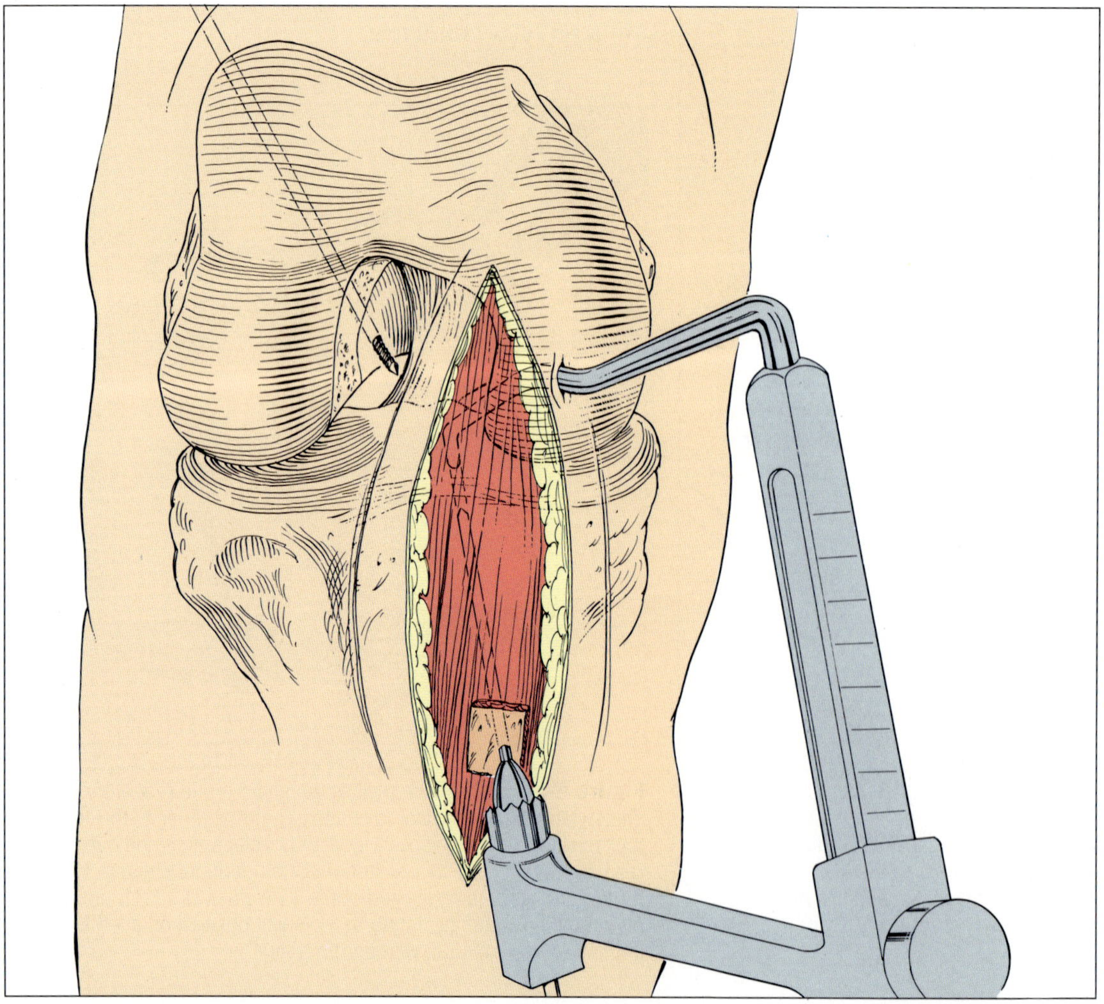

Figure 8-10. Pin placement on the tibial side. An osteoperiosteal window was created on the medial metaphyseal region of the tibia. Care was taken not to violate the superficial medial collateral ligament, the remaining portion of the medial third patellar tendon, and the pes anserine. The stylet is positioned in the middle third of the former anterior cruciate ligament insertion site. The goal of pin placement is to place this stylet centrally within the tibial eminence region so that when the knee is extended, the pin is posterior to the intercondylar apex by approximately 3 mm. In this illustration, we had not overreamed the femoral pin because we intended to perform isometry readings. (*From* Hardin, *et al* [32]; with permission.)

The knee is flexed 30° and the tibial guide is secured to the proximal tibial metaphysis, taking care to provide an adequate bone bridge between the tibial tunnel and tibial plateau. The guidepin is drilled under arthroscopic visualization (Fig. 8-10). When placed, the pin should be located 2 to 3 mm posterior to the intercondylar apex with the knee extended. If the position is not optimal, a parallel pin technique can be used to correct pin position. A common error is lateralization of the pin so that subsequent over-reaming of the tunnel results in a graft that impinges on the lateral wall. A cannulated drill is used to over-ream (Fig. 8-11). Cancellous bone is collected during tibial and femoral reaming for subsequent bone grafting of the patellar graft harvest site. A motorized synovial resector is introduced through the tibial tunnel, inferomedial portal, or patellar tendon rent to debride the intra-articular tibial opening. An arthroscopic rasp is placed through the tibial tunnel to chamfer the edges, which helps to eliminate areas of stress or impingement on the graft (Fig. 8-12).

Alternative Method of Femoral Tunnel Placement

Newer femoral aiming guides for pin placement in endoscopic ACL reconstruction that key off the posterior "over-the-top" position make determination of the anatomic position easier and more predictable. These aiming guides have a 7-mm offset that, when drilling with a 10-mm diameter reamer over the guidepin, allows a 2-mm posterior wall (Fig. 8-13). Using this method, the supracondylar femur preparation is performed but the femoral tunnel is not made. At this point, the tibial tunnel should be drilled first in the aforementioned fashion. The femoral aiming guide is then placed through the tibial tunnel and locked into place under arthroscopic visualization in the posterolateral corner. Occasionally, this is facilitated by having the knee drained "dry." A guidepin is then drilled several millimeters into the femur to mark this isometric point and then removed along with the aiming guide. The J-shaped aiming guide and

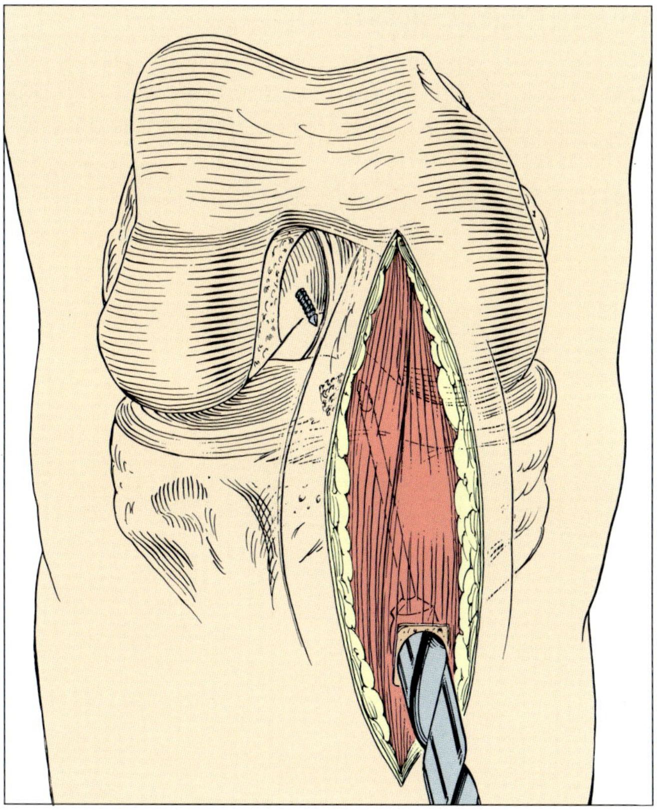

Figure 8-11. After appropriate placement of the pin, it is over-reamed with an appropriately sized reamer. (*From* Hardin, *et al* [32]; with permission.)

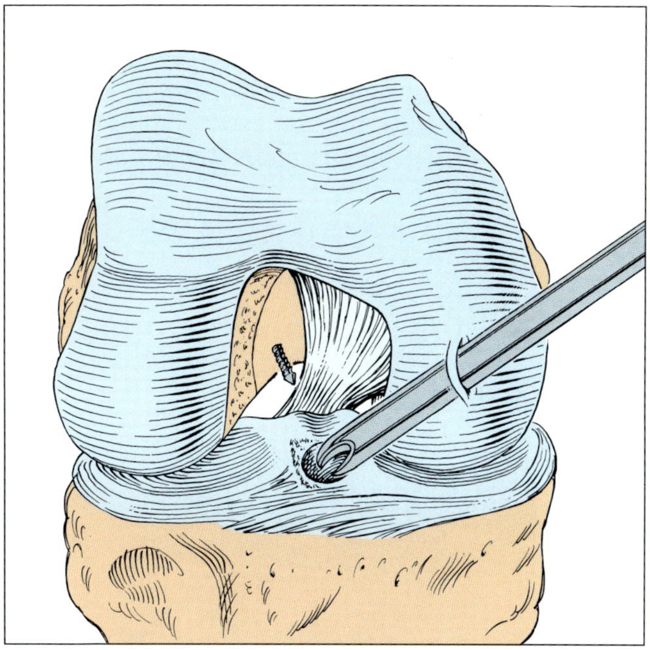

Figure 8-12. Intra-articular debris is cleared with an arthroscopic shaver. (*From* Hardin, *et al* [32]; with permission.)

rear-entry guide are then passed as noted previously. Instead of securing the rear-entry guide into a position 5 mm anterior to the "over-the-top" position, it is now secured under arthroscopic visualization into the hole previously made by the K-wire. A new guidepin is now introduced from outside-in and overreamed as described previously. This should further obviate the need for isometry testing. Using this technique, there is a slight difference in the exact location of the pin site (5 mm versus 7 mm). As noted, the goal of anatomic femoral tunnel placement is to leave a small 1- to 2-mm cortical bridge posteriorly. This apparent difference takes into consideration the divergent femoral tunnels that occur in outside-in versus inside-out techniques. For example, in using an outside-in technique, the starting position on the lateral femoral cortex can vary significantly provided the intra-articular entrance is anatomically placed.

Isometry Testing

If isometry testing is used, then the femoral tunnel has not been reamed at this point. The femoral guidepin is removed and a 22-gauge wire loop is placed through this hole intra-articularly and passed out of the knee through the tibial tunnel. It is then used to draw a suture retrograde through the tibia, knee joint, and the femoral tunnel. The suture is then secured proximally with a hemostat and distally into a Graf-Clancy strain gauge (Acufex Microsurgical, Mansfield, MA) which is secured into the tibial tunnel. The knee should not be subluxed anteriorly and the suture should be taut within the knee. The knee is then flexed from 0° to 90° and excursion of the strain gauge documented. If excursion exceeds 2.5 mm, the joint should be inspected arthroscopically to explain and remedy the possible nonisometric graft position. Possible impingement of the suture on the tibial or femoral tunnels should be noted. If isometry placement is correct, then the suture is removed and the guidewire is replaced manually and gently tapped into place with a mallet. A drill should not be used to replace the pin in order to prevent incorrect orientation of the pin. The pin is then overreamed as described above. There are limitations to isometry measurement because the reading is only as accurate as the isometer. Additionally, the entire graft is never completely isometric; different fiber bundles are isometric through different ranges of motion.

Graft Placement

Prior to graft passage, the tunnels are inspected and fine-tuning of the lateral femoral wall and notch is performed (Figs. 8-14 and 8-15). The bone-tendon-bone–free graft is passed antegrade through the

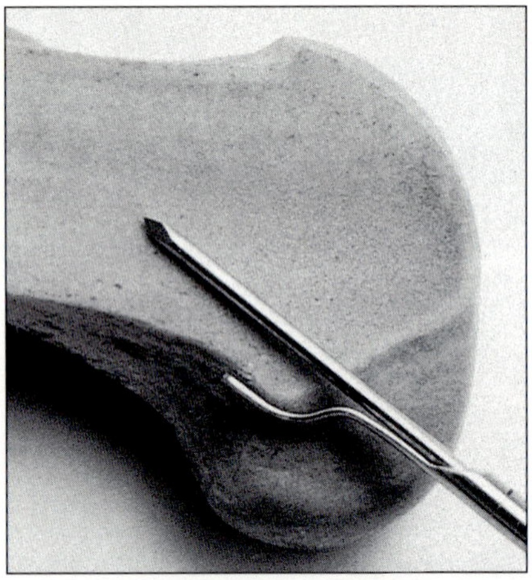

Figure 8-13. An alternative technique for determining placement of the femoral tunnel is the use of an offset guide. This guide keys off the "over-the-top" position. A 7-mm offset is used with placement of the pin and subsequent overreaming, leaving a 2-mm intact posterior cortex. The pilot pinhole is made and then the rear-entry guide positioner may be passed in the "over-the-top" position and its stylet introduced in the provisional pinhole formerly created.

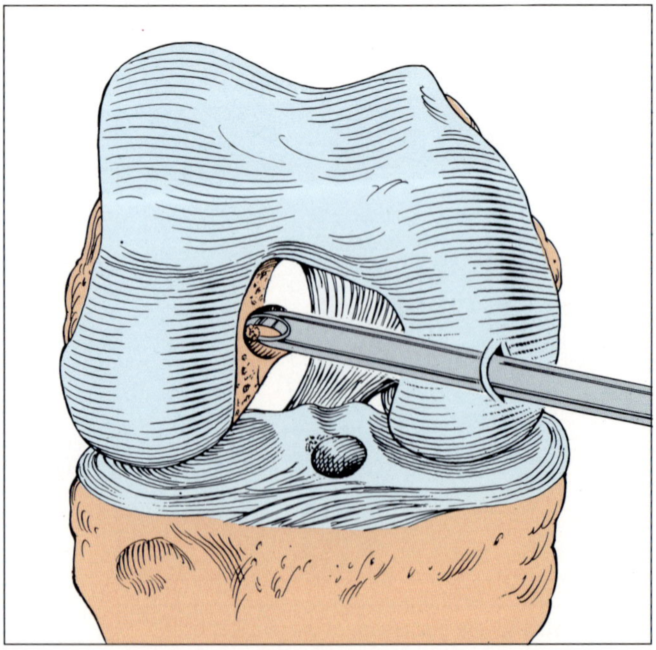

Figure 8-14. Prior to graft passage, tunnel entrances are inspected and fine-tuned. Phase 2 notchplasty may be performed at this time, chamfering the intra-articular entrance site, smoothing the lateral wall, and expanding the notch as needed. (*From* Hardin, *et al* [32]; with permission.)

femoral tunnel intra-articularly and finally into the tibial tunnel. With the knee positioned at 60°, a Yankauer suction tube can be passed retrograde through the knee. The tube can be clamped at the tibial and femoral ends, and gross isometry testing can be performed. Two wire loops can then be passed through the tube from proximal to distal and the suction tubing is removed for graft passage. The sutures on the tibial bone plug are passed through the wire loops and then passed in two groups through the knee. Alternatively, a commercial ligament graft passer (DePuy, Warsaw, IN) can be used.

The knee is maintained at 60° of flexion, and the tibial bone plug is passed under arthroscopic visualization through the joint and into the tibial tunnel (Fig. 8-16). An arthroscopic probe or grabber may be necessary to help manipulate the graft through the joint and around the potential obstructions of the PCL, intercondylar eminence, or lateral femoral wall. Once passage is complete, tension can be applied to both sides through the sutures and the graft probed to assess laxity. Laxity may imply incarceration in the tibial tunnel, requiring tibial hole enlargement with a synovial resector or burr. Orientation and tension

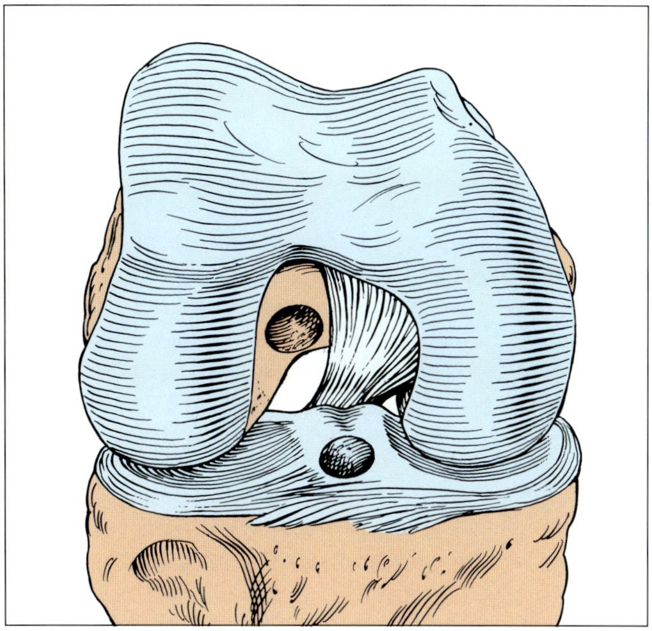

Figure 8-15. Central placement of the tibial tunnel entrance site at the 11-o'clock to 11:15 position on the femoral side. Note the small posterior cortex remaining on the femoral tunnel. (*From* Bach [8]; with permission.)

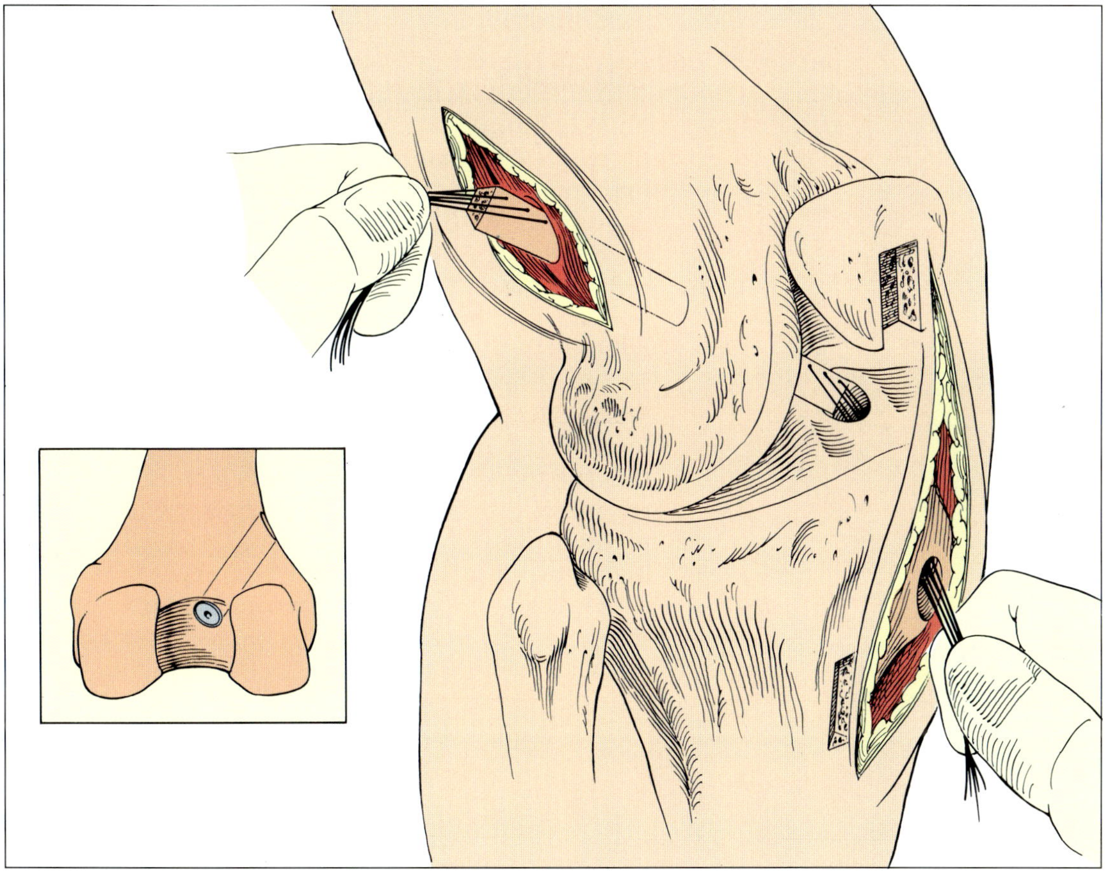

Figure 8-16. The graft is passed antegrade from the femoral tunnel intra-articularly and the tibial tunnel. This procedure should be viewed arthroscopically, because the tibial plug at times may impinge on the edge of the posterior cruciate or may be caught on the intra-articular edge of the tibial tunnel. The *inset* view once again depicts the close proximity of the femoral tunnel to the posterior cortex. (*From* Nogalski and Bach [34]; with permission.)

must be assessed in both flexion and extension, looking especially for impingement on the lateral femoral wall or anterior notch outlet.

Although a variety of devices are used for securing the graft (buttons, staples, and unicortical screws and posts) interference-fit cannulated Kurasaka screws (DePuy, Warsaw, IN) (Concept, Largo, FL) are preferred. The advantages are related to linear load resistance, stiffness, and maximum tensile strength [30]. However, several problems may occur with interference screw fixation, such as graft-screw length mismatch, tunnel-graft screw mismatch, tunnel-screw divergence, graft advancement, graft translocation, graft fracture, and suture laceration of the graft block [31].

The femoral side is secured first, using a 9-mm diameter screw. The graft cortex is directed laterally, placing the screw adjacent to the cortex, thus translating the graft medially. The knee is then cycled several times while isometric placement of the graft is checked. With the knee in full extension, a 9-mm screw is then placed anterior to the graft on its cortical surface to reduce the risk of intra-articular screw placement (Fig. 8-17). In contrast to many orthopedists, final fixation is performed in complete extension, rather than 20° to 30° of knee flexion. A posterior Lachman is not performed during fixation. Fixation in extension takes graft strain characteristics into consideration and minimizes the likelihood of overconstraining the knee. After placement of the screws, the arthroscope is replaced in the knee and the graft is probed for appropriate tension and possible impingement. The knee is placed through a full range of motion and a Lachman test should show 2 to 3 mm of translation with a firm endpoint. The pivot shift must be eliminated.

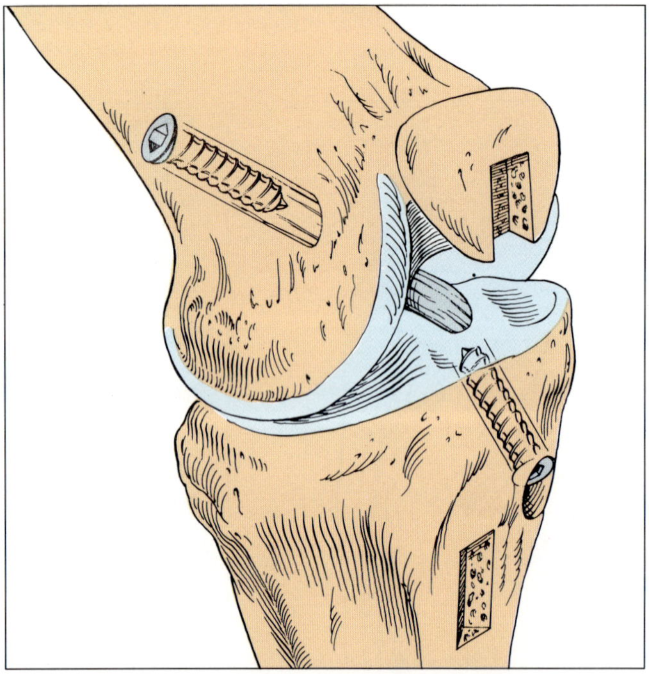

Figure 8-17. Fixation of the graft using interference-fit screws. The interference screw has been placed along the cortex on both the femur and tibia. The screw is placed on the anterior aspect of the tibial bone plug. (*From* Nogalski and Bach [34]; with permission.)

If the tourniquet has been inflated during the procedure, it is released at this time and meticulous hemostasis achieved. The osteoperiosteal flap on the tibia should be closed over the tibial plug. The patellar graft harvest site should be bone-grafted using bone from the tunnel reamings and contouring of the bone plugs. The patellar tendon rent and iliotibial band are closed using interrupted sutures. A small hemovac drain is placed intra-articularly through the superomedial pump portal. The skin is closed with a running subcuticular suture.

SUMMARY

This technique was used with minor modification between 1987 and 1991 by the senior author in approximately 250 knees [8,9•,10•]. Our clinical experience with our initial 75 patients following a minimum of 2 years revealed predictable stability (92% negative pivot shift), a low reoperation rate (which has been reduced to 2% with an early complete extension protocol), and a high patient subjective satisfaction rate (95%). In October 1991, we began a prospective study of endoscopic single-incision patellar tendon autografts. It is our opinion that the two-incision technique is a more predictable technique with fewer pitfalls than the endoscopic technique. Arthroscopy-assisted ACL surgery is a highly technically demanding technique that should be performed only by experienced arthroscopic surgeons. The two-incision technique is an excellent one that belongs in the surgical armamentarium of sports medicine knee ligament surgeons.

REFERENCES AND RECOMMENDED READING

Papers of interest, published recently, have been highlighted as:

- • Of special interest
- •• Of outstanding interest

1. Jones KG: Reconstruction of the anterior cruciate ligament using the central one third of the patellar ligament. *J Bone Joint Surg* 1970, 52A:1302–1308.
2. Noyes FR, Butler DL, Grood ES, *et al.*: Biomechanical analysis of human ligament grafts used in knee ligament repairs and reconstructions. *J Bone Joint Surg* 1984, 66A:344–352.
3. Clancy WG Jr., Graf BK: Arthroscopic meniscal repair. *Orthopedics* 1983, 6:1125–1129.
4. Clancy WG Jr., Thomsen E, Dueland RT, *et al.*: Anterior cruciate and posterior cruciate ligament reconstruction with patellar tendon utilizing a medial vascularized graft, lateral vascularized graft, and free patellar tendon graft. *Orthop Trans* 1987, 12:70.
5. Paulos LE, Butler DL, Noyes FR, *et al.*: intra-articular cruciate reconstruction: Replacement with vascularized patellar tendon. *Clin Orthop* 1987, 172:78–84.
6. Friedman MJ: Arthroscopic semitendinosis (gracillis) reconstruction for anterior cruciate ligament deficiency, in *Techniques in Orthopaedics*. Edited by Dorr L. Frederick, MD: Aspen Publishers; 1988:74–80.
7. Gomes JLE, Marczyk LRS: Anterior cruciate ligament reconstruction with a "loop" or double thickness of semitendinosus tendon. *Am J Sports Med* 1984, 12:199–203.
8. Bach BR Jr.: Arthroscopy-assisted patellar tendon substitution for anterior cruciate ligament insufficiency: Surgical technique. *Am J Knee Surg* 1989, 2:3–20.
9. • Nogalski M, Bach BR Jr..: Surgical treatment of acute ACL insufficiency. In *Knee Surgery*. Edited by Fu F, Harner C, Vince K, *et al.* Baltimore: Williams & Wilkins; 1994:679–730.

This chapter reviews the results of current surgical techniques used for anterior cruciate ligament reconstruction. Description of surgical techniques including single and two-incision arthroscopy-assisted patellar tendon autograft is reviewed.

10. • Bach BR Jr., Jones GT, Sweet F, *et al.*: Arthroscopic-assisted ACL reconstruction using patellar tendon substitution: Minimum two year follow-up study. *Am J Sports Med* 1994, 22:758–767.

This retrospective review of 62 patients studied at a minimum 2-year follow-up reports the authors' initial results using a two-incision arthroscopy-assisted technique without extra-articular augmentation. Clinical review includes information on the KT-1000 arthrometer, Cybex testing, Tegner, Lysholm, Noyes, a modified Hospital for Special Surgery rating scale, and functional scoring including single leg hop for distance, timed single leg hop, and vertical jump. Results revealed predictable stabilization, excellent motion recovery, minimal quadriceps deficits on Cybex testing, and a low reoperation rate.

11. Buss DD, Warren RF, Wickiewicz TL, *et al.*: Arthroscopically assisted reconstruction of the anterior cruciate ligament with use of autogenous patellar tendon grafts: Results after twenty-four to forty-two months. *J Bone Joint Surg* 1993, 75-A:1346–1355.
12. Gillquist J, Odensten M: Arthroscopic reconstruction of the anterior cruciate ligament. *Arthroscopy* 1988, 4:5–9.
13. Goble EM: Fluoroarthroscopic allograft anterior cruciate reconstruction. In *Techniques in Orthopaedics*. Edited by Dorr L. Frederick, MD: Aspen Publishers; 1988:65–73.
14. Bruchman WC, Bain JR, Bolton CW: Prosthetic replacement of the cruciate ligaments with expanded polytetrafluoroethylene. In *The Crucial Ligaments*. Edited by Feagin JA. New York: Churchill Livingstone; 1988:507–515.
15. Fowler PJ: Techniques using braided polypropylene as a ligament augmentation device. In *Techniques in Orthopaedics*. Edited by Dorr L. Frederick, MD: Aspen Publishers; 1988:81–85.
16. Friedman MJ: Gore-Tex anterior cruciate ligament reconstruction. In *Techniques in Orthopaedics*. Edited by Dorr L. Frederick, MD: Aspen Publishers; 1988:36–43.
17. Hill JA: Autograft, xenograft, and synthetic cruciate ligament reconstruction: State of the art. In *Arthroscopic Surgery*. Edited by Parisien JS. New York: McGraw Hill; 1988:205–212.
18. Springer SI: Anterior cruciate ligament substitution: Endoscopic technique. In *Arthroscopic Surgery*. Edited by Parisien JS. New York: McGraw Hill; 1988:213–220.
19. Sachs RA, Daniel D, Stone ML, *et al.*: Patellofemoral problems after ACL reconstruction. *Am J Sports Med* 1989, 17:760–765.
20. Sgaglione NA, Warren RF, Wickiewicz TL, *et al.*: Primary repair with semitendinosis tendon augmentation of acute ACL injuries. *Am J Sports Med* 1990, 18:64–73.
21. O'Brien SJ, Warren RF, Wickiewicz TL, *et al.*: The iliotibial band lateral sling procedure and its effect on the results of anterior cruciate ligament reconstruction. *Am J Sports Med* 1991, 19:21–25.
22. Marder RA, Raskind JR, Carroll M: Prospective evaluation of arthroscopically assisted ACL reconstruction: Patellar tendon versus semitendinosis and gracilis tendons. *Am J Sports Med* 1991, 19:478–483.
23. Morgan CD, Casscells SW: Arthroscopic meniscus repair: a safe approach to the posterior horns. *Arthroscopy* 1986, 2:2–12.
24. Warren RF: Arthroscopic meniscus repair. *Arthroscopy* 1985, 1:170–172.

25. Bach BR, Warren RF: "Empty wall" and "vertical strut" signs of ACL insufficiency. *J Arthroscopy* 1989, 5:137–140.

26. Kieffer DA, Lurnow RJ, Southwell RB, *et al.*: Anterior cruciate ligament arthroplasty. *Am J Sports Med* 1984, 12:301–312.

27. Anderson AF, Lipscomb AB, Liudahl KJ, *et al.*: Analysis of the intercondylar notch by computed tomography. *Am J Sports Med* 1987, 15:547–522.

28. Arnoczky SP, Warren RF: The microvasculature of the meniscus and its response to injury: an experimental study in the dog. *Am J Sports Med* 1983, 11:131–141.

29. Noyes FR, Butler DL, Grood ES, *et al.*: Biomechanical analysis of human ligament grafts used in knee ligament repairs and reconstructions. *J Bone Joint Surg* 1984, 66A:344–352.

30. Kurosaka M, Yoshiya S, Andrish JT: A biomechanical comparison of different surgical techniques of graft fixation in anterior cruciate ligament reconstruction. *Am J Sports Med* 1987, 15:225–229.

31. Bach BR: Technical pitfalls of Kurosaka interference screw fixation. *Am J Knee Surg* 1989, 2:76–82.

32. Hardin GT, Bach BR Jr., Bush-Joseph C, *et al.*: Endoscopic single incision ACL reconstruction using patellar tendon autograft: Surgical Technique. *Am J Knee Surg* 1991, 5:144–155.

33. Hardin GT, Bach BR Jr.: Distal rupture of the infrapatellar tendon. *Am J. Knee Surg* 1992, 5:140–143.

34. Nogalski MN, Bach BR Jr.: Acute Anterior Cruciate Ligament Injuries. In *The Knee*. Edited by Fu F, Harner C, Vince K. Baltimore: Williams & Wilkins; 1994: 717–718.

9

CHAPTER

Anterior Cruciate Ligament Reconstruction With Quadrupled Semitendinosus Autograft

THOMAS D. ROSENBERG AND THOMAS J. PAZIK

Arthroscopically assisted anterior cruciate ligament (ACL) reconstruction has achieved wide application and is no longer considered a new technique. Advances in instrumentation and skills have encouraged the successful incorporation of arthroscopic ACL reconstruction techniques into general orthopedic practices. The technique allows for improved intra-articular visualization of associated meniscal and chondral lesions, precise notchplasty, accurate tunnel placement, intraoperative strain measurements, dynamic assessment for graft impingement, and minimization of morbidity.

Despite wide acceptance, several controversies persist in relation to patient selection, graft selection, surgical techniques, and rehabilitation protocols. Patellar tendon bone-tendon-bone (BTB) autografts that insult the extensor mechanism are in use predominantly. Misconceptions concerning the use of hamstring tendons for ACL reconstruction have persisted despite new evidence to the contrary. These misconceptions are 1) mechanical properties of the hamstring grafts are inferior, 2) hamstring constructs stretch out over time, and 3) tendon-to-bone healing (a requirement for both hamstring and BTB constructs) is insufficient for accelerated rehabilitation protocols [1].

Noyes and coworkers [2] reported that a 14-mm BTB patellar tendon graft represented 168% of ACL strength and that a single semitendinosus strand represented 70% of ACL strength. Extrapolation from Noyes' data is necessary to estimate commonly used autograft configurations. A 10-mm BTB graft would represent approximately 120% of ACL strength. Assuming that doubling a graft produces equal tension in both strands, a doubled semitendinosus graft would represent 140% of ACL strength and a quadrupled construct may exceed 200% of ACL strength. Noyes' study also demonstrated that the semitendinosus has a stiffness almost identical to that of the ACL, whereas the central third patellar tendon is 3.76 times stiffer. Woo and Adams [3] have emphasized the importance of graft stiffness and ultimate load to failure in the function of an effective ligament substitute. Early reports of suboptimal stability achieved by hamstring grafts can be attributed to the use of single or double constructs and nonphysiometric graft positioning.

Although interference screw fixation has been heralded as a primary advantage of BTB reconstruction, major advocates of the BTB graft use sutures and buttons for fixation, and it appears that the advantage of interference screws for rigid initial fixation has been exaggerated. Indeed several recent reports, including our own series, have demonstrated that superior stability is achieved when using a quadrupled semitendinosus graft (Maeda and coworkers, Paper presented at the AOSSM Interim Meeting, New Orleans, 1994; Rosenberg and coworkers, Unpublished data; Waller and coworkers, Paper presented at the Australian Orthopaedic Association, 1994). Although interference screws provide good initial fixation for BTB grafts, improved methods for graft fixation have been developed with comparable pull-out strength (Rowden and coworkers, Paper presented at the Australian Orthopaedic Association, 1994), which allow early range of motion and weight bearing for hamstring constructs.

Biologic fixation and incorporation are more important. Optimal graft size, stiffness, tissue compatibility, positioning, graft-to-tunnel conformity, and the method of postoperative rehabilitation contribute to biologic fixation. Rodeo and coworkers [4] studied tendon-to-bone healing in a dog model, revealing a steady progression in tendon-to-bone pull-out strength from 2 to 6 months postoperatively. Fixation failure occurred before 8 weeks and graft failure occurred thereafter. Sharpey-like fibers were noted at the bone interface in 8-week specimens. Importantly, tendon-to-bone healing may be less optimal for patellar tendon grafts that do not fill the tibial tunnel. "Windshield wipering" of the graft and synovial fluid ingress may occur with patellar tendon grafts, especially in the tibial tunnel.

Sachs and coworkers [5] have shown that the three most common complications following ACL surgery—quadriceps weakness, flexion contracture, and anterior knee pain—are strongly interrelated. Advancements in preoperative and postoperative protocols have been reported to decrease the incidence of postoperative extensor mechanism morbidity in ACL reconstruction using patellar tendon autografts [6,7]. Despite aggressive rehabilitation, however, extensor mechanism dysfunction has continued to compromise postoperative outcomes [8•]. Earlier, we reported persistent radiographic, strength, and functional extensor mechanism deficits after patellar tendon autograft reconstructions in patients treated postoperatively with a moderately aggressive rehabilitation protocol (Rowden and coworkers, Paper presented at the Australian Orthopaedic Association, 1994). In a recent prospective study, Re and coworkers (Paper presented at the Australian Orthopaedic Association) demonstrated significant differences between the incidence of postoperative anterior knee pain in autogenous patellar tendon reconstruction (47%) and hamstring reconstruction (14%). Yasuda and coworkers [9••] demonstrated a residual 30% quadriceps deficit in female patients having undergone BTB reconstructions.

The senior author, Thomas D. Rosenberg, and Benjamin Graf have developed a proximal anchoring device, the EndoButton (Acufex Microsurgical, Mansfield, MA) (Fig. 9-1) that provides secure femoral fixation for endoscopic ACL reconstruction using tendon or BTB grafts. A quadrupled semitendinosus autograft is usually used because of its ease of harvest, enhanced graft properties, and minimal morbidity. This technique has been used in over 500 ACL reconstructions with no known instance of fixation failure and with results that compare favorably with established techniques.

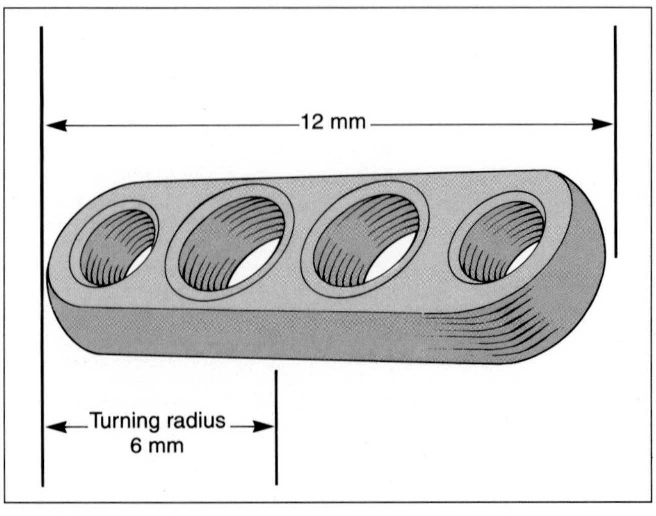

Figure 9-1. The EndoButton (Acufex Microsurgical, Mansfield, MA), a titanium proximal femoral graft anchoring device.

TECHNIQUE

A padded tourniquet is placed on the proximal thigh and then placed within an arthroscopic leg holder. The well leg is abducted, flexed at the hip and knee, placed in a padded support, and the end of the table is flexed completely. After routine sterile preparation and draping, the leg is exsanguinated and the tourniquet is inflated to 300 mm Hg. Alternatively, the procedure can be accomplished without a tourniquet by using an arthroscopic pump. The tourniquet may be briefly utilized for improved visualization during graft harvest, then deflated, and a pump is used for the arthroscopic portion of the procedure.

A superomedial outflow portal is created and is used initially to inject 30 cm^3 of 0.25% bupivacaine hydrochloride with epinephrine solution. Accurate control of knee flexion is critical throughout the procedure. Full-length surgical gowns are used to maintain sterility. The surgeon sits on a stool with the limb controlled by placing the patient's foot on the surgeon's thigh. Rolling forward or backward on the stool, the surgeon carefully controls knee flexion and extension.

For confirmed grade III ACL tears necessitating reconstruction, semitendinosus harvest is completed prior to developing arthroscopic portals. A 5- to 6-cm vertical incision is made over the anteromedial tibial, beginning 2 to 3 cm distal to the joint line and 1 cm medial to the tibial tuberosity. The sartorius aponeurosis is identified and the underlying semitendinosus and more proximal gracilis are palpated. The sartorius aponeurosis is fenestrated in line with its distal fibers with a scalpel and Metzenbaum scissors, exposing the underlying semitendinosus tendon. Working proximally, digital palpation allows isolation of the semitendinosus from the gracilis at the naturally occurring separation 5 to 8 cm proximal to their insertions. A curved hemostat and then a small penrose drain are placed around the semitendinosus to allow positive identification and tensioning for disinsertion from the tibia. Sharp division of the proximal and distal margins of the semitendinosus, while carefully avoiding the underlying medial collateral ligament, usually permits the tendon to be digitally popped off its tibial insertion, preserving maximal tendon length. A #5 (#2 for smaller patients) Ticron whip stitch is placed at five or six levels in the distal tendon, providing control of the free end.

With traction applied to the tendon, the deep fascial bands and attachments to the medial gastrocnemius fascia can be identified and divided with Metzenbaum scissors. The finding of a distal fascial attachment confirms the correct identification of the semitendinosus, as does the repalpation of the proximally lying gracilis. Premature transection of the tendon may occur without release of these fascial attachments. With the knee flexed 50° to 70°, gentle traction is maintained on the tendon while a closed-end tendon stripper is advanced proximally in line with the tendon (Fig. 9-2). An open-end tendon stripper has a greater chance of prematurely amputating the tendon. Generally, a free graft with a length between 24 and 40 cm is obtained. The tendon is transferred to the back table where a quadrupled construct is prepared concurrent with the intra-articular tunnel preparation. The sartorius expansion is then reapproximated with a 0-0 Vicryl suture (Ethican, Somerville NJ).

The graft is prepared on the back table by the surgeon or an assistant while the surgeon proceeds with the intra-articular portion of the procedure. Muscle remaining on the proximal tendon is removed by scraping with a #5 or #6 curette or with a medium or large Cobb periosteal elevator. The proximal end is thin and may be folded over a few millimeters prior to tubularizing with a baseball stitch of 2-0 or 3-0 Vicryl

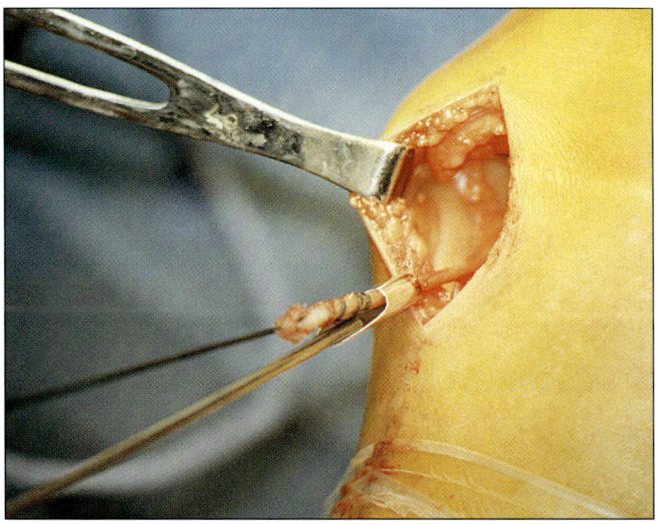

Figure 9-2. The semitendinosus is harvested through a vertical anteromedial incision. Control of the distal tendon is provided by a Ticron whip stitch (American Cyanamid Co., Danbury, CT) as the tendon stripper is advanced proximally.

on a tapered needle. Overall tendon length is measured and the graft length is determined by calculating one quarter of the overall tendon length. With a properly harvested tendon, it is rare to find inadequate tendon length for use as a quadrupled graft. Required minimum tendon length for use as a quadrupled graft is approximately 22 cm in a small patient, allowing 20 to 25 mm for intra-articular length and a minimum of 15 mm within both the tibial tunnel and femoral socket. The necessary graft length increases with the size of the patient, *eg*, a large individual requires a minimum tendon length of 26 to 27 cm. This allows 30 to 35 mm for intra-articular length and 15 to 20 mm within each bone tunnel. If the semitendinosus is too short for use as a quadrupled graft, the gracilis can be harvested and doubled semitendinosus and doubled gracilis grafts can be used. Another excellent option is a tripled semitendinosus graft that leaves the gracilis intact.

Graft preparation is performed on a graft preparation board (Fig. 9-3). The tendon is sharply divided exactly in half on the board. A #5 Ticron suture (#2 for smaller patients) on a tapered needle is whip-stitched in each end of the grafts using holding clamps to secure the grafts during suture placement. The two grafts are then each doubled over to produce a quadrupled construct. A 6-mm polyester tape is placed through both grafts and the graft diameter is determined with sizing tubes (Fig. 9-4). The polyester tape is then placed through the two central holes of the EndoButton but is not tied at this time. A #5 Ticron suture is placed through the leading EndoButton holes and a #2 Ticron suture is placed through the trailing hole. The EndoButton is placed within the EndoButton clamp in preparation for tying the polyester tape at the appropriate suture span length after the femoral channel is completed and measured.

The anterolateral portal is incised 1 cm above the joint line immediately adjacent to the patellar tendon, and the anteromedial portal is created 1 cm above the joint line slightly (5 to 8 mm) off the patellar tendon. Systematic diagnostic arthroscopy is completed without addressing meniscal or chondral pathology at this time. Excision of the ligamentum mucosum and fatpad are performed as necessary to facilitate viewing of the intercondylar region. The tibial stump of the ACL is preserved partially to guide tibial tunnel placement.

The intercondylar notch is evaluated. Anatomic narrowing or encroachment of osteophytes necessitates notch expansion to prevent graft impingement along the lateral femoral condyle and on the roof in terminal extension. Notchplasty allows improved identification of the femoral attachment site. The extent of notchplasty is determined by individual anatomy with some degree of notch enlargement required in most cases. Viewed from the anterolateral portal, the distal outlet of the notch is best visualized in 45° to 60° of flexion and the proximal outlet at 90°. Notchplasty gouges inserted through the anteromedial portal remove bone at the superior and lateral aspects of the notch, and fragments are removed with grasping forceps. Curettes and a power abrader are used to contour the intercondylar notch to its optimal configuration while carefully protecting the posterior cruciate ligament. With the knee flexed 90°, the notchplasty is carried to the proximal outlet. The "over-the-top" location is identified, however, the proximal outlet is not generally expanded.

Next, the tibial tunnel is prepared using the endoscopic aimer, a guidepin, and cannulated drills. The

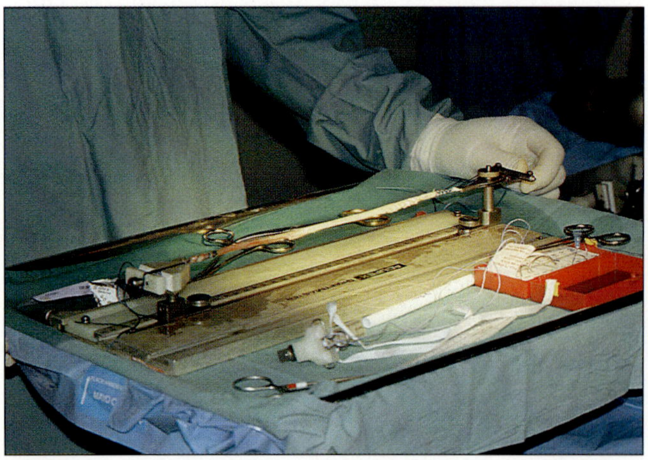

Figure 9-3. Graft preparation is facilitated by using a graft preparation board. Holding clamps secure the graft during suture placement.

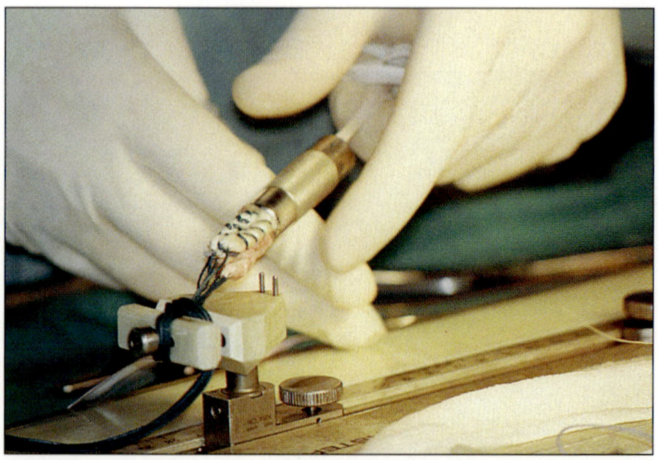

Figure 9-4. The four ends of the graft are evened and held with a clamp while polyester tape is passed through the looped graft ends. Graft-sizing tubes are passed over the looped end to determine the graft diameter.

pretibial periosteum is vertically incised with electrocautery, beginning at the superior margin of the gracilis insertion and progressing 2 to 3 cm proximally adjacent to the infrapatellar tendon. Limited periosteal elevation is performed with an elevator at the anteromedial tibial guide entry site. The endoscopic aimer is usually adjusted to either the *ENDO* or 45° position and the guidetip is positioned intra-articularly through the anteromedial portal. This endoscopic orientation produces an ovoid intra-articular aperture that more closely approximates the anatomic ACL footprint on the tibia than the more circular, less anatomic aperture produced with a more vertical tunnel. The guidepin is typically angled at 45° with the tibia when viewed laterally. A more vertically-oriented tibial tunnel may preclude optimal femoral access and necessitate a lateral incision to develop a femoral tunnel.

The guidetip is impaled in the ACL stump so that the guidepin enters the joint in the center of the tibial ACL stump. We prefer a tibial guide with the aiming line directed at the guide's elbow 7 mm up from the guide's tip, which provides a more visible target (Fig. 9-5). The guidetip is positioned with the tip impaling the posterior fibers of the tibial stump, which provides guidepin placement in the center of the tibial stump. Prior to guidepin insertion, the knee is usually extended with the tibial guide in place to evaluate the relationship of the guide's aiming line to the intercondylar notch. With optimal guidepin positioning, 5 to 6 mm of clearance between the pin and the roof of the notch should be observed. Precise guidepin position is demanded and if necessary the pin is reinserted until both optimal position and direction are confirmed. A cannulated drill corresponding to the size of the graft is used to drill the tibial tunnel to just breaking through the intra-articular cortex. A 5.5-mm synovial resector is placed through the tibial tunnel to remove debris. Proper tunnel orientation will permit endoscopic instrumentation to the "over-the-top" region of the femur with the knee maintained near 90° flexion. The femoral anatomic attachment site is identified and the ACL footprint is studied, confirming the "over-the-top" drop-off point with a probe.

A point 2 to 3 mm distal to the "over-the-top" position in the footprint is identified and marked using a pilot pin. Strain is now premeasured using the Isotac (Acufex Microsurgical, Mansfield, MA) (Fig. 9-6). The Isotac suture is passed through a centering plug and the strain gauge is positioned into the tibial tunnel. With the knee flexed to 45°, the slack is taken out of the sutures. The sutures are then secured to the isometer in the zero position. The isometer spring is released, and the knee is moved through a range of motion, demonstrating the strain pattern for the center of the proposed femoral attachment site. An optimal

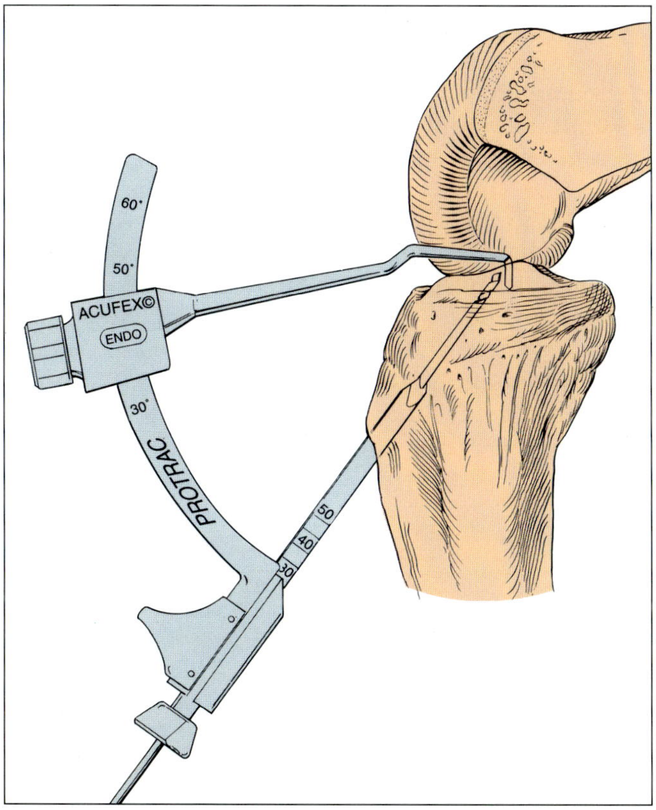

Figure 9-5. The tibial guidewire is set on *ENDO* and positioned within the posterior fibers of the tibial anterior cruciate ligament footprint. The guidewire is typically angled at 45° with the tibia when viewed laterally. (*Adapted from* Rosenberg and Graf [12]; with permission.)

reading reveals a zero to 1-mm change in length with flexion from 45° to 110° and 2- to 3-mm elongation from 45° to 0°. Strain can be viewed as a percentage of elongation or shortening. Isometer strain gauge measurements are anticipated to be slightly higher in taller patients.

A guidepin is inserted at the selected femoral point and advanced 2 to 3 cm into the femur while maintaining the knee at 90° of flexion. A calibrated, cannulated, endoscopic drill bit sized to match the graft's diameter is manually placed through the tibial tunnel and abutted against the femur. Intra-articular graft length is estimated from the calibration lines on the drill bit. The length of graft contained within the femoral socket (the graft insertion length) is determined by taking half of the remaining graft length after subtracting the intra-articular length from the overall prepared graft length. Femoral socket depth is drilled 6 mm deeper than the graft insertion length to allow for a turning radius of the EndoButton. A passing pin is advanced through the tibial tunnel, femoral socket, and the anterolateral femoral cortex. The 4.5-mm cannulated drill bit is used to overdrill the passing pin to produce a passing channel in the femoral socket. A depth gauge measures the total femoral channel length precisely.

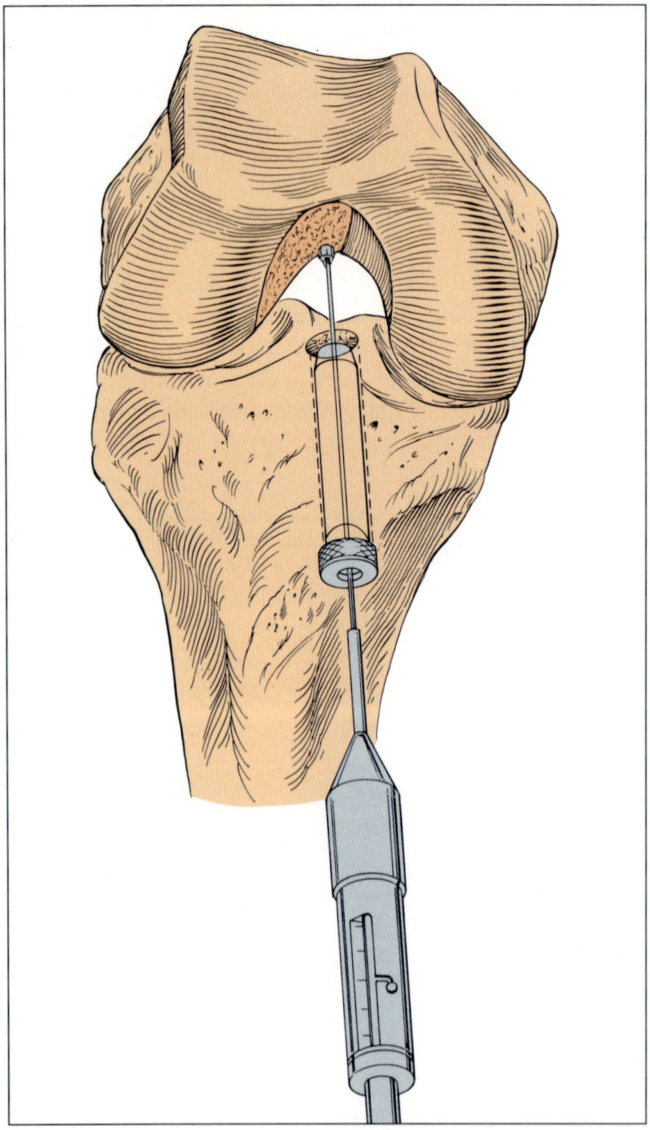

Figure 9-6. The Isotac (Acufex Microsurgical, Mansfield, MA) with centering plug and isometer strain gauge is positioned at the proposed femoral attachment site. The knee is taken through a range of motion. Strain measurements are taken to confirm optimal femoral positioning. (*Adapted from* Rosenberg and Graf [12]; with permission.)

Graft preparation can now be completed by tying the 6-mm polyester tape at its calculated length (Fig. 9-7). The suture span length is determined by subtracting the graft insertion length from the total femoral channel length. The graft preparation board facilitates positioning and measurement as the polyester tape is tied with four square throws.

While an assistant completes graft preparation, meniscal and chondral pathology are addressed. Meniscal repair is performed for unstable repairable tears using a single cannula inside-out technique with accessory posteromedial or posterolateral incisions. Thorough excoriation is vigorously performed to remove all fibrin and synovial debris from both sides of the tear and the adjacent meniscosynovial junction. Stable peripheral tears are thoroughly excoriated to facilitate a healing response even though suturing may not be required. Unstable, irreparable tears are excised to a stable, tapered rim.

While maintaining 90° of knee flexion, a passing pin is placed through the tibial tunnel, femoral socket, quadriceps, and overlying skin, while counterpressure is applied to the thigh with a retractor (Fig. 9-8). The #5 and #2 Ticron sutures are threaded through the eyelet of the passing pin, which is extracted proximally, bringing the sutures out through the thigh. The #5 Ticron suture is used as a leading suture to pull the EndoButton and graft construct proximally into the joint while controlling slack in the trailing #2 Ticron suture (Fig. 9-8) (*top inset*). The graft is viewed arthroscopically to confirm seating is completely in the femoral socket, where a graft marker line can be observed even with the internal femoral aperture, and the graft is felt to be firmly in place. The trailing #2 Ticron suture is pulled to rotate the EndoButton external to the femur, whereupon an abrupt shift is usually felt (Fig. 9-8) (*bottom inset*). The graft is firmly pulled in a distal direction, confirming that the EndoButton has locked the graft in place.

With tension applied to the distal graft sutures, the knee is taken through a range of motion to arthro-

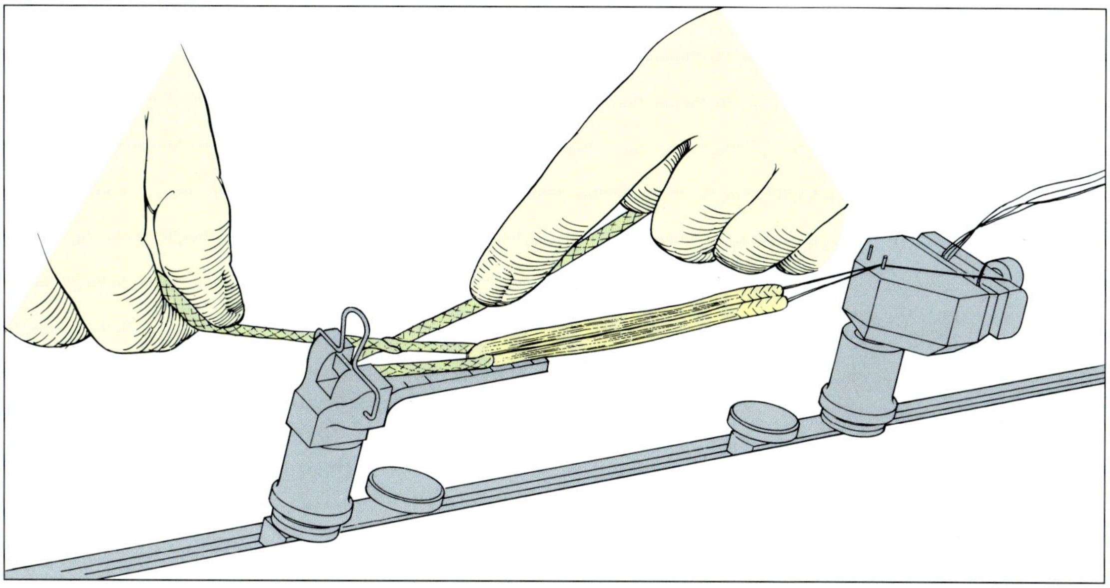

Figure 9-7. Graft preparation is completed. The graft preparation board facilitates positioning and measurement as the polyester tape is tied with four square throws at the calculated suture span length. (*Adapted from* Rosenberg and Graf [12]; with permission.)

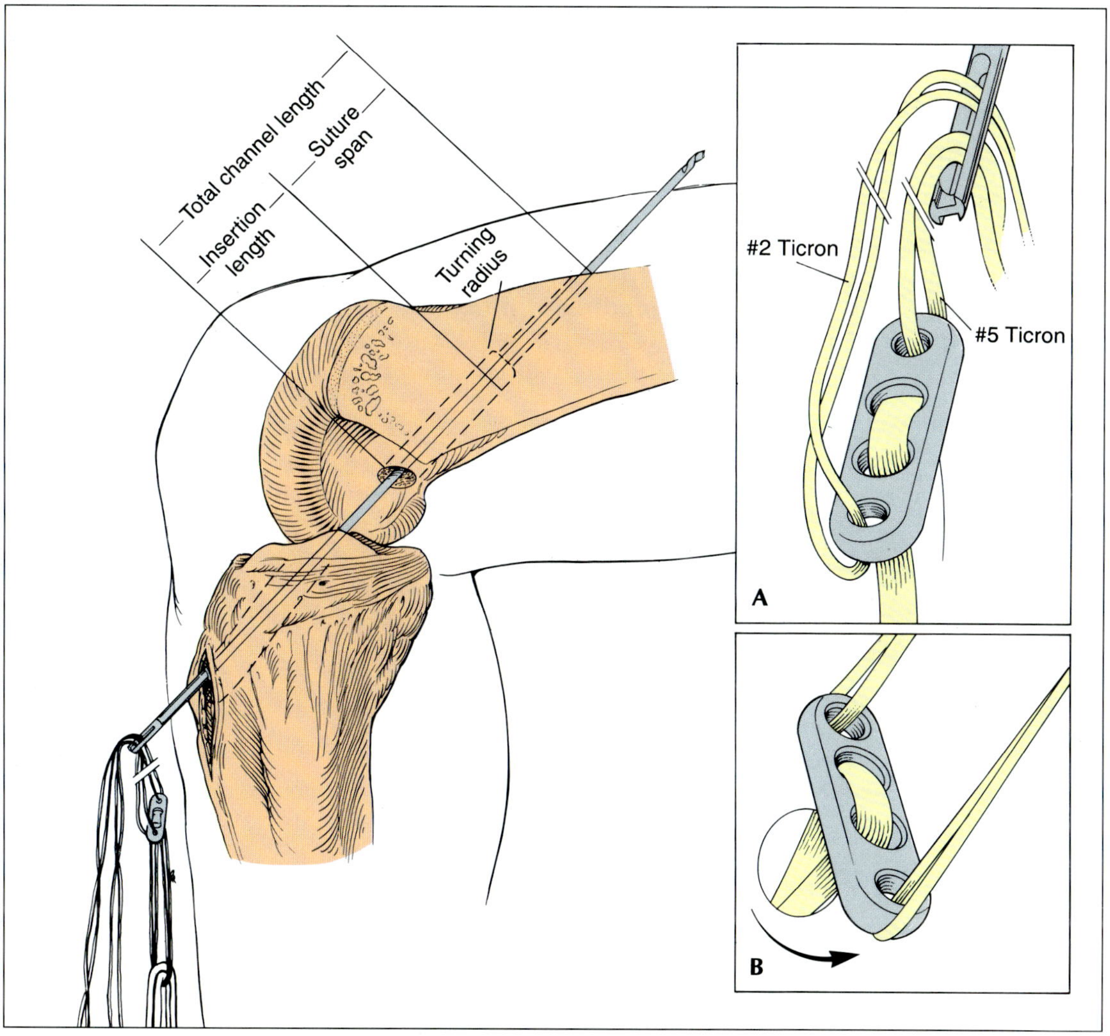

Figure 9-8. The completed graft-EndoButton (Acufex Microsurgical, Mansfield, MA) construct is passed proximally into position with the passing pin piercing the quadriceps and skin proximally. **A**, A #5 Ticron suture (American Cyanamid Co., Danbury, CT) is used to lead and pass the EndoButton. A trailing #2 Ticron suture rotates the EndoButton after exiting the anterolateral femoral cortex. **B**, The #2 Ticron suture is pulled to rotate the EndoButton external to the femur. (*Adapted from* Rosenberg and Graf [12]; with permission.)

scopically confirm the absence of graft impingement. If slight impingement is noted, the notch can be slightly enlarged with curettes or an abrader. A single cortex is drilled perpendicular to the anteromedial tibial with a 2.5-mm drill bit (approximately 1 cm distal to the tibial tunnel outlet) for placement of a self-tapping unicortical cancellous fixation post, which is incompletely advanced into position. The graft is tensioned at 20° to 30° of knee flexion and the matched Ticron sutures are secured around the fixation post, which is then fully tightened (Fig. 9-9).

FEMORAL BISOCKET TECHNIQUE

Sapega and coworkers [10] and Covey and coworkers (Paper presented at the 38th Orthopaedic Research Society, Washington, 1992) have suggested that certain limited deviations from isometry are physiologic and consistent with more anatomically correct reconstructions. This approach to graft placement might be more appropriately termed as physiometric rather than isometric. During passive motion, the bulk of the normal ligament demonstrates 2 to 3 mm of elongation (tightening) in the last 20° of extension. Often, this physiometric relationship can be best achieved by using a bisocket technique to spread out the femoral attachment site along the axis of the native ACL. In a large patient with a wide proximal outlet, centering the entire graft at the most isometric spot does not optimize physiometric graft behavior. In such patients, the bisocket technique more closely reproduces the normal femoral footprint and creates anteromedial and posterolateral fiber bundles that more nearly replicate the physiometric behavior of the native ACL.

In a recent dog study, Rodeo and coworkers [4] demonstrated progressive ingrowth of bone into a tendon implanted in a bone tunnel, creating an attachment between bone and tendon morphologically identical to Sharpey's fibers, and most likely mediated by pluripotential mesenchymal cells of bone marrow origin. Hoffman (Personal communication) has demonstrated a similar regeneration of Sharpey's fibers in humans. Whiston and Walmsley [11] implanted rabbit tendons into bone and demonstrated that graft repair and remodeling is mediated by fibroblasts infiltrating from the periphery toward the central core. Geometric alteration of the graft from a circular to bicircular configuration probably provides a biologic advantage for graft incorporation and remodeling by increasing the bone-to-tendon surface area and decreasing the diameter of the graft.

Two separate double-stranded graft-EndoButton constructs are constructed from each half of the semitendinosus. Graft preparation is begun in the same way as described for the single socket technique by placing a whip stitch in each end. The two semitendinosus halves are individually looped over a 6-mm polyester tape that is passed through the central holes of an EndoButton. Next, #5 and #2 Ticron sutures are threaded through the peripheral holes to provide leading and trailing sutures. Graft preparation is completed by tying the polyester tape at the calculated suture span length, which is determined by measure-

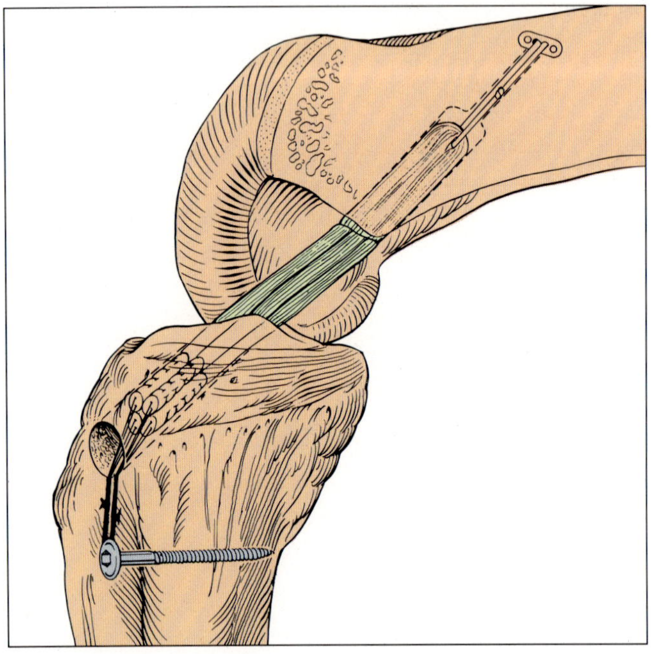

Figure 9-9. The distal end of the graft is tensioned with firm manual tension and secured over a fixation post. (*Adapted from* Rosenberg and Graf [12]; with permission.)

ments of the femoral sockets as described for the single-socket technique.

Two femoral positions are selected at approximately the 11:30 and 10-o'clock positions (right knee) and isometry is measured at least for the superior point (Fig. 9-10A and 9-10B). The graft constructs are usually 6 to 7 mm in diameter, and the femoral sockets are reamed accordingly, with the surgeon recognizing that the cross-section of two 7-mm sockets is equivalent to one 10-mm socket. Each femoral socket is completed as described for the single-socket technique. When the two graft-EndoButton constructs have different diameters, insertion is facilitated by passing the larger graft into the superior socket, securing it proximally with the EndoButton, and then passing the second graft. Range of motion is completed while observing proper graft tension pattern and absence of impingement. The grafts are tensioned separately and tied over a single fixation post. Because the bisocket technique utilizes two EndoButtons and two polyester tapes, pull-out strength is increased. For this technique, Rowden and coworkers, (Paper presented to the Australian Orthopaedic Association, 1994) have demonstrated that the ultimate tensile load at time zero is 688± 59 N compared with 461± 118 N for patellar tendon BTB grafts secured with interference screws.

Postoperative Rehabilitation

Postoperative protocols emphasize early return of function consistent with current understanding of graft incorporation and remodeling during the process of ligamentization. The standard protocols for isolated ACL reconstruction is shown in Figure 9-11. Postoperative rehabilitation is varied as necessitated by concomitant procedures, such as meniscal repair or microfracture arthroplasty. Meniscal repairs are usually immobilized in a postoperative brace for 2 weeks following surgery. Rarely is return of motion or anterior knee pain problematic.

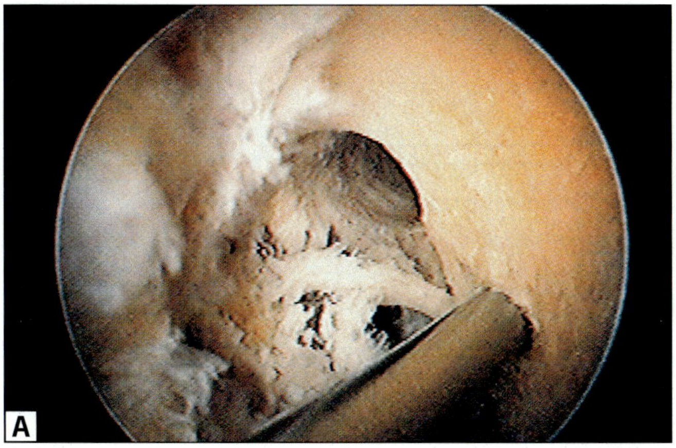

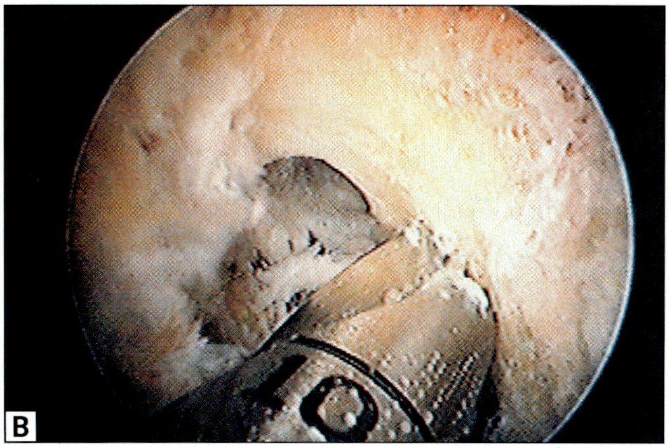

Figure 9-10. **A**, **B**, The femoral bisocket is prepared with the first guidepin placed at the 12:30 position for a left knee. After reaming the first socket, the second guidewire is positioned 2 to 3 mm inferior to the edge of the first socket, then overdrilled to the calculated depth. Sockets are each completed with a 4.5-mm passing channel and measurements are taken permitting accurate graft insertion.

Accelerated anterior cruciate ligament protocol

Activities/daily living	Week 1	2	3	4	5	6	7	8	Month 3	4	5	6	9	12
Shower without brace			→	→	→	→	→	→	→	→	→	→	→	→
Sleep without brace					→	→	→	→	→	→	→	→	→	→
Break down brace (Must have adequate quad)					With good quad, minimal edema, and good body composition.								→	→

☒ Use postoperative or sports brace to control range of motion during exercise. Extension and flexion degrees indicate brace settings that generally permit 10˚ more extension than actual setting.

Range of motion	Week 1	2	3	4	5	6	7	8
Passive								
Extension/flexion		Progress as tolerated						0/140
Patellar mobilization (superior/inferior, medial/lateral glides)	→	→	→	→	→	→	→	→

Brace locked at 10˚ for first 6 weeks. Unlock brace for passive range-of-motion exercise 3 times/day for 20–30 minutes then re-lock brace at 10˚

Extension

Lie on stomach and lower leg into extension

Sit on firm surface and place 5–10 lbs above knee

Flexion

Lie on back; use gravity to slide foot down wall

While sitting use gravity and opposite leg to bend knee

Brace settings	Week 1	2	3	4	5	6	7	8	Month 3	4	5	6	9	12
Weight bearing	As tolerated		→	→	→	→	→	→	→	→	→	→	→	→
Ambulation brace settings														
Extension/flexion	10/10	→	→	10/120	→	→	→	→	→	Discontinued for walking after 12 weeks				

Strength training	Week 1	2	3	4	5	6	7	8	Month 3	4	5	6	9	12
☒ Isometric co-contraction (Hams/quads) Set hams, then quads (electric stimulation may be used)	10/10	→	→	→										
☒ Leg raises Weight applied at level of proximal tibia	10/10	→	→	→	→	→	→	0/0						
☒ Hamcurls seated - passive extension		10/90	10/100	10/110	→	→	→	→	→	→	→	→	→	→
☒ Hip isotonics Resistance above knee		10/10	10/10	10/90	→	→	→	→						
☒ Mini-squat/leg press/toe rise		30/90	→	→	→	→	→	→	→	20/90	→	→	→	→
Cycling - Stationary Remove brace, adjust seat height for extension limit		Well leg	20˚ ext	→	→	→	→	→	→	→	→	→	→	→
Cycling - Outdoor Adjust seat height for extension limit						Level ground only			Seated hill climb		Standing hill climbs			

Figure 9-11. Postoperative protocol for isolated anterior cruciate ligament reconstruction. BAPS—balance and proprioception system; KAT—kinesthetic awareness trainer; UBE—upper body ergometer. (*continued*)

Balance/coordination	Week 1	2	3	4	5	6	7	8	Month 3	4	5	6	9	12
☒ BAPS/KAT/sandunes/Rhomberg test/tape touch			30/90	30/120	10/120	→	→	→	→	→	→	→	→	→
☒ Profitter								30/120	30/120	20/120	→	→	→	→
☒ Sport cord lateral agility				40/120	30/120	20/120	20/120	→	→	→	→	→	→	→

Conditioning	Week 1	2	3	4	5	6	7	8	Month 3	4	5	6	9	12
UBE (upper body conditioning)	→	→	→	→	→	→	→	→	→	→	→	→	→	→
☒ Swimming (refer to pool protocol)			30/90	→	→	→	30/120	20/120	20/120	10/120	→	→	→	→
☒ Walking (100% weight)			10/120	→	→	No Brace	No Brace	→	→	→	→	→	→	→
☒ Stairmaster				30/120	20/120	20/120	→	→	→	→	→	→	→	→
☒ Cross-country ski machine				30/120	30/120	20/120	→	→	→	→	→	→	→	→
☒ Rowing				30/120	30/120	20/120	→	→	→	→	→	→	→	→
☒ Run/jog										20/120	→	→	→	→

	Week 1	2	3	4	5	6	7	8	Month 3	4	5	6	9	12
☒ **Isokinetics**								30/90	30/90	20/90	20/90	10/90	→	→

Anterior shear pad is placed 2" above mid-shaft of the tibia
Start with high speeds, 180° and up
Seated position for flexion and extension
Extension limit controlled by brace or machine

Power training ☐ Yes ☐ No	Week 1	2	3	4	5	6	7	8	Month 3	4	5	6	9	12
☒ Low repetitions - leg press/squats/hamcurls										20/90	20/90	10/90	→	→

Not recommended if serious articular cartilage damage is present. (Refer to operative report.)

Note to Physical Therapist:

Remove brace for passive range of motion.

If extension falls behind goals use:
- Active assisted knee extension
- Ambulation with no brace after 6 weeks
- Vaulting galt after 7 weeks

If no progress or patient falls behind more than 2 weeks on ROM, contact physician's office.

Fit sports brace approximately 6 months post-operative
- Thigh circumference (measured 7" above mid-patella) should be within 1/2" of opposite leg
- Set brace with 20° extension stop

To Return to Sports:

Minimum of 6 months postoperative
No swelling
Quadriceps strength 85% of opposite knee
Hamstring strength 90% of opposite knee
Hop distance 85% of opposite knee
Range of motion 0° to 140°

To return to sports: wear sports brace for 12 months

Figure 9-11. *(continued)*

References and Recommended Reading

Recently published papers of particular interest have been highlighted as:

- • Of interest
- •• Of outstanding interest

1. Howell SM: Arthroscopically assisted technique for preventing roof impingement of an anterior cruciate ligament graft illustrated by the use of an autogenous double-looped semitendinosus and gracilis graft. *Operative Techniques in Sports Med* 1993, 1:58–65.

2. Noyes F, Butler DL, Grood ES, *et al.*: Biomechanical analysis of human ligament grafts used in knee-ligament repairs and reconstructions. *J Bone Joint Surg* 1984, 66A:344–352.

3. Woo SL-Y, Adams DJ: The tensile properties of human anterior cruciate ligament (ACL) and ACL graft tissues. In *Knee Ligaments* Edited by Daniel DM, Akeson WH, O'Connor JJ. New York: Raven Press; 1990:279–289.

4. Rodeo SA, Arnoczky SP, Torzilli PA, *et al.*: Tendon-healing in a bone tunnel: a biomechanical and histologic study in the dog. *J Bone Joint Surg* 1993, 75A:1795–1803.

5. Sachs RA, Daniel DM, Stone ML, *et al.*: Patellofemoral problems after anterior cruciate ligament reconstruction. *Am J Sports Med* 1989, 17:760–765.

6. Shelbourne KD, Nitz P: Accelerated rehabilitation after anterior cruciate reconstruction. *Am J Sports Med* 1990, 18:292–299.

7. Shelbourne KD, Wilckens JH, Mollashby A, *et al.*: Arthrofibrosis in acute anterior cruciate ligament reconstruction: the effect of timing of reconstruction and rehabilitation. *Am J Sports Med* 1991, 19:332–335.

8.• Rosenberg TD, Franklin JL, Baldwin GN, *et al.*: Extensor mechanism function after patellar tendon graft harvest for anterior cruciate ligament reconstruction. *Am J Sports Med* 1992, 20:519–526.

Ten patients undergoing bone-tendon-bone anterior cruciate ligament reconstruction underwent a detailed postoperative evaluation that included isokinetic testing, functional testing, radiographic evaluation, and axial computed tomography. Despite achieving ligamentous stability, patients still experienced persistent weakness, functional deficits, axial computed tomography deficits, patellar chondrosis, and pain.

9.•• Yasuda K, Yasumitsu O, Yoshie T, *et al.*: Quantitative evaluation of knee instability and muscle strength after anterior cruciate ligament reconstruction using patellar and quadriceps tendon. *Am J Sports Med* 1992, 20:471–475.

A postoperative evaluation of 65 patients undergoing anterior cruciate ligament reconstruction with central one third patellar and quadriceps tendon demonstrated persistent quadriceps strength deficit. Quadriceps weakness may be caused by extensor mechanism impairment resulting from graft harvest.

10. Sapega AA, Moyer RA, Schneck C, *et al.*: Testing for isometry during reconstruction of the anterior cruciate ligament. *J Bone Joint Surg* 1990, 72A:259–267.

11. Whiston TB, Walmsley R: Some observations on the reaction of bone and tendon after tunneling of bone and insertion of tendon. *J Bone Joint Surg* 1960, 42B:377–386.

12. Rosenberg TD, Graf B: *Endoscopic Technique for ACL Reconstruction With Pro-Trac Tibial Guide: EndoButton Fixation.* Mansfield, MA: Acufex Microsurgical, Inc.; 1991.

10

CHAPTER

Posterior Cruciate Ligament Arthroscopic Techniques

JOSHUA PORT
DOUGLAS W. JACKSON

Arthroscopically assisted posterior cruciate ligament (PCL) reconstruction has not experienced the widespread application presently seen with reconstruction of the anterior cruciate ligament (ACL). The history of PCL surgery dates back to reports in 1917 and 1919 by Hey-Groves [1,2] who used a semitendinosus tendon that was freed distally and passed first through the posterior capsule then through a tunnel directed toward the medial femoral epicondyle. The proximal semitendinosus was then sutured to the semimembranosus at the level of the tibia.

Mayo Robson [3] in 1903 published a report of ligament (ACL and PCL) repair in an acutely dislocated knee. Since then, various techniques to reconstruct the PCL-deficient knee have appeared in the literature as single cases or as series with small numbers and short follow-up. In 1975, Meyers and coworkers [4] reviewed 33 of 53 patients with traumatic knee dislocations and reported better results in those patients with acute repair of all ligaments. Hughston and coworkers [5] reported follow-up on 29 of 32 repairs of acute PCL injuries and recommended acute repair over late reconstruction. In 1982, follow-up of PCL reconstructions in which the medial head of the gastrocnemius was used showed no improvement in objective stability, however, improvement was reported in patient function [6]. Clancy and coworkers [7] reported using central third patellar tendon autografts in 1983 with 11 of 13 patients described as having good to excellent results from reconstruction for chronic PCL deficiency. Similarly, good to excellent results were reported in 10 reconstructions performed in the acutely injured knee.

ANATOMY

The PCL is the larger of the two cruciate ligaments and is completely covered by a synovial sleeve. It averages 38 mm in length and 13 mm in width with the knee in extension [8]. Cross-sectional data obtained via laser micrometer show that the PCL increases in size as it goes from its tibial to its femoral insertion, in contradistinction to the ACL. Further, the PCL is at least 1.5 times as large as the ACL from midsubstance to the femoral insertion. A midsubstance cross-sectional area of the PCL at 30° of knee flexion measured 40.9 mm in a cadaveric specimen (Harner, Paper presented at AAOS, San Francisco, 1993).

The orientation of the PCL is vertical in the frontal plane and 30° to 45° when angled forward in the sagittal plane [8]. The ligament is described as consisting of two bands: anterolateral and posterome-

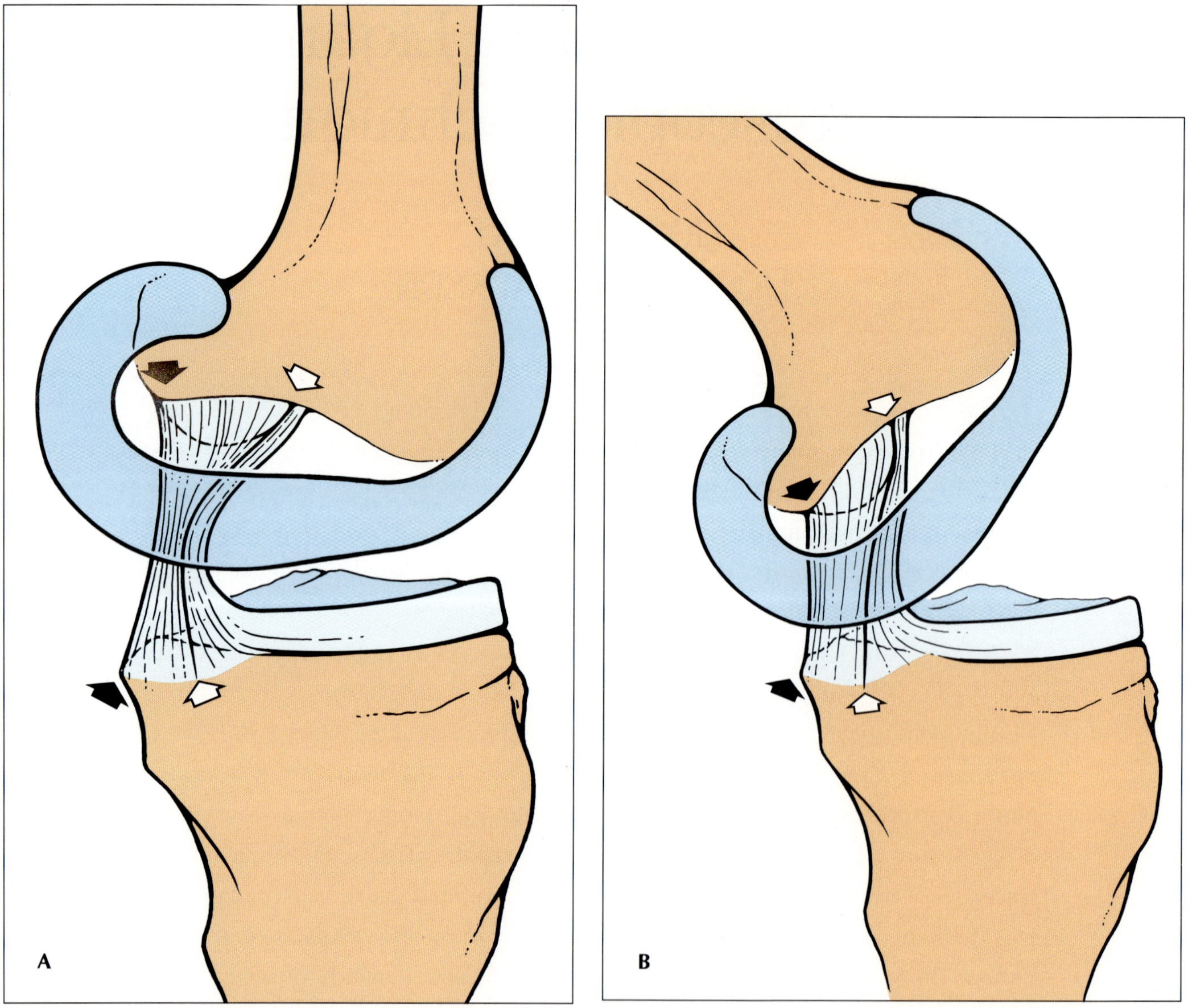

Figure 10-1. **A**, **B** Lateral view of the posterior cruciate ligament illustrating the continuum of fibers that comprise the anterolateral and posteromedial bands. *Black arrows* denote the posteromedial bundle that is most taut in extension and relaxes with flexion. *White arrows* denote the anterolateral bundle that is lax in extension and tightens in flexion. It is the anterolateral band that confers the majority of stability against posteriorly directed force in the clinically significant position of knee flexion.

dial that are named for the attachments of the bundles on the femur (anterior or posterior) and the tibia (medial or lateral). The fibers of the ligament are a continuum rather than two distinct structures. In extension, the thinner posteromedial bundle is taut. With flexion, the thicker anterolateral portion of the PCL tightens with a concomitant decrease in tension of the posteromedial fibers [9] (Fig. 10-1). The femoral insertion is in the form of a circle segment on the posterior aspect of the lateral surface of the medial femoral condyle. The span is approximately 32 mm in the anteroposterior dimension and extends as distal as 3 mm proximal to the articular cartilage [8,10] (Fig. 10-2). The tibial insertion is on the sulcus between the two plateaus, starting just posterior to the articular surface of the tibia and extending approximately 1 cm below (Fig. 10-3). The PCL spans up to 13 mm in the medial to lateral dimension [8,10].

The ligament of Humphry is the smaller of the two meniscal-femoral ligaments associated with the PCL and is located anterior to the PCL. It arises from the posterior horn of the lateral meniscus and inserts at the distal extent of the PCL attachment to the medial femoral condyle. The ligament of Wrisberg is larger than the ligament of Humphry and is posterior to the PCL. It arises from the posterior horn of the lateral meniscus and inserts on the medial femoral condyle at the anterior edge of the PCL, just anterior to the anterior lateral bundle. The presence of either or both of the meniscal-femoral ligaments is somewhat variable and has been reported to be between 35% and 100% in humans [9,11]. When present, the meniscal-femoral ligaments may play a role as secondary restraints to posterior translation after the PCL is sectioned [12•].

The posterolateral or arcuate ligamentous complex functions mainly as the primary restraint to external rotation of the tibia on the femur, but it is also a secondary stabilizer to posterior translation of the knee. The arcuate ligament complex is comprised of the LCL, the popliteus, the arcuate ligament, and the lateral head of the gastrocnemius [13,14]. The iliotibial band and the extensor mechanism play secondary roles in terms of posterior stability. The anatomy and biomechanics of the iliotibial band, the extensor mechanism, the posterolateral corner, and their relationship to posterior knee instability goes beyond the scope of this chapter.

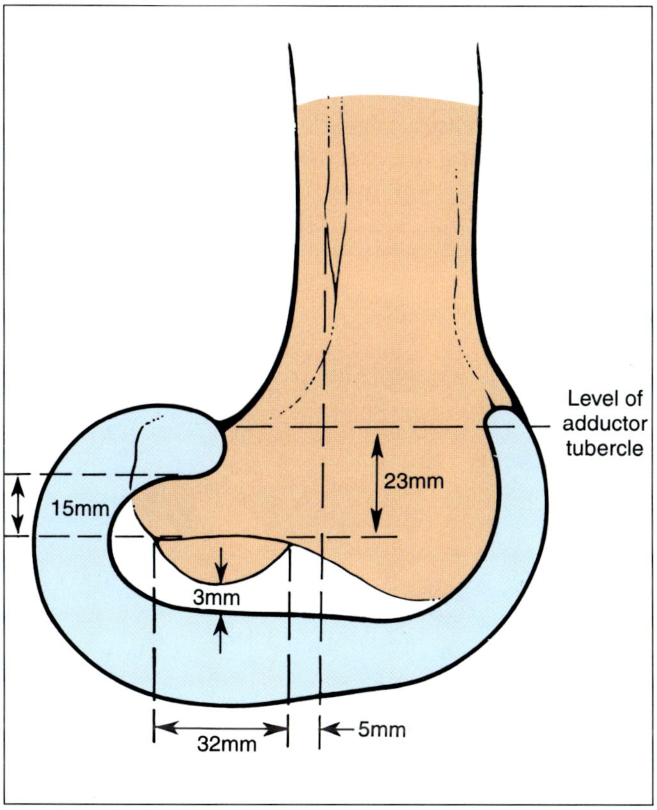

Figure 10-2. The femoral origin of the posterior cruciate ligament is in the form of a circle segment. The average dimensions and position of the insertion are noted.

BIOMECHANICS

Butler and coworkers [15] determined that the PCL is the primary restraint and accounts for as much as 95% of the resistance to posterior tibial translation. Selective cutting studies of the PCL-posterolateral structures suggest that the PCL has a maximum load to failure of approximately 2,000 N [16]. It is the primary restraint to posterior translation in all positions of the motion arc from full extension to 90° of flexion. Isolated sectioning of the PCL increases posterior translation to the greatest degree at 75° to 90° of knee flexion [17,18]. In the arc 0° to 30° to flexion, isolated PCL section produces a minimal amount of translation that is equal to the amount produced by isolated section of both the lateral collateral ligament (LCL) and the lateral ligamentous complex [17]. The PCL has no effect on varus-valgus or external rotation of the tibia if the LCL and the lateral ligamentous complex are intact [12•,17].

Combined sections of the LCL-lateral ligamentous complex and PCL significantly increase posterior tibial translation, varus angulation, and external rotation at all angles of flexion. Varus angulation increases slightly with isolated section of the LCL and further with subsequent section of the arcuate ligamentous complex. Significant varus angulation of up to 30° at 60° of knee flexion results from PCL section following prior sectioning of the LCL-lateral ligamentous complex [17]. External tibial rotation is increased at all angles, 0° to 90°, if the LCL-lateral ligamentous complex is cut. Isolated cutting of the PCL results in no increase in external rotation. Combined section of the PCL after prior sectioning of the LCL and lateral ligamentous complex shows an increase in external rotation at 60° to 90° of knee flexion, but no increase in external rotation in the motion arc from 0° to 30° [17]. This finding has clinical significance because an increase in external rotation seen with 0° to 30° of knee flexion reflects incompetence of the LCL and lateral ligamentous complex structures.

Isolated medial collateral ligament sectioning does not increase valgus angulation in full extension. Combined PCL and medial collateral ligament sectioning increases valgus laxity at all angles of knee motion, including full extension [17].

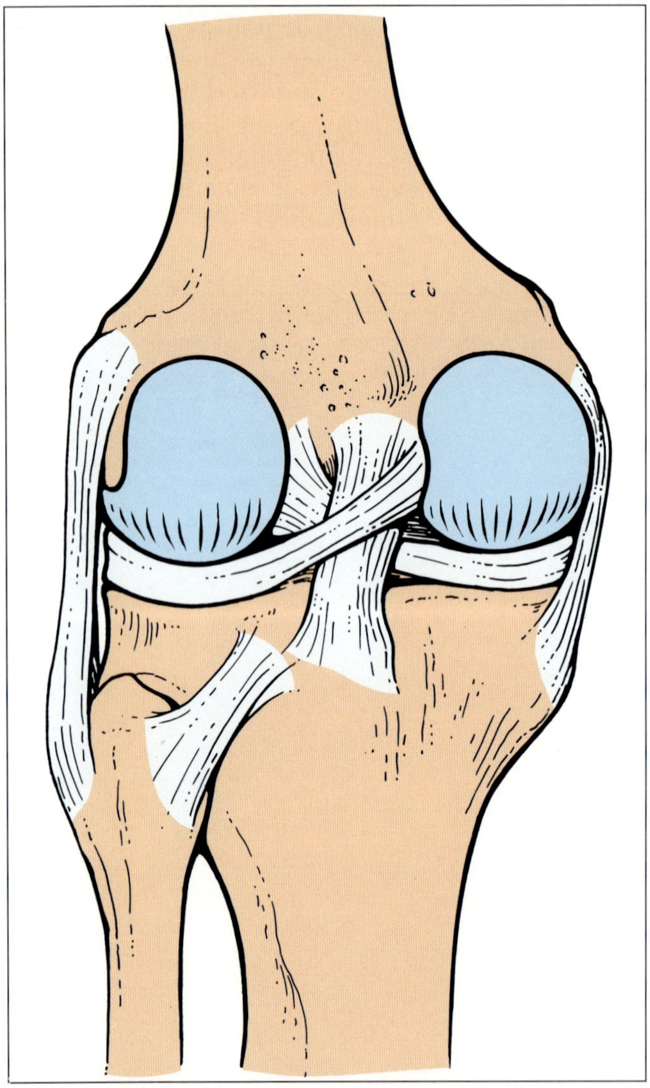

Figure 10-3. The tibial insertion of the posterior cruciate ligament is posterior on the sulcus between the medial and lateral tibial plateaus. The insertion starts just inferior to the articular surface and spans greater than 1 cm below.

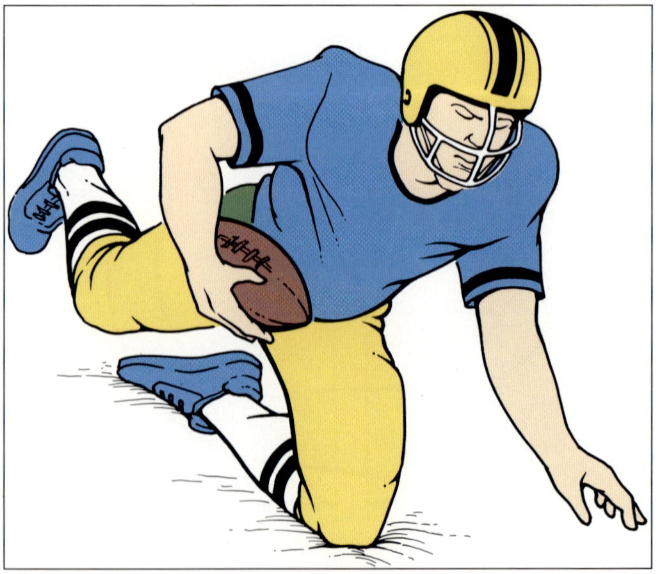

Figure 10-4. In the athlete, a fall onto a flexed knee with the foot in plantar flexion can result in an isolated posterior cruciate injury.

Clinical Evaluation

History

The frequency of recognized PCL injuries is less than that of recognized ACL injuries. Patients with chronic PCL deficiency have fewer complaints of instability. Chronic PCL-deficient patients may develop patellofemoral and medial compartment pain secondary to degenerative changes. These patients often have difficulty climbing stairs, kneeling, and bending. The history of the mechanism of injury is an important key to diagnosis in an isolated PCL tear. The two most common mechanisms are a direct blow from a car dashboard to the anterior tibial surface with the knee flexed and a fall (often from a motor scooter) onto a flexed knee [19•]. In the athletic population, a fall onto a flexed knee with a plantar flexed foot is a common cause of an isolated PCL injury [20] (Fig. 10-4). After suffering a tear of the PCL, the patient often recognizes that he or she has had a significant knee injury but, unlike an ACL tear, there is minimal effusion and no significant sensation of instability. Often, no "pop" is heard and the patient is usually able to ambulate.

Physical examination

The hallmark of the physical examination of PCL insufficiency is the absence of the normal 8- to 10-mm anterior tibial femoral step-off with the knee flexed at 90° (Fig. 10-5). Another physical finding is the asymmetric posterior sagging of the tibial tubercle compared with the uninvolved limb that is noted with the patient's knees and hips flexed at 90° with the examiner supporting the ankles (Fig. 10-6). The 90° quadriceps active test is performed with the patient supine and the hips flexed at 45°. The knees are flexed at 90° and the foot is supported flat on the table by the examiner. With an intact PCL, the contraction of the quadriceps occurs along a posteriorly directed course from the tibial tubercle to the patella, and tibial motion is approximately 0 to 2 mm posterior. With a PCL injury, the tibia sags posteriorly and the line of force from the tibia to the patella is directed anteriorly. With quadriceps contraction, anterior tibial translation results [21] (Fig. 10-7).

A posterior drawer test should be performed at both 30° and 90° of knee flexion. Isolated PCL injuries show increased posterior drawer at 90° of knee flexion but not increased posterior tibial translation at 30°. Injury to the posterolateral corner structures alone show an increased posterior translation with the knee flexed at 30°, and if the PCL is intact, this translation does not increase with further knee flexion. Combined PCL, LCL, and lateral ligamentous complex injuries show significantly increased posterior drawer at all angles of knee flexion.

The examiner must accurately assess the resting position of the tibia to avoid interpreting the laxity as a false-positive anterior drawer. Grading of posterior laxity has been scaled from 1+ (up to 5 mm of transla-

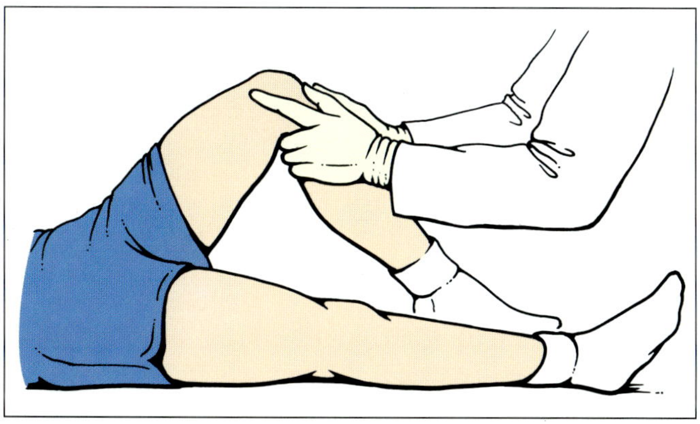

Figure 10-5. The tibial femoral step-off should be palpable in the supine patient with the knee flexed to 90°. The examiner should palpate the anterior joint line in the resting position and then perform anterior and posterior drawer testing. Comparison must be made with the opposite leg.

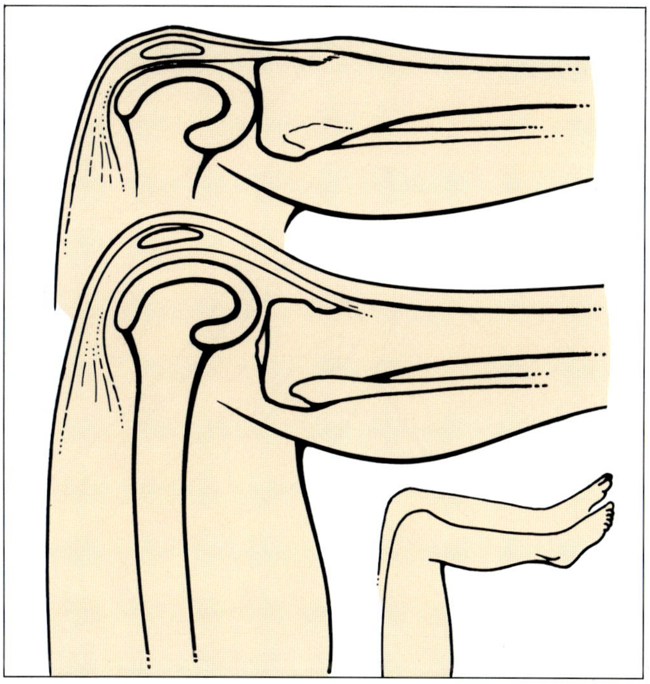

Figure 10-6. The sag sign, illustrated here on the right knee, is seen when comparing the tibial tubercle heights with the knees and hips flexed to 90° and the examiner supporting the patient's ankles. The posteriorly subluxated tibia as drawn is responsible for the difference in the knee contours.

tion), 2+ (6 to 10 mm), to 3+ (greater than 10 mm) [14]. In general, grade 2 laxity allows the tibia to subluxate posteriorly so that the anterior tibia is flush with the femoral condyles at 90° of knee flexion. Grade 3 laxity is subluxation of the tibia posterior to the femoral condyles in the same position. Some chronic PCL laxity will not further translate from the resting subluxated position. Muscular guarding may make an accurate examination more difficult. The end point of the posterior drawer examination should be noted by the examiner as soft or firm. It is crucial to compare all findings with the opposite extremity, especially in the individual with generalized ligamentous laxity.

Isolated PCL injuries will not increase varus or valgus displacement or internal and external rotation of the tibia upon manual testing. The uninjured knee has the smallest varus or valgus displacement in full extension that increases as knee flexion increases to

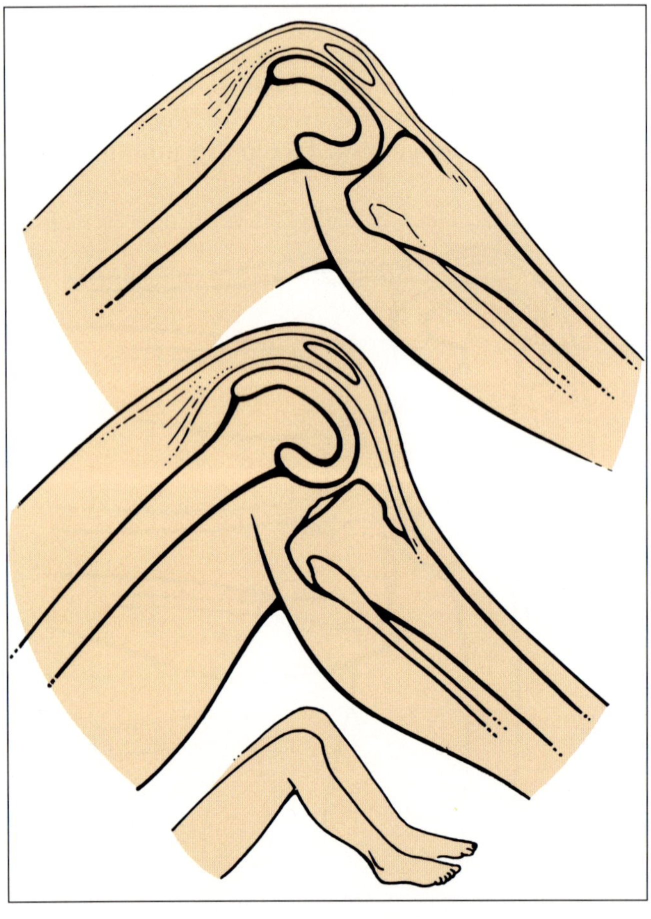

Figure 10-7. The quadriceps active test is performed with the knee at 90° of flexion. The posteriorly subluxated tibia of the posterior cruciate ligament (PCL)-deficient knee (*top*) is pulled forward when the quadriceps are contracted (*bottom*). In the PCL-intact knee, there is no significant motion of the knee with quadriceps contraction in this position.

90°. Increased varus-valgus displacement in flexion beyond that of the uninvolved limb indicates a collateral ligament injury. Increased varus-valgus laxity in full extension indicates combined injuries to the cruciates as well as the collaterals [21].

The neurovascular structures about the knee must also be carefully examined, especially in the acutely injured knee. Cruciate injuries with combined lateral ligamentous complex injuries often have injury to the peroneal nerve. Knee dislocations have an increased risk for vascular injury and nerve injury and merit an arteriogram if suspicion of an arterial injury exists even in the presence of palpable distal pulses.

Roentgenograms

Plane radiographs of the PCL-deficient knee should include a 30° anteroposterior flexion weightbearing view, a lateral view, a Merchant view, and an intercondylar notch view. In the chronic PCL-deficient knee, these views allow roentgenographic evaluation of patellofemoral or medial compartment arthrosis. Acute fractures at the tibial insertion of the PCL are best seen on the lateral view of the knee.

Magnetic Resonance Imaging

The PCL is well visualized on modified sagittal plane images. These images are obtained with the foot externally rotated at 20°. The PCL should appear dark with low-signal intensity on T_1 and T_2 imaging (Fig. 10-8). Often the ligament of Humphry (anteriorly) and the ligament of Wrisberg (posteriorly) can be visualized. Magnetic resonance (MR) imaging is very accurate in documenting acute PCL injuries [22]. A high-intensity signal is seen at the site of the ligament injury (Fig. 10-9). Often effusion is present, although rarely to the extent seen with acute ACL injuries. Thorough MR imaging assessment should include examination for concurrent injuries to the collateral ligaments, ACL, and articular cartilage. T_2 imaging can reveal associated bone edema that may be indicative of more extensive trauma to the overlying articular cartilage (Fig. 10-10). Over a period of 6 months to a year, the signal of an injured PCL may revert back to a low intensity indistinguishable from normal (Fig. 10-11). As techniques of imaging articular cartilage improve, MR imaging may become more useful in the chronic PCL-deficient knee to evaluate the extent of arthrosis.

TREATMENT

The natural history of isolated tears to the PCL has not been completely documented. Early reports showed good to excellent results with nonoperative treatment

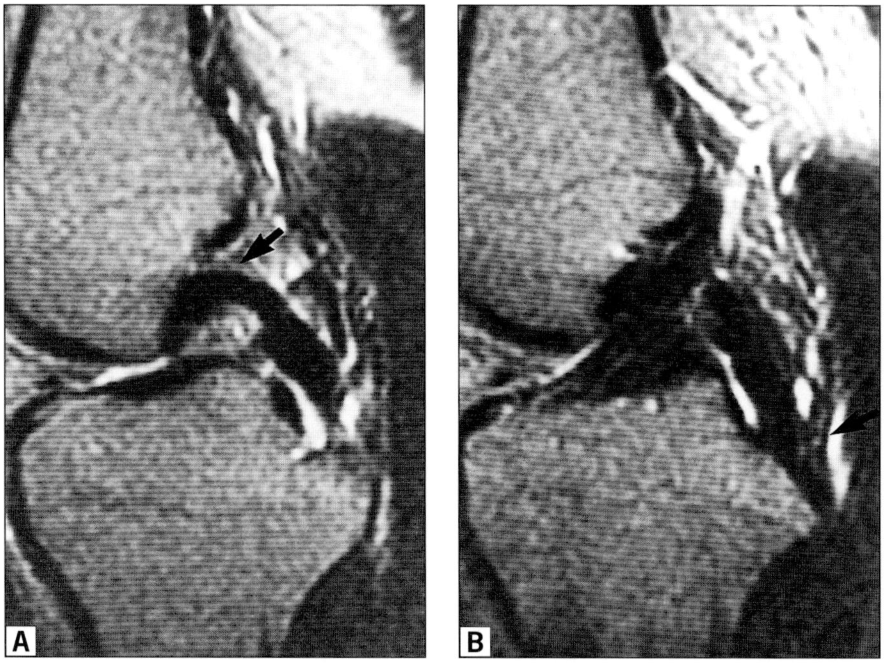

Figure 10-8. T_2-weighted images of intact posterior cruciate ligament. Note the dark black signal throughout the ligament and the visualization of both the **A**, femoral and **B**, tibial insertion sites (*arrows*). The contour is smooth and regular and the width is thick.

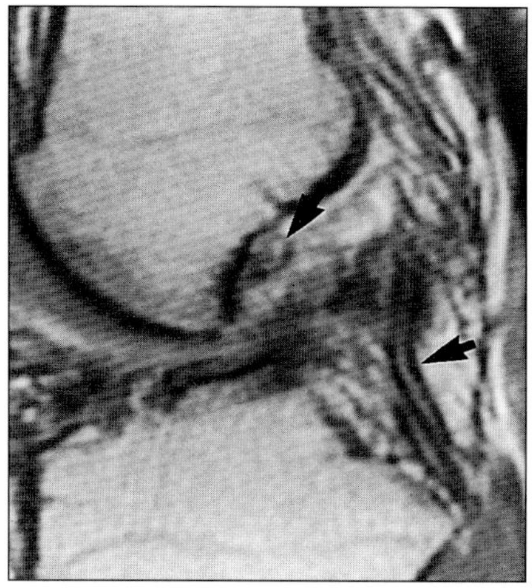

Figure 10-9. Proton density sagittal spin-echo image of a patient with acute anterior cruciate ligament and posterior cruciate ligament (PCL) tears. Note the absence of ligament in the anatomic site of the PCL. There is suggestion of an abnormally thin ligament signal at both the femoral and tibial insertions of the PCL (*arrows*). There is midsubstance decontinuity suggestive of a midsubstance tear of the PCL.

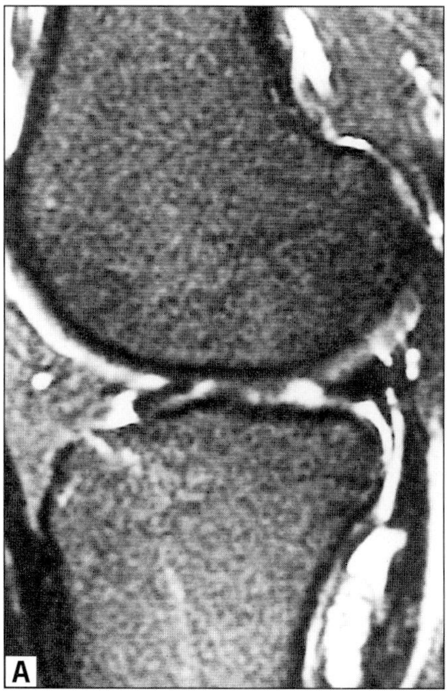

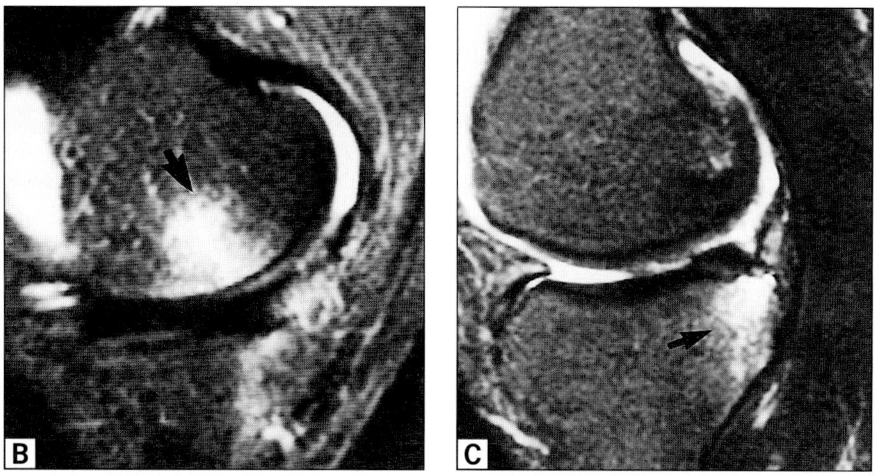

Figure 10-10. Fat saturation fast spin-echo images are shown that allow examination for marrow abnormalities. **A**, A normal study showing a homogeneous gray signal throughout the distal femur and proximal tibia. **B**, Image consistent with bone contusion of the distal femur with increased marrow signal denoting the zone of injury (*arrow*). **C**, The matching lesion of bone contusion in the proximal tibia (*arrow*). The diagnosis of bone contusion requires clinical correlation as similar signal changes are seen representing fibrovascular marrow changes in the elderly patient with degenerative arthritis. The signal increase in the acutely injured knee is thought to represent bleeding and contusion from trabecular microfracture.

[24–26]. Longer term follow-up in these patients demonstrated pain that necessitated secondary surgical procedures. Few returned to sports. More recently, it has been documented that nonoperative treatment of PCL tears has significant morbidity [27,28•;29] Kennedy and Grainger [30] noted significant degenerative changes occurring at an average of 5 years after PCL injury treated nonoperatively. These changes were most significant in the medial compartment. The natural history of nonoperatively treated lesions has not yet been fully defined. Specific treatment recommendations and surgical indications will remain controversial until the natural history of nonoperative and operative outcomes are clarified.

Grade I injuries to the PCL are defined as 5 mm or less of posterior tibial translation with the knee flexed to 90°. Parolie and Bergfeld [23] noted that isolated lesions often decrease up to 5 mm in anteroposterior translation with the knee at 90° if the tibia is internally rotated. Tightening with internal rotation indicates that the posterolateral corner is intact.

Grade I posterior cruciate injuries probably cannot be improved on with current surgical techniques. Grade II lesions have up to 10 mm of posterior translation. In this position, the tibia rests flush with the femoral condyle. Isolated lesions will tighten with internal rotation. Grade II lesions in athletic, lower energy injuries have been noted to tighten somewhat during the healing process and may end up nearer to grade I laxity with nonoperative management. In general, the level of disability and symptomatology, patient demands and expectations, and the degree of posterior laxity must be carefully considered in formulating treatment recommendations to a patient. In addition, once surgery is indicated, the results of present techniques must be better able to document improvement. The residual posterior instability after reconstruction may not represent an improvement for the patient. The present limitations and variations in successful reconstruction of the PCL must be kept in mind prior to committing the patient to PCL reconstructive surgery.

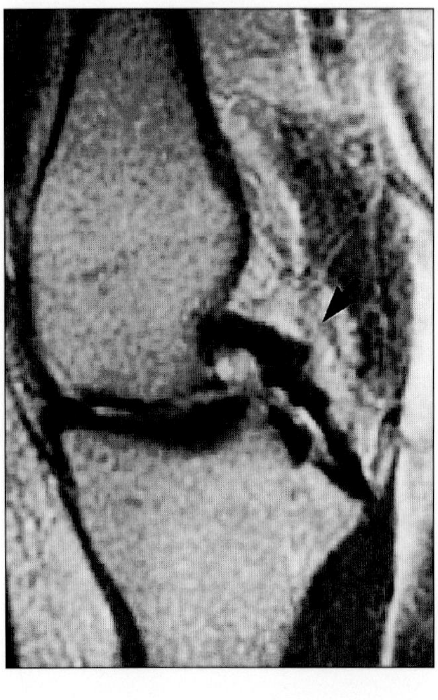

Figure 10-11. Proton density sagittal image of a chronic posterior cruciate ligament (PCL) injury of over 2 years duration. The contour of the PCL is normally smooth; here it is irregular. The signal, however, is of normal intensity (*arrow*). This is an example of how the signal of PCL injuries may revert to normal over time.

Surgery in chronic grade III lesions and knees that have been dislocated with resultant injuries to both cruciate ligaments are those most commonly reconstructed. With significant grade III posterior laxity, often other injuries, especially to secondary structures, exist and must be carefully evaluated. It is important that these injuries be addressed at the time the PCL is reconstructed. The patient should be re-examined preoperatively, intraoperatively, and before closure to determine if any remaining laxity exists. With knee dislocations, reconstruction of the PCL is often performed at the same time as ACL reconstruction. In these cruciate reconstructions, we prefer to tension and fix the PCL graft prior to tensioning and fixation of the ACL graft. The PCL is tensioned with the knee at 70° of flexion and the tibial-femoral step-off should be re-established prior to fixation.

Acute grade III injuries of the PCL, especially in the higher demand patients, are a relative indication for reconstruction of the PCL. Grade I isolated tears in our hands, even in high-demand patients, currently are being treated nonoperatively. Nonoperative treatment of the acute PCL injury requires progressive and focused rehabilitation. The medial compartment and the patellofemoral joint are potential future problems. We prefer to involve the patient in understanding the importance of monitoring symptoms and changes. The initial focus is on re-establishing range of motion with the emphasis on obtaining full extension. After motion is re-established, quadriceps strengthening is initiated and then maintained on a long-term basis.

SURGICAL TECHNIQUE

Prior to surgery, when the patient is under anesthesia, evaluation and documentaion of the posterior ligamentous and other associated laxities is recorded. A video arthroscopy of the injured knee is performed through the standard arthroscopic portals. This evaluation of the knee includes documenting the status of the articular cartilage, menisci, cruciate ligaments, and patellar tracking. If amenable to treatment, associated intra-articular pathology is addressed prior to the PCL reconstruction. Preparation of the femoral and tibial attachment sites requires visualization of these areas. The adjacent soft tissue and remaining PCL is debrided using a full-radius resector. A curette or knife may be helpful. A bony notchplasty may be performed if necessary. Adequate visualization of the underlying bone at the tibial attachment site of the PCL requires special attention to detail. The attachment lies on the posterior surface of the tibia, in the sulcus between the medial and lateral tibial plateaus. It is difficult to view and debride this area at the same time from the anterior portals. A 30° arthroscope placed through the intercondylar notch from an anterior portal will allow visualization of the insertion of the PCL in some patients. We prefer a 70° arthroscope that is passed through the intercondylar notch for more distal visualization. Alternatively, a 30° or 70° arthroscope placed through a separate posteromedial portal allows complete visualization of the tibial insertion of the PCL as it is debrided.

We prefer a posteromedial portal for instrumentation to debride the PCL and prepare the tunnel site. This debridement is viewed with a 70° arthroscope passed through the anterolateral portal. When using posterior medial and lateral portals, care must be taken to avoid damaging the saphenous vein or nerve, the popliteal neurovascular bundle, and the peroneal nerve. An 18-gauge spinal needle is helpful to locate the desired entry point, angle, and direction for the eventual posterior portal. With the knee flexed to 90°, the saphenous nerve moves anterior and nearer to the joint line. The selection of these portals can be made under direct visualization with the arthroscope passed through the intercondylar notch. A full-radius resector is then inserted from the posteromedial or posterolateral portal to resect the stump of the PCL. A curved curette or periosteal elevator passed through the intercondylar notch can be used to elevate the posterior capsule from its tibial attachment. Sufficient soft tissue and capsule are removed to allow visualization and selection of the site for the osseous tunnel. The capsule and PCL insertion are intimately related at the distal aspect of the PCL attachment. It is important to elevate the posterior capsule from the residual PCL for additional protection during drilling of the tibial osseous tunnel.

SELECTION OF ISOMETRIC POINTS

It has been estimated through computer modeling that isometry is more sensitive to changes in the femoral attachment site than at the tibial attachment site [30,31]. The isometric position on the femur is located within a bullet-shaped zone. The center of the zone is 11.3 mm back and 6 mm down from the intersection of the femoral trochlear groove with the roof of the intercondylar notch. The zone has an anteroposterior dimension of 3.3 mm and a superoinferior dimension of 10.6 mm [32]. Attachment sites in this zone produce length changes less than 3 mm throughout an arc of motion. Isometry is less sensitive to changes in the tibial attachment site. Anatomic positioning of the tibial tunnel on the posterior sloping sulcus between the two condyles has been desired. Intraoperative isometry measurements are dependent on the gravitational condition under which the limb is tested [33]. Attention to positioning of the knee joint must be considered if an isometer is used during PCL reconstruction. The PCL has a broad femoral attachment that is a continuum of fibers. It has been described as having an anterolateral and posteromedial portion. The objective is to recreate the anterolateral portion of the PCL. This thicker portion of the ligament contains the fibers that are tightest in flexion and are primarily responsible for the stability of the tibia against posterior translation with the knee flexed (Fig. 10-1). The patient with PCL instability has the greatest problem when the knee is in flexion. The posteromedial bundle is thinner and more isometric but is taut in extension, thus it does not provide the requisite stability in flexion. Because we prefer to duplicate the anterolateral bundle with our graft, we prefer to be slightly more anterior on the femoral tunnel placement and more lateral on the tibial tunnel placement.

The guidepin is placed in the tibia with an arthroscopic drill guide. There are several guide systems available. The guide should allow length measurement, protect the surrounding soft tissues, and provide an accurate and reproducible selection of the target for the drill. In addition, we prefer to confirm placement and angle of the guidepin in the tibia using a fluoroscopic image intensifier. The penetration of the pin, drill, or curette through the posterior tibial cortex is done by hand and under direct arthroscopic visualization (Fig. 10-12).

We prefer to place the tibial pin through a short anterolateral skin incision. If a patellar tendon autograft has been harvested, we extend that excision slightly distal and lateral. Anteromedial incisions are used by some surgeons. The advantage of an anterolateral incision is that the graft fixation device can be placed deep under the musculature and may not be as prominent or palpable. Fixation devices on the medial tibial surface often require a second procedure for removal. The proximal tibial soft tissue is raised subperiosteally at the desired entry point. The drill guide is positioned through the anteromedial portal. The arthroscope may be placed through the posteromedial portal to directly view the placement of the guidewire. This placement may be checked on fluoroscopy. The drill guide should be oriented at approximately 45° to the long axis of the tibia. The tibial guidepin is then drilled through the tibia to a depth that perforates the posterior cortex at the anatomic insertion of the ligament. In general, this pin parallels the posterior flare of the tibia and proximal tibiofibular joint (Harner, Paper presented at AAOS, San

Francisco, 1993). It is important to avoid allowing the drill to "walk" from the desired point of entry in the tibia. Particularly from the lateral side of the tibia, the drill can skive off the tibial surface and progress between the tibia and fibula. Posterior penetration of the soft tissue in this position is of concern. A tapping technique, a sharp drill, an oscillating drill, or a predrilled starting hole can reduce the likelihood of the drill walking. The aim is to create a tunnel that skirts along, but does not perforate through, the posterior metaphyseal tibial flare and exits at the distal portion of the anatomic insertion of the PCL. A cannulated drill is then used to drill the tibial tunnel. We prefer to confirm the position of the drill under fluoroscopic guidance.

The potential for neurovascular injury during PCL reconstruction using the arthroscopic-assisted technique is greatest during the drilling of the tibial tunnel. It is important to understand the unique anatomy of the distal insertion of the PCL to minimize hazardous consequences. Distally, the posterior portion of the PCL is confluent with the posterior capsule and periosteum. The anteroposterior diameter of the tibia narrows abruptly distal to the PCL insertion. It is this anatomic configuration of the posterior aspect of the proximal tibia that makes a distal exit of the drill bit a potential problem. Square-shaped shoulders on the drill bit are potentially more hazardous (Fig. 10-13) [14].

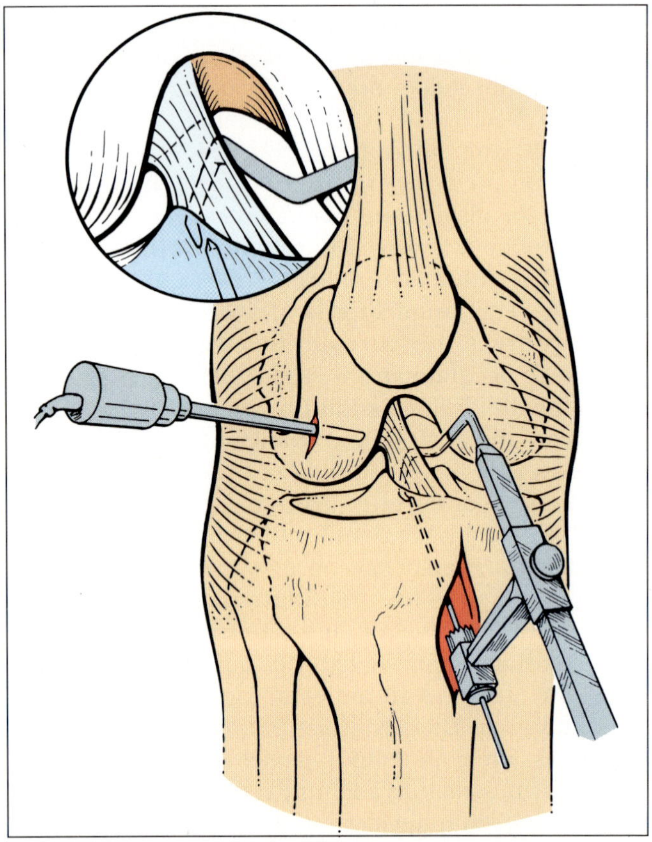

Figure 10-12. Proper position of the guidewire for the tibial tunnel requires the drill guide to be firmly seated at the anatomic insertion of the posterior cruciate ligament 1 cm caudal to the articular surface posteriorly. The angle is approximately 45° and parallels the slope of the posterior tibial cortex. The ideal position is slightly lateral of midline as the anterolateral bundle is the one being reconstructed. We prefer to place the tunnel through an anterolateral incision as shown. Observation of proper positioning of the guide can be via a 70° arthroscope from the anterolateral portal as shown, or with a 30° arthroscope from the posteromedial portal. Confirmation by fluoroscopic examination is strongly recommended.

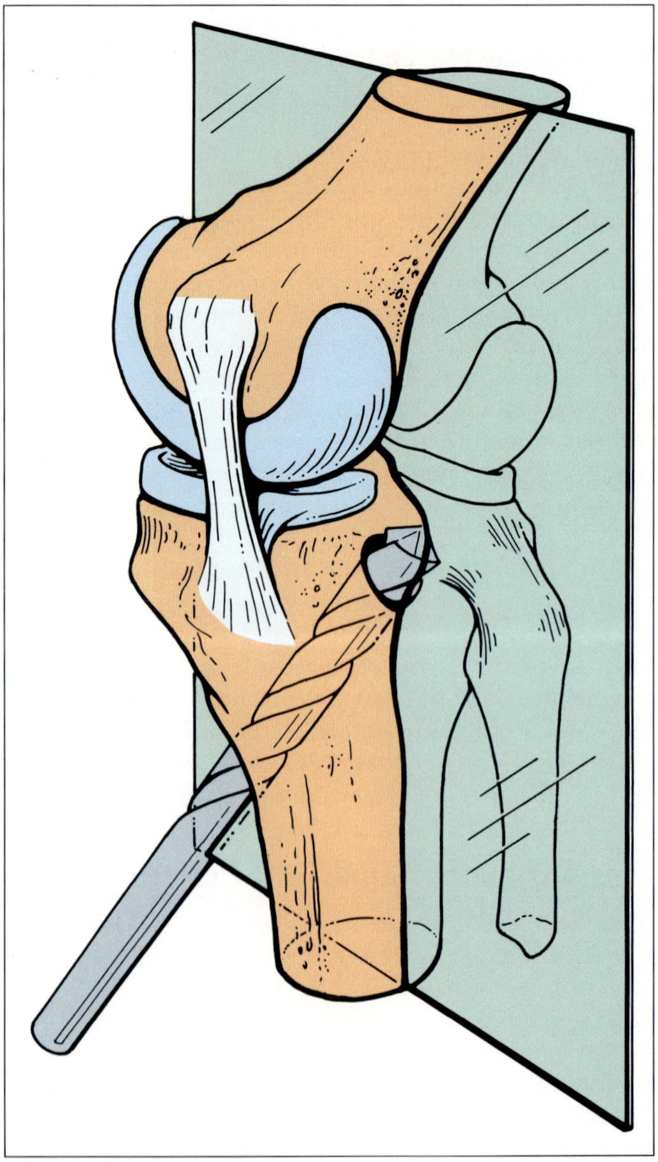

Figure 10-13. A drill with squared shoulders is potentially hazardous as premature exit through the posterior cortex places the drill in close proximity to the neurovascular structures.

The sciatic nerve divides into the tibial and common peroneal nerve in the distal third of the femur. As the tibial nerve enters the popliteal fossa, it is superficial and lateral to the popliteal artery and vein. At the level of its insertion, only the posterior capsule separates the PCL from the popliteal artery, vein, and the tibial nerve (Fig. 10-14). Between the heads of the gastrocnemius, muscular branches of the tibial nerve supply the gastrocnemius, soleus, plantaris, and popliteus muscles. As the tibial nerve reaches the level of the joint line, it is immediately adjacent to the popliteal artery. Distally, the tibial nerve passes deep to the arch of the soleus, closely applied to the popliteus. Once distal to the popliteus, the nerve supplies the soleus, tibialis posterior, flexor digitorum longus, and flexor hallucis longus.

In the arthroscopically assisted technique for PCL reconstruction, the tip of the drill bit exits the posterior tibial cortex in close proximity to the neurovascular structures (Fig. 10-15). At this level, the risks of injury are increased as a result of unexpected penetration of the drill bit owing to the anatomic configuration of the proximal tibia. Damage to the neurovascular structures may occur in several ways. The sharp edges of the drill bit may lacerate the popliteal artery directly or blunt trauma may cause an intimal injury. Nerve palsy may occur as a result of direct trauma, excessive traction, ischemic injury associated with popliteal artery injury, and by compression from a hematoma. This hematoma may accumulate as a result of adjacent soft-tissue injury and bleeding. To minimize the problems, it helps to completely elevate or debride the soft tissues of the tibia for good visualization. This includes not only the shelf of the tibia, but also the entire area where the tip of the drill bit may exit. It has been our experience that scar tissue formation in chronic cases as a result of previous PCL surgery, severe trauma, or both makes elevation and debridement more difficult and increases the potential for neurovascular injury. Once soft tissue has been cleared and the tunnel is being drilled, we prefer the drill bit to be visualized arthroscopically and its exit protected with a retractor, a finger, or both. A drill bit with tapered shoulders, such as the acorn drill bit, may be less likely to cut into or tear the adjacent soft tissues and thus less likely to damage neurovascular structures [34]. As the drill bit exits along the angled posterior cortex, a tapered configuration makes it less likely for the drill to grab the asymmetric cortical surface and lunge forward.

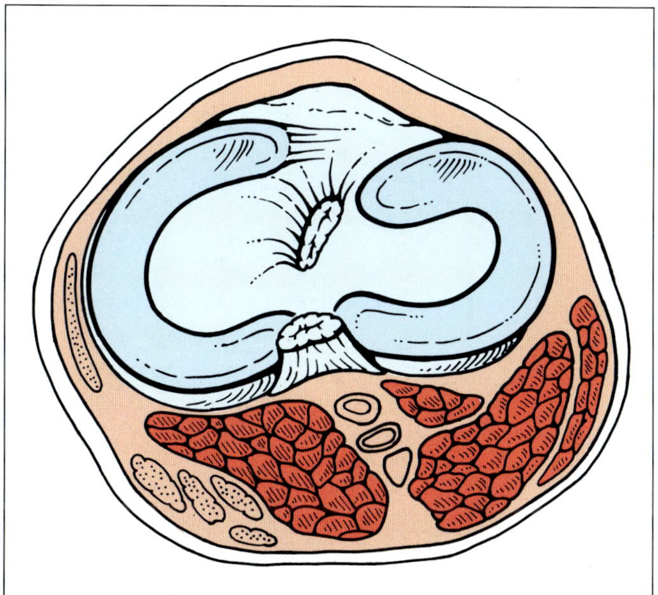

Figure 10-14. At the level of its insertion, only the posterior capsule separates the posterior cruciate ligament from the popliteal artery and vein, and the tibial nerve.

Our preference is to penetrate and enlarge the opening of the posterior tibial cortex by hand using a curette. This is done progressively and under direct vision. Some authors have proposed using an oscillating drill in favor of the standard drill to minimize risks associated with power-driven drill bits. Regardless of the technique, it is important to drill the tibial tunnel with great manual control and under direct vision, either arthroscopically or with fluoroscopic guidance.

The femoral bone tunnel is drilled over a guidepin after dissection of the starting point. We prefer a longitudinal incision midway between the medial femoral epicondyle and the beginning of the articular surface on the medial aspect of the anterior femur. The optimal position in terms of minimizing graft divergence would be to drill a tunnel just off the articular margin of the femur. However, this may weaken the remaining subchondral bone distal to the drill and may possibly play a role in the collapse of the tunnel or in the development of avascular necrosis. The vastus medialis is incised longitudinally and retracted proximally. The guidepin is placed in the position midway between the femoral epicondyle and the articular surface of the femur using commercially available drills. The tip of the drill guide is positioned in the joint in a previously chosen point depending on the size of the eventual osseous tunnel. We prefer this placement to measure the radius of the tunnel plus 2 mm back from the articular cartilage margin and to be at the axilla of the roof of the notch. Following placement of the femoral guidewire, a cannulated drill system is used to create the femoral tunnel of desired size. The osseous tunnels in the femur and tibia are chamfered using a bone rasp or Gore smoother. It is important to avoid sharp tunnel edges because graft abrasion can ensue and damage collagen. The tunnels become divergent through the range of motion of the knee. Sharp edges at the entrance to these bony tunnels can be deleterious to the graft.

Placement and Fixation of the Graft

We prefer to pass our grafts from proximal to distal. This is subject to surgeon preference and may be determined by the type of graft and the length and shape of the desired bone plugs. We pass a red rubber catheter through the tibial tunnel and grasp it intra-articularly with an arthroscopic grasper. The catheter is then advanced into the joint and passed out through the femoral tunnel. We affix the red rubber catheter to a Gore smoother and then retrograde these through the femoral tunnel. The Gore smoother is then used for smoothing and chamfering the tunnels. The sutures in the end of the graft can be placed through the eyeloop at the end of the Gore smoother and passed from the femoral tunnel through and out the tibial tunnel from proximal to distal. Regardless of the graft used, it is important that the bone plug or graft material being passed is of a smaller diameter than the tibial tunnel. We lubricate the graft with sterile lubricant to facilitate passage. The graft is then passed with a smooth steady motion with tension held on both ends. If the passage of the graft is difficult, the graft is removed and the arthroscope is replaced to view the tunnels. Most often, inadequately debrided soft tissue around the tunnels hinders graft passage. Often with an Achilles allograft or a bone–patellar-tendon–bone allograft or autograft, one end of the bone plug can be fashioned larger than the tunnel for press-fit fixation in the femur (Fig. 10-16). If this is the case, the bone plug is pulled into position until secure. Impaction may be necessary to fully engage the bone plug into the tunnel. Tension is placed on the graft while the knee is placed through a range of motion. The graft must be carefully inspected to ensure proper placement and the absence of impingement or abrasion.

Normal PCL tension has been poorly characterized [35•]. Graft tensioning must take into account the difference between the two bundles of the PCL. In general, most authors prefer tensioning the graft with the knee at 70° of flexion because they are attempting to recreate the anterolateral bundle of the PCL. It is our practice to preload and then cycle our PCL grafts in place prior to fixation. The amount of tensioning of the PCL graft has not been precisely established, but we attempt to apply between 8 and 10 lbs of tension to the graft at fixation. We re-establish the tibial step-off and tension the graft at its greatest excursion.

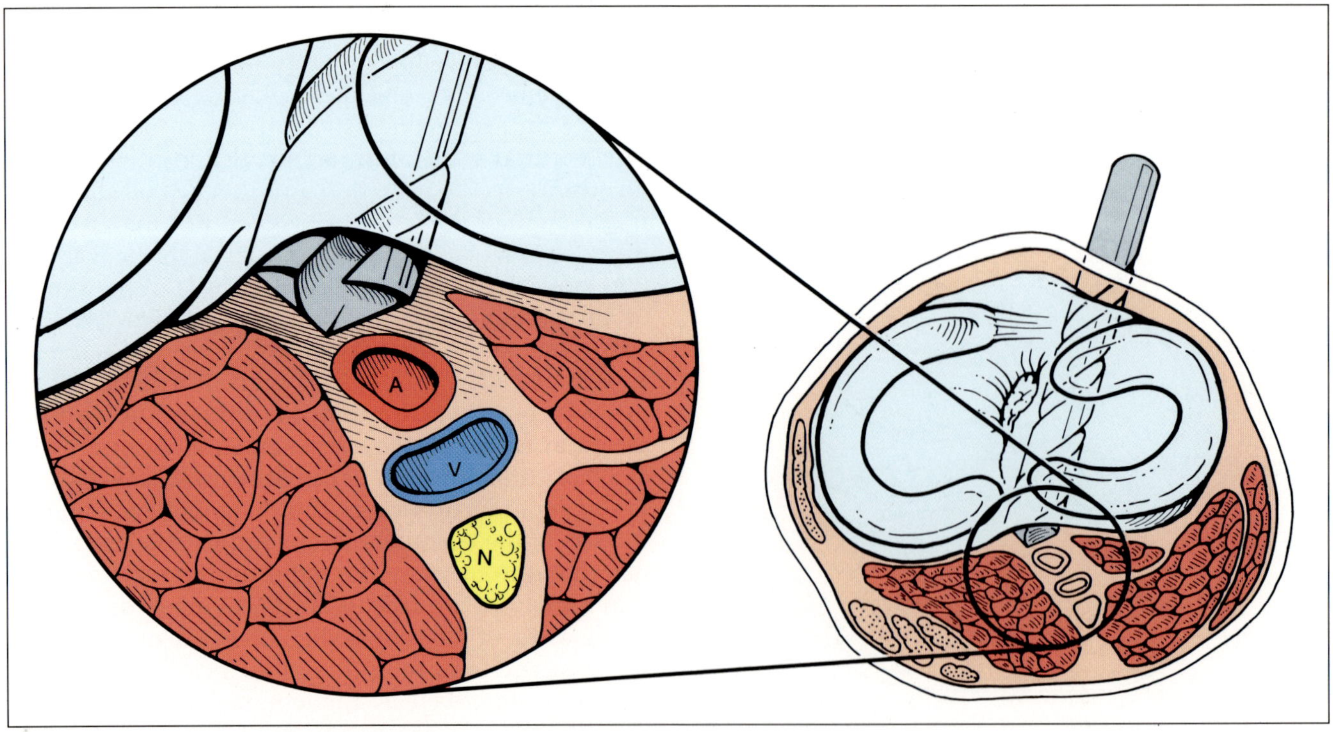

Figure 10-15. Axial section at the level of the posterior cruciate ligament insertion demonstrates the relationship of the neurovascular structures and their proximity to the exit point of the drill bit.

Fixation of the graft is highly dependent on the graft material. Available options include interference screws, staples, screw and soft-tissue washers, or sutures tied over a post. The most common choices of grafts for PCL reconstruction are a bone–patellar-tendon–bone allograft, an autograft, or an Achilles tendon allograft (Fig. 10-17). These grafts can be well fixed using a press-fit construction in the femur or tibia. We prefer to obtain a press-fit on the femoral side. The bone of the graft is tapered to a larger size of at least 2 mm greater than the bony tunnel and is compressed with hand instrumentation. It is then impacted into position and should be able to be pulled tight and resist migration into the joint. The ideal position of the collagen of the graft is with the bone flush with the subchondral bone of the medial femoral condyle. Interference screw fixation can be used in the femoral tunnel if desired.

Distal fixation can be accomplished with an interference screw with bone–patellar-tendon–bone grafts (Fig. 10-18). Alternatively, the interference screw fixation can be augmented by tying sutures over a post. Another option is tying sutures over a post alone. If an Achilles allograft is used, options include staples, soft-tissue screws and washers, tying sutures over a post, or some combination of the above (Fig. 10-19).

There are several important points in terms of graft fixation. The knee should be positioned at 70° for tensioning at the longest excursion of the graft to avoid capturing the joint with resultant loss of flexion. It is important to re-establish and maintain the normal tibial step-off. Some form of fixation should be used that will hold the graft in position long enough for the biologic incorporation of the graft into the entrance and bony tunnel.

Graft Selection

The ideal graft for cruciate ligament reconstruction should meet several criteria:

1. The graft should have sufficient tensile strength to withstand the loads and forces seen during knee function.
2. Fixation of the graft material should be simple and secure.
3. The graft should be available in the necessary sizes.
4. The graft should not have an associated immunologic response.
5. The graft should be sterile and not transmit any disease or infection.
6. Acquisition of the graft should cause minimal additional morbidity to the procedure.
7. The graft should have the durability to last a sufficient length of time.

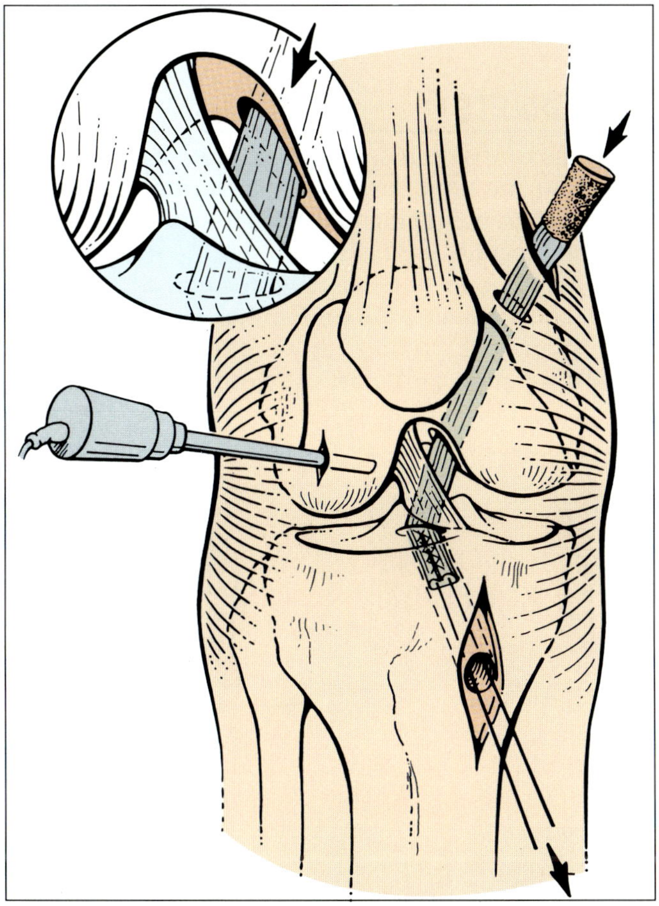

Figure 10-16. A trapezoidal or cone-shaped bone plug 2 mm larger than the diameter of the femoral tunnel can be passed as illustrated for a press-fit of the femoral side. Lubrication of the graft with sterile lubricant facilitates graft passage.

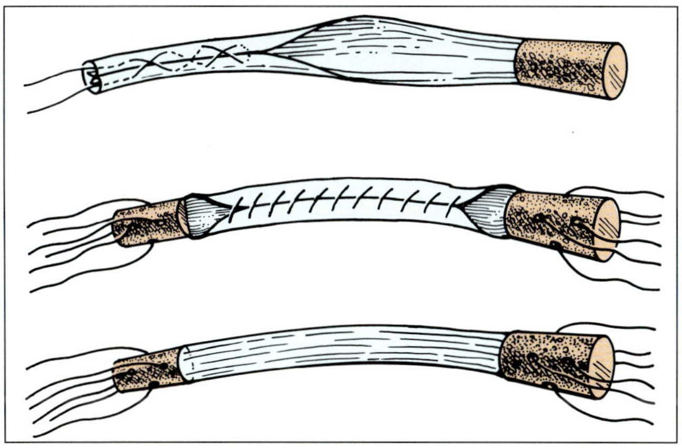

Figure 10-17. The most commonly used grafts and their preparation are illustrated: Achilles allograft (*top*), patellar tendon allograft (*middle*), and patellar tendon autograft (*bottom*). Patellar tendon autograft can also be fashioned for press-fit in the femur with the larger of the bone plugs being harvested from the tibial side.

No one graft is available today that clearly stands out in all situations and meets all of these criteria. This is evidenced by the variety of grafts currently in use. Each graft has advantages and disadvantages.

AUTOGRAFTS

Autografts include all of the different tissues that may be harvested from the patient. They are the most popular grafts used for cruciate reconstruction today. The most common ones for PCL reconstruction are the central third of the patellar tendon and the semitendinosus tendon. The tensile strength and stiffness of these grafts varies. Bone–patellar-tendon–bone autografts for ACL reconstruction have been considered the gold standard with which others are compared. Clancy [7] initially recommended a sandwich of two bone–patellar-tendon–bone autografts for PCL reconstruction or a combination of one autograft and one allograft. He now uses a single 10-mm autograft of patellar tendon. Autografts used for PCL reconstructions transfer tendon collagen to replace the ligament collagen. Tendons have collagen that is oriented and organized differently, is composed of parallel fibers, and functions under different dynamic loading. Some authors have suggested that a ligamentization occurs following transplantation. The autograft at the time of harvesting has living fibroblasts. The survival of the viable fibroblast in the transplanted autografts has been questioned. It appears that few if any of the cells survive, however, they are rapidly replaced by fibroblast-appearing cells that are likely of synovial origin. The revascularization and incorporation process is well underway within the first few weeks and progresses over the next several months. Authors disagree on when the reconstructed PCL reaches its maximum maturation. Most patients do not reach their maximum functional recovery for 6 to 12 months. Some see improvement into the second postoperative year.

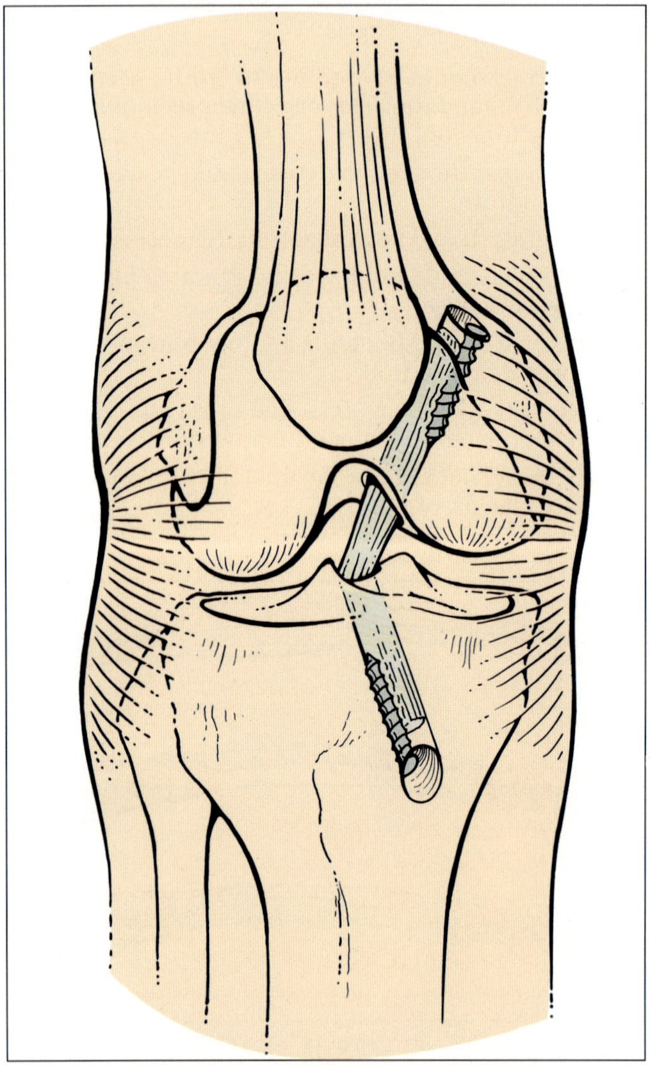

Figure 10-18. Interference screw fixation of a bone–patellar-tendon–bone autograft.

ALLOGRAFTS

Allografts consist of tissue obtained from different individuals of the same species. This alternative to autografts is currently being extensively treated. The most popular allografts used at the present time are Achilles tendon and bone–patellar-tendon–bone allografts for PCL reconstruction. Allografts offer an advantage in that their use avoids any complications from harvesting of an autograft. Allografts have the same

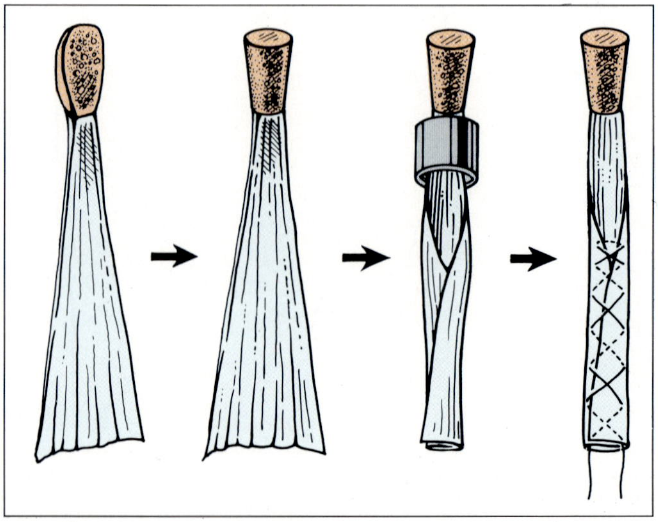

Figure 10-19. Sizing and preparation of an Achilles tendon allograft.

potential for revascularization and incorporation as the autografts. The initial tensile strength of the allograft material is similar to autografts. Replacement of the PCL with a PCL allograft has some theoretical biomechanical and biologic advantages. The technical aspects of this surgery would require selective tensioning and positioning of the fibers. This is currently not possible. Drawbacks of allografts include delayed incorporation and the potential of disease transmission. Immunogenicity of the grafts can be significantly reduced by freezing. Freeze drying can reduce those autogenicities still further. It appears that neither of these preparations clinically alters the mechanical properties of the graft, although immunogenic reactivity of fresh-frozen and freeze-dried allografts within the joint is undergoing investigation. In addition, secondary sterilization techniques such as selective solvents and irradiation are currently being used. Further works are necessary before allografts can be considered the preferred choice over autografts for cruciate ligament reconstruction. Long-term follow-up results are still being accumulated to answer some questions on allografts in comparison with autografts.

Artificial Ligaments

The major concern with prosthetic ligaments is their long-term durability. If the substitute is to act as a prosthesis, it must show little abrasion externally or internally. In addition, it should not produce particulate matter that is irritative to the intra-articular environment. Artificial ligaments have potential advantages. Their tensile strength meets or exceeds that necessary to replace the cruciate ligaments. Secure fixation is immediate and allows rapid mobilization and rehabilitation. Prosthetic ligaments eliminate the problems with immunogenicity and transmission of disease. They also eliminate the potential morbidity related to the autograft donor site. The prosthetic ligaments are readily available in various sizes and in unlimited supplies. A prosthetic ligament that replaces the PCL and has good long-term survival is not clinically available at this time.

Complications Following Cruciate Reconstructions

Any presentation of surgical techniques requires discussions of potential complications. Complications following arthroscopically assisted PCL surgery can be divided into three categories: 1) General complications common to surgical procedures about the knee; 2) specific complications related to the cruciate reconstruction; and 3) complications related to the graft procurement.

General complications common to surgical procedures include infection, thrombophlebitis, skin necrosis, hematoma and hemarthrosis, sensory nerve damage, tourniquet palsy, reflex sympathetic dystrophy, peroneal palsy, and vascular injury. When these occur, early recognition and treatment will minimize their effect.

Specific complications related to PCL reconstruction include failure to regain full extension or full flexion (or both), patellofemoral complications, graft impingement, inadequate graft fixation, and failure to re-establish the desired stability.

Failure to regain full range of motion following reconstruction can be related to graft placement or a generalized arthrofibrosis about the joint. Aggressive postoperative physical therapy is helpful in preventing contractures. If the range of motion plateaus in the postoperative phase, arthroscopic intervention and gentle manipulation should be considered.

Graft impingement and capturing the joint are complications unique to ligament reconstructions. Careful selection of the location of the tunnels combined with adequate notchplasty and measurements of graft excursion will limit the frequency of these complications. Improper tensioning of the graft will result in either continued instability or capturing of the joint.

Conclusions

Arthroscopic management of PCL injuries has gradually evolved to its present state. Skilled surgeons have used knowledge in the development of new instruments and techniques that have advanced the frontiers of PCL reconstruction and have made arthroscopic management of PCL injuries of the knee possible. These techniques are now applicable on a more widespread basis. Arthroscopic treatment of the PCL is based on a systematic approach. With continued evolution and refinement of techniques, surgical results will continue to improve and complications will be minimized. Improved instrumentation, simpler techniques, and better grafts loom on the horizon. The ideal cruciate graft is not currently present. Advances in graft technology will dramatically affect PCL surgery in the future.

REFERENCES AND RECOMMENDED READING

Papers of interest, published recently, have been highlighted as:

- • Of special interest
- •• Of outstanding interest

1. Hey-Groves EW: Operation for the repair of the crucial ligaments. *Lancet* 1917, 2:674–675.

2. Hey-Groves EW: The crucial ligaments of the knee joint: their function, rupture, and the operative treatment of the same. *Br J Surg*, 1919-1920, 7:505–515.

3. Robson AWM: Ruptured crucial ligaments and their repair by operation. *Ann Surg* 1903, 37:716–718.

4. Meyers MH, Moore TM, Harvey JP, Jr.: Follow-up notes on articles previously published in the Journal of Traumatic Dislocations of the Knee Joint. *J Bone Joint Surg* 1975, 57:430–433.

5. Hughston JC, Bowden JA, Andrews JR, *et al.*: Acute tears of the posterior cruciate ligament. Results of operative treatment. *J Bone Joint Surg* 1980, 62:438–450.

6. Kennedy JC, Galpin RD: The use of the medial head of the gastrocnemius muscle in the posterior cruciate deficient knee. Indications — Technique—*Results*. *Am J Sports Med* 1982, 10:63–72.

7. Clancy WG, Shelbourne KD, Zoellner GB, *et al.*: Treatment of knee joint instability secondary to rupture of the posterior cruciate ligament. Report of a new procedure. *J Bone Joint Surg* 1983, 65:310–322.

8. Girgis FG, Marshall JL, Monajem ARS: The cruciate ligaments of the knee. *Clin Orthop* 1975, 106:216–231.

9. Brantigen OC, Voshell AF: The mechanics of the ligaments and the menisci of the knee joint. *J Bone Joint Surg* [Am] 1941, 23:44–66.

10. Warren RJ, Arnoczky SP, Wickiewicz TL: Anatomy of the knee. In *The Lower Extremity and Spine in Sports Medicine* Edited by Nicholas JA, Hershman EB, St. Louis, MO: Mosby-Yearbook; 1986:657–694.

11. Heller L, Langman J: Meniscofemoral ligaments of the human knee. *J Bone Bone Joint Surg* [Am] 1979, 61:56–62.

12.• Cooper DE: Posterior cruciate ligament reconstruction: the anatomic and biomechanical basis. *Operative Techniques in Sports Med* 1993, 1:89–98.

An excellent presentation of the important biomechanics of the posterior and posterolateral structures of the knee. Cutting studies are summarized.

13. Baker CL, Jr., Norwood LA, Hughston JC: Acute posterolateral rotatory instability of the knee. *J Bone Joint Surg* [Am] 1983, 65:614–618.

14. Hughston JC, Andrews JR, Cross MJ, *et al.*: Classification of knee ligament instabilities. Part 1. The medial compartment and cruciate ligaments. *J Bone Joint Surg* [Am] 1976, 58:159–172.

15. Butler DL, Noyes FR, Grood ES: Ligamentous restraints to anterior-posterior drawer in the human knee. *J Bone Joint Surg* [Am] 1980, 62:259–270.

16. Kennedy JC, Hawkins RJ, Willis RB: Tension studies of human ligaments. Yield point, ultimate failure, and disruption of the cruciate and collateral ligaments. *J Bone Joint Surg* [Am] 58:350–355.

17. Gollehon DL, Torzilli PA, Warren RF: The role of the posterolateral and cruciate ligaments in the stability of the human knee. *J Bone Joint Surg* [Am] 1987, 69:233–242.

18. Grood ES, Stowers SF, Noyes FR: Limits of movement in the human knee: the effects of sectioning the PCL and posterolateral structures. *J Bone Joint Surg* [Am] 1988, 70:88–97.

19.• Rubinstein RA, Jr, Shelbourne KD: Diagnosis of posterior cruciate ligament injuries and indications for nonoperative treatment. *Operative Techniques in Sports Med* 1993, 1:99–103.

Review of history and physical examination in the evaluation of posterior cruciate ligament injuries. Classification discussed with respect to treatment options.

20. Trickey EL: Rupture of the posterior cruciate ligament of the knee. *J Bone Joint Surg* [Br] 1968, 50:334–341.

21. Noyes FR, Grood ES: Diagnosis of knee ligament injuries: In *The Crucial Ligaments. Diagnosis and Treatment of Ligamentous Injuries about the Knee*. Edited by JA Feagin, Jr. New York: Churchill Livingstone; 1988:261–286.

22. Fischer SP, Fox JM, Del Pizzo W, *et al.*: Accuracy of diagnoses from magnetic resonance imaging of the knee. *J Bone Joint Surg* [Am] 1991, 73:2–10.

23. Parolie JM, Bergfeld JA: Long term results of nonoperative treatment of isolated posterior cruciate ligament injuries in the athlete. *Am J Sports Med* 1986, 14:35–38.

24. Fowler PJ, Messieh SS: Isolated posterior cruciate ligament injuries in athletes. *Am J Sports Med* 1987, 15:553–557.

25. Torg JS, Barton TM, Pavlov H, *et al.*: Natural history of the posterior cruciate ligament deficient knee. *Clin Orthop* 1989, 246:208–216.

26. Clancy WG, Shelbourne KD, Zoellner GB, *et al.*: Treatment of knee joint instability secondary to rupture of the posterior cruciate ligament. *J Bone Joint Surg* [Am] 1983, 310–332.

27. Cross MJ, Powell JF: Longterm follow-up of the posterior cruciate ligament rupture. A study of 116 cases. *Am J Sports Med* 1984, 12:292–297.

28.• Keller PM, Shelbourne KD, McCarroll JR, *et al.*: Nonoperatively treated isolated posterior cruciate ligament injuries. *Am J Sports Med* 1993, 21:132–136.

Retrospective review of 40 patients with posterior cruciate ligament injuries treated nonoperatively. Study suggests that nonoperative treatment may not be as effective as once thought.

29. Kennedy JC, Grainger RW: The posterior cruciate ligament. *J Trauma* 1967, 7:367.

30. O'Connor J, Shercliff T, Fitzpatrick D, *et al.*: Geometry of the knee. In *Knee Ligaments: Structure, Function, Injury, and Repair*. Edited by Daniel DM, Akeson WH, O'Connor JJ. New York: Raven;1990:163–199.

31. Sidles JA, Larson RV, Garinni JL: Ligament length relationships in the moving knee. *J Orthop Res* 1911, 6:593–610.

32. Grood ES, Hexey MSD, Lindenfield TN: Factors effecting the region of most isometric femoral attachments. Part 1: the posterior cruciate ligament. *Am J Sports Med* 1989, 17:197–207.

33. Sapega AA, Moyer RA, Schneck C, *et al.*: Testing for isometry during reconstruction of the anterior cruciate ligament. *J Bone Joint Surg* [Am]. 1990, 72:259–268.

34. Jackson DW, Proctor CS, Simon TM: Arthroscopically assisted PCL reconstruction: a technical note on potential neurovascular injury related to drill bit configuration. *Arthroscopy* 1990, 9:224–227.

35.• Harner CD, Miller MD: Graft tensioning and fixation in posterior cruciate ligament surgery. *Operative Techniques in Sports Med* 1993, 1:115–120.

Reconstruction: Important hazards are discussed. Thorough review of author's technique and reasoning behind graft tensioning in posterior cruciate ligament.

11

CHAPTER

The Frozen Shoulder

JAMES C. ESCH

Frozen shoulder is a primary shoulder condition that presents itself with various degrees of pain and restricted range of motion. Arthroscopy enables early diagnosis in patients with pain. Some patients benefit from arthroscopic excision of contracted structures from the glenohumeral joint and subacromial bursa.

HISTORY

Duplay [1] in 1872 introduced the term *periarthrite scapulohumeral*, theorizing that the pathology was in the periarticular tissue of the shoulder. Codman [2] coined the term *frozen shoulder*. Codman said that this shoulder disability was difficult to define, difficult to treat, and difficult to explain from the point of view of pathology. This statement still rings true today. Neviaser [3] used the term *adhesive capsulitis* based on his arthrographic findings. Structures that are implicated as causative include subacromial bursitis, biceps tendinitis, rotator cuff tendinitis, subacromial adhesions, biceps adhesions, intra-articular adhesions, subsynovial inflammation, coracohumeral ligament, and capsular retraction. Lundberg [4] introduced the idea of primary and secondary causes, with the latter including rotator cuff tears, impingement, and calcified bursitis.

Clinical Presentation

Symptoms

The typical patient is a woman between 40 and 70 years of age with a severely painful shoulder "frozen" at her side. Intense night pain and sleep deprivation is common. Functional limitations include stretching overhead, reaching behind the back, and combing one's hair.

Other patients are a diagnostic challenge because they present this condition with lesser degrees of pain and limitation of motion. An atypical patient with early frozen shoulder is a 47-year-old man who presents with a very painful shoulder and a positive impingement sign. He is unable to play recreational tennis and has not improved with exercise and medications. Diagnostic arthroscopy shows diffuse synovitis, subacromial bursitis, and a smooth rotator cuff on both the bursal and articular side.

Physical Findings

Restriction of active and passive range of motion, especially rotation and abduction, are characteristic. Abduction limitation ranges from 35° to 145° with absent rotation. The combined restriction of motion is because shoulder elevation represents a combination of glenohumeral and scapulothoracic motion, with the former contributing two thirds of the motion. Elevation requires external rotation for the greater tuberosity to clear the acromion as the arm passes from 80° to 120°. Pain is mild within the patient's arc of motion. The pain is worse if the examiner attempts to passively increase motion.

Radiographic Findings

Routine radiographs are normal. Arthrography shows a diminished capsular space, irregular joint outline, and variable filling of the biceps tendon sheath [5].

Natural History

Traditional teaching claims that the frozen shoulder runs a self-limiting natural course of about 2 years [6–9]. However, many patients are unwilling to wait 2 years because they cannot work or participate in recreational activities.

Other studies present a less optimistic outlook. Lloyd-Roberts [10] reported residual symptoms in 33% of 27 patients at 18 months. Meulengracht [11] found 23% of 65 patients with pain and limited motion at 3-year follow-up. Sixty-one percent of Reeves' 41 patients had restricted motion at 5-year follow-up [12]. Shaffer and coworkers [13•] examined 62 patients at an average 7-year follow-up. Thirty-four percent of the patients had bilateral involvement. Sixty percent of the shoulders displayed some degree of restriction compared with sex and age-matched control patients. Thirty percent showed some restriction when compared with the opposite shoulder. Seven patients had some mild function limitation.

There are classically three clinical phases of frozen shoulder (Table 11-1) [14]. The lengths of the painful (freezing), stiffening (frozen), and thawing stages are variable.

Differential Diagnosis

Frozen shoulder is a primary condition. Diabetic patients frequently develop a frozen shoulder, and in these patients the condition occurs at a younger age, is less painful, is often bilateral, and has a poorer prognosis. Causes of secondary shoulder stiffness include rotator cuff diseases, fracture-dislocation residuals, calcific tendinitis, and osteoarthritis. Cervical spine lesions, autoimmune disease, chest wall tumors, thyroid disorders, Parkinson's disease, cerebral vascular accident, adult head injury, and myocardial infarction are other causes of frozen shoulder.

Table 11-1 Clinical phases of frozen shoulder

Phase	Time, *mo*	Symptoms
I Painful	2–9	Insidious onset of pain with progressive loss of motion
II Stiffening	4–12	Pain with progressive loss of motion, muscle atrophy
III Thawing	6–9	Pain subsides, motion gradually returns over 1 to 3 years

PATHOLOGY

Lundberg [4] evaluated the shoulder capsule from 14 patients with a frozen shoulder. Histology showed increased fibrous tissue, fibroblasts, and vascularity but an unchanged synovial lining and no inflammatory cell infiltrate.

Ozaki and coworkers[15] operated on 17 patients who had recalcitrant adhesive capsulitis. At surgery, contracture of the coracohumeral ligament and rotator interval was the main cause of the restricted glenohumeral movement. Histologic studies showed fibrosis, hyalinization, and fibrinoid degeneration in the contracted connected tissue. Fibrosis of the subsynovial tissue and an absence of the synovial cell on the joint side of the rotator interval was present. Resection of these tissues relieved pain and restored motion.

Nobuhara and coworkers [16] evaluated 1219 patients with a frozen shoulder of whom 37 had surgery. Patients who did not have a posttraumatic condition improved. Nobuhara felt that a frozen shoulder started with subacromial bursitis disrupting the normal external rotation of the greater tuberosity as it cleared the acromion in the 90° to 120° arc. Next, contracture of the coracohumeral ligament limited external rotation. Surgical procedures consisted of resection of the coracohumeral ligament, coracoacromial ligament, and the anterior acromion.

Kieras and Matsen [17] treated 12 refractory frozen shoulders, including seven diabetic patients, by open lysis of subdeltoid adhesions, release of the coracohumeral ligament, subscapularis lengthening, and anteroinferior capsular release. Pain decreased and all patients returned to work. Average forward flexion improved from 73° to 132°, and average external rotation improved from 5° to 45°.

Hazleman [18] felt that previous studies reported advanced pathology but missed the mild nonspecific synovitis observed by arthroscopy during the first 12 weeks of disease. He also noted thickening of the subacromial bursa with the surrounding soft tissues friable and hypervascular. Shoulder capsular tissue from a patient with frozen shoulder showed fibroblast and myoblast proliferation identical to that seen in Dupuytren's disease; vascular changes suggested diabetic microangiopathy [19]. Hazleman suggested that future studies in frozen shoulder may show abnormalities at a cellular level, with malfunction in fibroblast recruitment and cytokine growth factor production and release.

Hannafin and coworkers [20•] performed capsular biopsies on 15 patients with a frozen shoulder. They described three phases according to clinical symptoms: examination under anesthesia, arthroscopy, and pathology (Table 11-2). Vascular inflammatory synovium characterizes the early phase. The fibroplasia seen in stages 2 and 3 has not been previously reported. With progression of the disease, this stage 1 synovitis provokes a progressive fibroblastic response in the underlying capsule, resulting in diffuse capsular fibroplasia, thickening, and contracture.

ARTHROSCOPIC OBSERVATIONS

Haeri and Maitland [21] saw no intra-articular adhesions in 21 patients who underwent an arthroscopic examination for frozen shoulder. These patients were in the late stage of the disease.

Detrisac and Johnson [22] reported marked synovitis in the superior foramen to the subscapularis bursa. This obscured viewing medially along the subscapularis tendon. Because of the usual internal rotation contracture, the axillary pouch appeared

Table 11-2 Stages of frozen shoulder*

Stage	Clinical	Examination under anesthesia	Arthroscopy	Histology
1	Pain, limited range of motion	Full range of motion	Diffuse vascular synovitis	Vascular inflammatory synovitis, normal capsule
2	Pain, limited range of motion	Limited range of motion	Diffuse vascular synovitis	Hypervascular synovial hyperplasia, diffuse capsular fibroplasia
3	Mild pain, marked loss of motion	Marked loss of motion	Minimal synovitis	Minimal synovial hyperplasia, capsular fibroplasia with scar formation

From Hannafin and coworkers [20]; with permission.

smaller than normal. The pouch assumed a more normal appearance after manipulation restored external rotation. Inspection after manipulation revealed hemorrhage in the anterior-inferior capsule.

Uitvlugt and coworkers [23•] evaluated 21 shoulders by arthroscopy followed by manipulation. Arthroscopy did not show intra-articular adhesions, articular cartilage atrophy, or degenerative changes. Synovitis originating from the subscapularis bursa was the principal arthroscopic finding. Infrequent observations were vascular synovitis of the rotator cuff and biceps tendon. Arthroscopic evaluation after manipulation showed hemorrhage in the anterior wall along its inferior aspect and along the inferior glenohumeral ligament. Manipulation did not cause a rotator cuff tear.

Neviaser [24,25] defined four stages of arthroscopic changes in adhesive capsulitis (Table 11-3). The hallmark is early synovitis with capsular contracture in the later stages. Stage 1 imitates rotator cuff impingement because pain is the main complaint and motion is normal.

Wiley [26] treated 37 frozen shoulder patients by arthroscopy followed by manipulation. Pain relief was striking and there were no complications. The arthroscopic appearance was uniform—a patchy vascular reaction around the biceps, the upper border of the subscapularis, and the opening into the subscapularis bursa. Biopsy showed nonspecific vasculitis without specific inflammatory changes. Joint capacity reduction was another finding. No patient had adhesions obliterating the infraglenoid recess. Wiley [26] reminds us that "such findings at routine arthroscopy should alert the surgeon to a diagnosis of frozen shoulder if the clinical presentation has been subtle."

Poehling noticed patchy vascular collections around the subscapularis and biceps with dense subscapular adhesions (Poehling, paper presented at the Eighth Annual Meeting, Arthroscopy of the Shoulder, San Diego, 1991). He saw neither obliteration of the infraglenoid recess nor intra-articular adhesions. He did not find changes in the subacromial space.

I [27•] have observed diffuse synovitis with local collections around the biceps tendon and rotator interval (Figs. 11-1 and 11-2). Inspection of the subscapularis recess from the anterior approach nicely displays this synovitis (Fig. 11-3). In the later stage,

Table 11-3 Arthroscopic stages of frozen shoulder*

Stage	Pathology	Physical	Treatment
1	Low-lying fibrinous synovitis, no capsular contracture	Pain, normal range of motion	Physical therapy
2	Increased synovitis with fibrinous adhesions and capsular contracture	Pain, restricted range of motion	Physical therapy, then manipulation
3	Subsiding synovitis and increased capsular contracture	Less pain, loss of motion	Physical therapy, then manipulation
4	Only capsular contracture, no intra-articular process	Loss of motion, pain at the extremes of motion	Physical therapy, then manipulation

**Data from Neviaser [24] and Neviaser [25].*

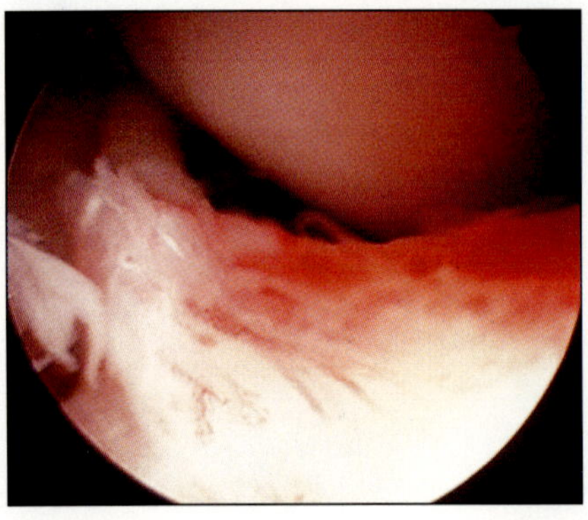

Figure 11-1. Early stage synovitis at the biceps attachment to the superior labrum. Arm suspension causes minimal distraction of the glenohumeral joint space.

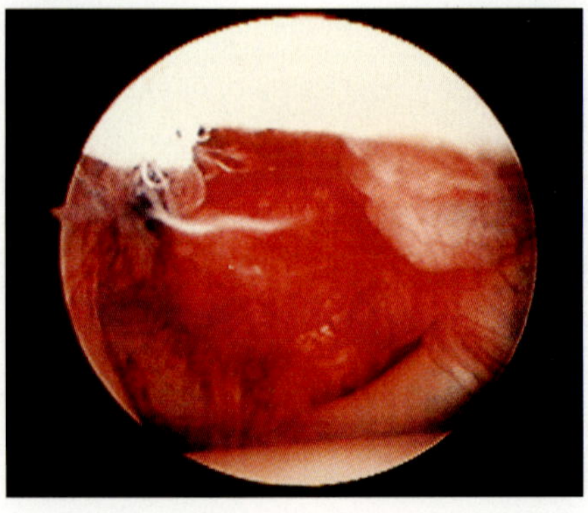

Figure 11-2. Synovitis in the rotator interval superior to the subscapularis tendon.

firm, dense adhesions between the subscapularis and the middle glenohumeral ligament can be seen (Fig. 11-4). The inferior recess is usually small, especially in individuals with restricted motion. Manipulation tears these adhesions that the surgeon then removes with a synovial resector under arthroscopic control. Subacromial bursoscopy shows a proliferative chronic bursitis (Fig. 11-5).

Patient Selection for Manipulation or Surgery

Patient Presentation

I find that patients fall into one of four groups (Table 11-4). Women who present with a painful shoulder arc of motion limited to less than 90° and frequently only 45° are the most common group. I teach circumduction exercises at the first office visit. Overhead bar and pulley exercises are done during the next 2 weeks at home. The majority of patients obtain greater than 90° to 135° at 4 weeks and recover completely in 3 to 6 months. If motion does not increase past 90° at 4 to 6 weeks, I consider manipulation under anesthesia with arthroscopy. I tell patients that motion will increase immediately, but pain will not abate for 3 to 4 weeks. Motion usually increases past 135° at 3 months with almost full recovery at 12 months.

Two groups of patients present with abduction limited to 90° to 135°. Most recover rapidly with exercises. Another group of patients does not improve with exercises and are candidates for evaluation by arthroscopy. Frequently, these are men with articular cartilage fragmentation of the humeral head and glenoid reflecting early osteoarthritis of the shoulder. Loss of motion and pain is due to osteoarthritis. Diagnostic arthroscopy differentiates osteoarthritis from idiopathic frozen shoulder.

Surgical Indications

Lack of progressive improvement after a few months of an exercise program is an indication for manipulation. Analgesics, nonsteroidal anti-inflammatory drugs, intra-articular steroids, and ice complement the exercise program. The patient is evaluated for

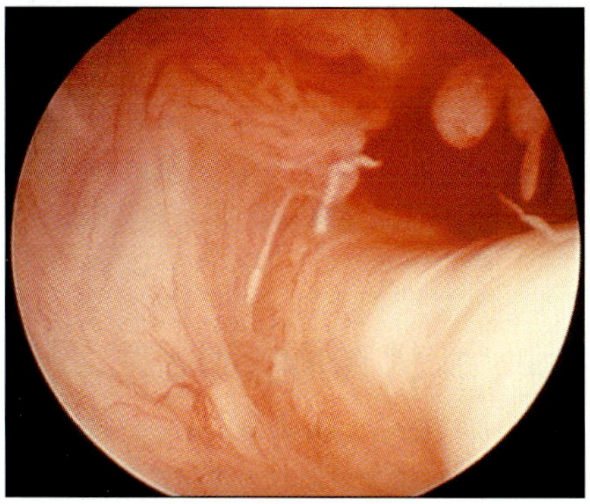

Figure 11-3. Viewing the subscapularis recess from anterior shows the early synovitis about the subscapularis tendon.

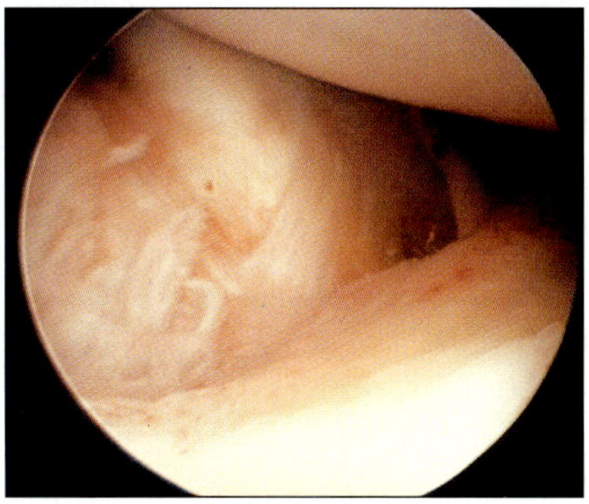

Figure 11-4. Adhesions in the rotator interval next to the subscapularis tendon.

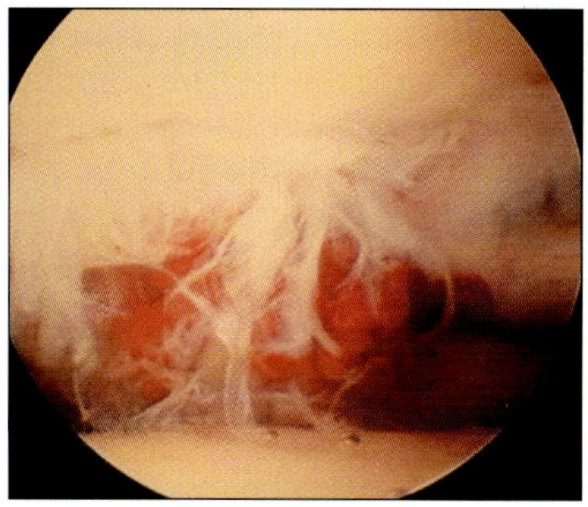

Figure 11-5. Subacromial bursoscopy shows exuberant bursitis. The rotator cuff is below and the acromion above.

Table 11-4 Patient groups with adhesive capsulitis

Motion	Response to exercise	Decision
Abduction < 45°–90°	Rapid improvement	Well 3–6 months without treatment
Abduction < 45°–90°	No improvement 4–6 wks	Manipulate with or without arthroscopy
Abduction 90°–135°	Rapid improvement	Well 3–6 months without treatment
Abduction 90°–135°	No improvement	Suspect primary osteoarthritis, perform diagnostic arthroscopy

secondary causes of stiffness. Manipulations in diabetic patients give satisfactory results but require a longer recovery period. Head injury patients with a frozen shoulder have a poor prognosis following manipulation. I treated one patient who presented with bilateral frozen shoulders after an adult head injury. He obtained a good result with one shoulder and a poor result with the other shoulder.

Clinical management of the frozen shoulder by hydraulic distention, under local anesthesia, is another treatment method [28]. Similarly, arthroscopy may work because it distends the joint [29].

SURGICAL TREATMENT

Three options are available for surgical treatment: 1)manipulation under anesthesia, 2)manipulation under anesthesia followed by arthroscopy, and 3)arthroscopic excision of adhesions.

Manipulation Under Anesthesia

The patient receives a general anesthetic plus a supraclavicular block for postoperative pain control. With one hand, the physician grasps the patient's arm just below the axilla, creating a short lever arm, while the other hand stabilizes the scapula. Slowly the arm is moved into forward flexion using a smooth, firm, and continuous force. A definite audible and palpable change in tissue resistance occurs as the arm passes through an 80° to 120° arc. If the tissues do not yield after 1 min of continuous pressure, closed manipulation is abandoned. After obtaining full forward flexion, the arm is gently stretched into external rotation with the arm at the side and at 90° of abduction. Finally, it is stretched into internal rotation. The rotational stresses are done with gentle pressure because humeral fractures are possible with the long lever arm. Fareed [28] calculated the torque magnification across the glenohumeral structures to be 11 times the force generated at the elbow. Some authors prefer to manipulate the arm initially into external rotation, followed by abduction, flexion, adduction, and internal rotation [30].

Johnson [31•] prefers to do a "50% manipulation." He manipulates the stiff arm to gain at least 50% of the decreased range of motion in all planes, using the opposite shoulder as a control. There were less palpable and audible tearing sensations. Arthroscopic inspection after manipulation showed capsular hemorrhage. Johnson says that the patient awakens with minimal discomfort, but a noticeable increase in motion. A home exercise program follows.

Manipulation Under Anesthesia Followed by Arthroscopy

For this technique, manipulation precedes diagnostic arthroscopy (Esch, paper presented at the Closed Meeting of American Shoulder and Elbow Surgeons, Williamsburg, 1993). A manipulation is done under anesthesia as described previously. Then a standard 4.0 arthroscope is inserted from the posterior portal, followed by an anterior arthroscopic portal. The arthroscopic findings in 40 patients were glenohumeral synovitis and hemorrhage due to rupture of anterior structures (capsule at the rotator interval, middle glenohumeral ligament, and inferior glenohumeral ligament). The subacromial bursa showed an exuberant subacromial bursitis, which was occasionally hemorrhagic.

Arthroscopic Excision of Adhesions

A complete diagnostic arthroscopy is possible but tedious. The joint is entered with the standard 4.0 arthroscope or a smaller 2.7 arthroscope. Usual findings are exuberant anterior synovitis about the biceps tendon and anterior capsule, small joint space, and a small axillary fold (Table 11-5, Figs. 11-1–11-3, Fig.

Table 11-5 Arthroscopic pathology in the frozen shoulder

Structure	Findings	Treatment
Anterior triangle	Diffuse synovitis, scar, and contracture of coracohumeral ligament	Synovectomy excise scar and coracohumeral ligament, manipulate
Subscapularis bursa	Dense adhesions	Excise adhesions
Axillary recess	Diffuse synovitis and contracture	Synovectomy and manipulation
Subacromial bursa	Chronic bursitis and adhesions	Subacromial decompression

11-6). A second portal is created anteriorly just superior to the subscapularis tendon using the Wissinger rod technique.

The arthroscope is moved to the anterior portal. The subscapular bursa is then inspected for adhesions (Fig. 11-7). A synovial resector resects the subscapularis bursa adhesions and the anterior capsule above the glenoid equator (Figs. 11-8 and 11-9). The middle glenohumeral ligament is then resected while preserving the inferior glenohumeral ligament (Figs. 11-10 and 11-11).

Another option is to view the anterior capsule while manipulating the arm first into full overhead elevation, then into external rotation. I have observed capsular rupture by direct anterior viewing while manipulating the arm.

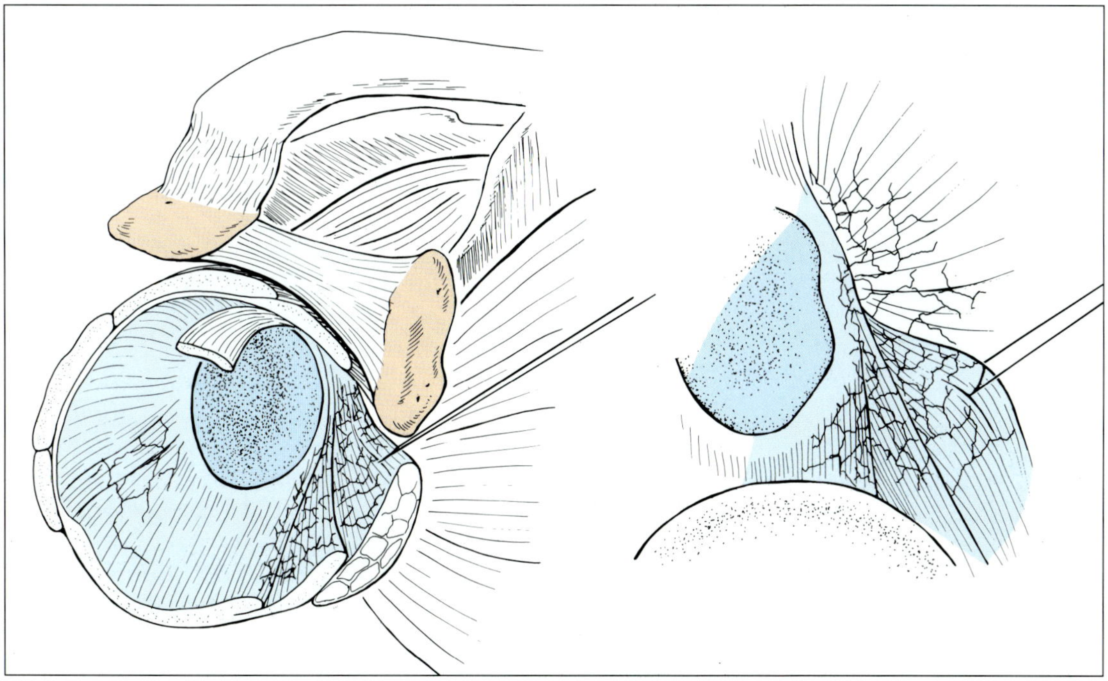

Figure 11-6. Early stage synovitis. A suture features the subscapularis synovitis by pulling the subscapularis tendon away from the middle glenohumeral ligament.

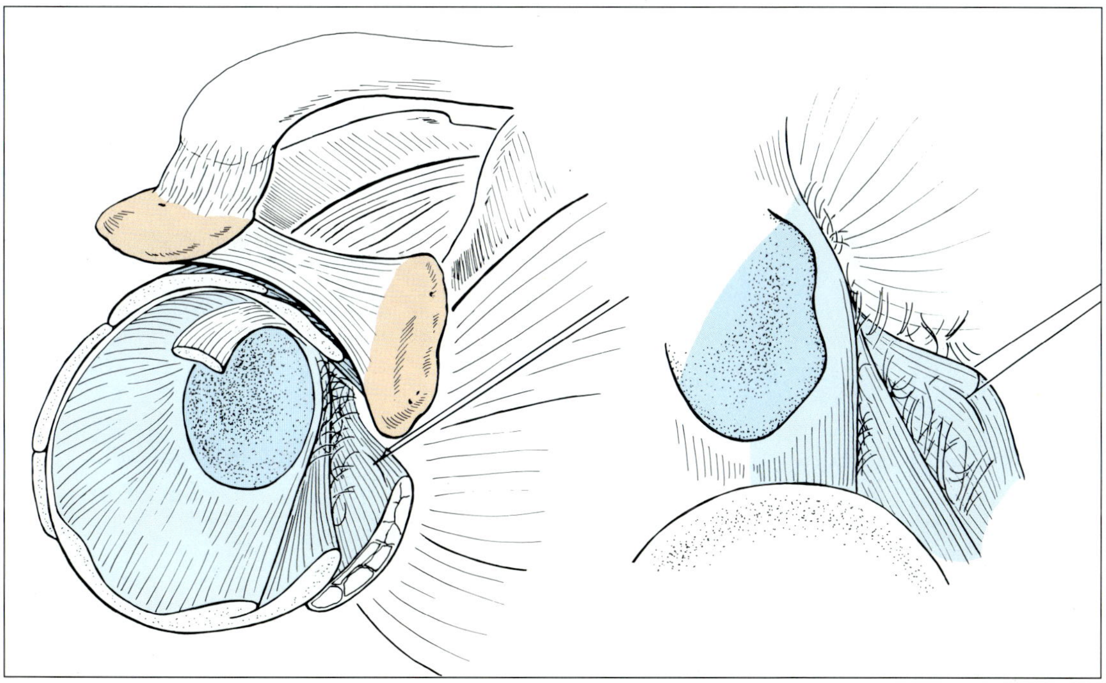

Figure 11-7. Adhesions obliterate the subscapularis space.

Subacromial bursoscopy shows exuberant bursitis (Fig. 11-5). The rotator cuff inspection reveals either an intact or partial tear. An arthroscopic subacromial decompression is done unless the subacromial bursa appears normal. The coracoacromial ligament is resected inferiorly to the coracoid (Fig. 11-12). The coracohumeral ligament is viewed coursing from the coracoid to the anterior edge of the supraspinatus. A switching stick left in the anterior glenohumeral portal helps orientation. The coracohumeral ligament should be probed and inspected while the arm is rotated externally. If the coracohumeral ligament is contracted, the ligament should be resected with a basket forceps.

In summary, surgery consists of arthroscopic resection of the following structures: 1)rotator interval; 2)middle glenohumeral ligament; 3)subscapularis bursa; 4)subacromial bursectomy; 5)anterior acromioplasty if type II or III acromion; 6)excision of coracoacromial ligament; and 7)excision of coracohumeral ligament. Active and passive exercises are begun immediately.

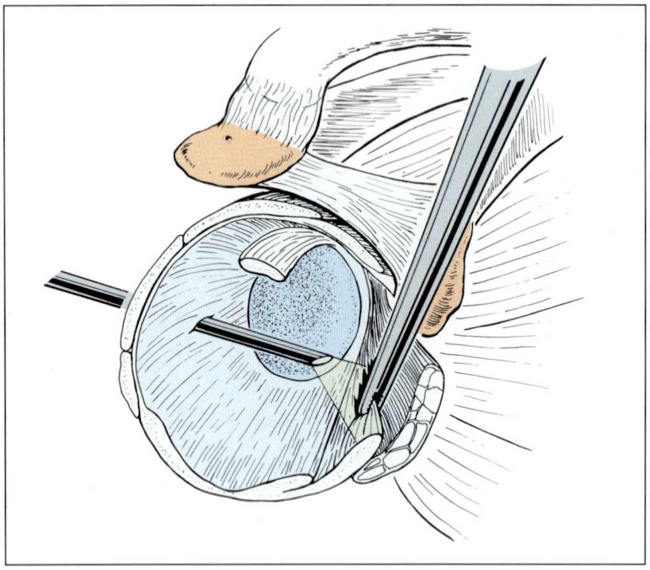

Figure 11-8. A synovial resector resects the adhesions and middle glenohumeral ligament.

POSTMANIPULATION EXERCISES

The patient is discharged after instructions in postoperative exercises, with emphasis on the need to move the arm continuously. Passive forward flexion begins immediately, so the patient immediately sees the gain in motion. When the arm block subsides, the patient should do 10 repetitions of circumduction exercises each hour. The continuous passive motion machine should be used as much as possible.

Continuous ice reduces swelling and pain. The circulating pump for local cold therapy uses a cooling pad and an ice water supply. Incorporate the pad into the postoperative dressing. Oral analgesics and nonsteroidal anti-inflammatory drugs control pain.

The patient attends physical therapy daily during the first postoperative week. The patient should immediately begin circumduction, overhead bar, and door pulley exercises at 10 to 20 repetitions each hour.

The patient requires continuous reassurance during the first 3 months after manipulation. Tell patients preoperatively that although their motion increases after manipulation, the pain does not subside until 3 to 6 weeks. Over the next year motion improves, but permanent loss of 20° of forward flexion, internal rotation, and external rotation is usual. Patients will feel their motion is excellent.

Complications of manipulation include humeral fractures, rotator cuff ruptures, dislocations, and traction nerve injuries.

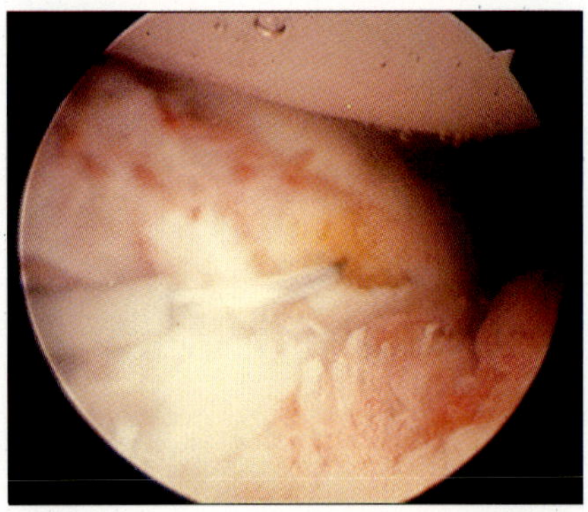

Figure 11-9. Electrocautery resecting the adhesions in the rotator interval between the subscapularis and supraspinatus.

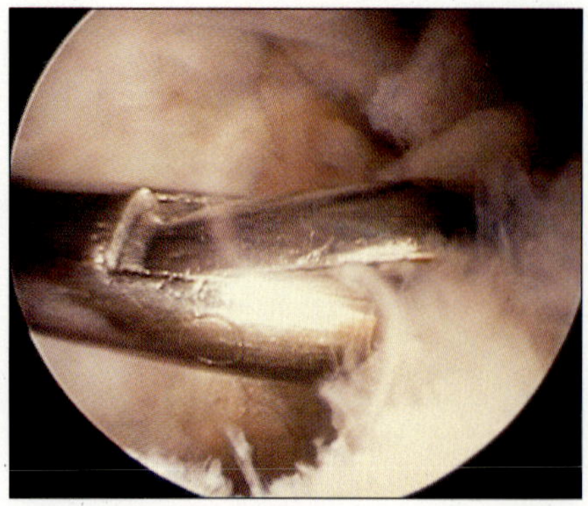

Figure 11-10. A basket forceps resecting the middle glenohumeral ligament.

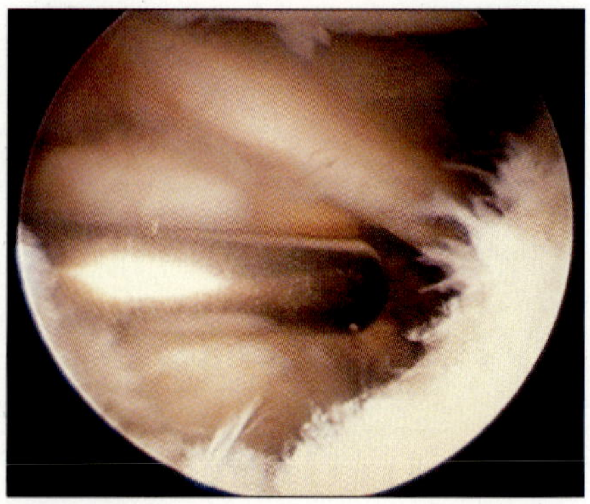

Figure 11-11. Completed resection of adhesions exposing the subscapularis tendon and muscle.

RESULTS

Haggart [32] reported 95% excellent or good results following manipulation in 97 patients with no reported complications.

Ogilvie-Harris and Wiley [33] reported generally successful results in 81 patients with a frozen shoulder. Approximately half the cases were idiopathic, but in 14 there was also mild osteoarthritis, and in 17 a partial tear of the rotator cuff. Diabetic patients and patients with associated intra-articular pathology obtained poorer results.

Wiley [26] reported striking pain relief in 37 patients treated by arthroscopy and manipulation. Abduction recovery varied as follows: 2 weeks (one patient), 4 weeks (four patients), 6 weeks (one patient), 8 weeks (nine patients), 12 weeks (five patients). The remaining 17 patients recovered more slowly: three recovered within 6 months, and the others in 1 to 2 years.

Hill [34] manipulated 17 frozen shoulders in 15 patients who did not respond to physical therapy. Seven of 10 patients were unable to work before manipulation and returned to work at an average of 2.6 months after manipulation. All returned to normal lifestyles sooner than the reported natural history would suggest.

Parker [35] reported 20 excellent or good results (91%) in 22 patients. Two of the three recurrences were in diabetic patients. One patient had a transient posterior deltoid paralysis.

Bradley [36] reported significant improvement in motion and pain relief for 15 patients evaluated by arthroscopy followed by manipulation. One patient with diabetes did not improve to the same levels as others.

I have had successful results in 10 patients treated by arthroscopic excision of adhesions. However, it took 1 year for a complete pain-free recovery of elevation and internal rotation.

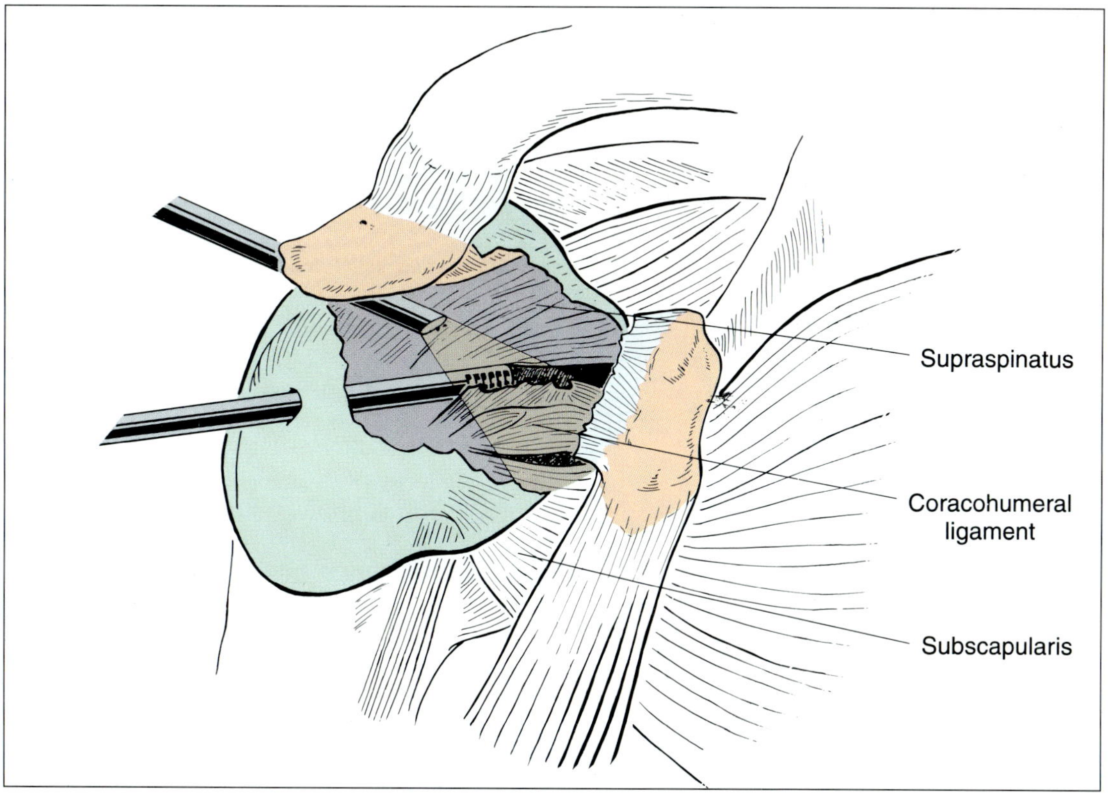

Figure 11-12. Resection of the subacromial bursa and acromioplasty. The coracoacromial ligament is trimmed down to the coracoid. The coracohumeral ligament is inspected coursing from the coracoid to the rotator interval and is resected if tight.

REFERENCES AND RECOMMENDED READING

Papers of interest, published recently, have been highlighted as

- • Of special interest
- •• Of outstanding interest

1. Duplay ES: De la periarthrite scapulohumeral et des raideurs de l'epaule qui en son la consequence. *Arch Gen Med* 1872, 20:513.
2. Codman ED: *The Shoulder*. Boston: Thomas Todd; 1934:216.
3. Neviaser JE: Adhesive capsulitis of the shoulder. *J Bone Joint Surg* 1945, 27:211–222.
4. Lundberg BJ: The frozen shoulder. *Acta Orthop Scand* 1969, 119(suppl):1–59.
5. Neviaser JS: Arthrography of the shoulder joint. *J Bone Joint Surg* [Am] 1962, 44:1321–1330.
6. Gray RG: The natural history of "idiopathic" frozen shoulder. *J Bone Joint Surg* [Am] 1978, 60:564.
7. Watson-Jones R: Simple treatment of stiff shoulders. *J Bone Joint Surg* [Br] 1963, 45:207.
8. Withers RJW: The painful shoulder: Review of one hundred personal cases with remarks on the pathology. *J Bone Joint Surg* [Br] 1949, 31:414–417.
9. Rowe CR, Leffert RD: Idiopathic chronic adhesive capsulitis ("frozen shoulder"). In *The Shoulder*. Edited by Rowe CR. New York: Churchill-Livingstone; 1988:159.
10. Lloyd-Roberts GC, French PR: Periarthritis of the shoulder, a study of the disease and its treatment. *BMJ* 1959, 1:1569–1571.
11. Meulengracht E, Schwartz M: Course and prognosis of periarthritis humeroscapularis. *Acta Med Scand* 1952, 143:350.
12. Reeves B: The natural history of the frozen shoulder syndrome. *Scand J Rheumatol* 1975, 4:193.
13. • Shaffer BS, Tibone JE, Kerlan RK: Frozen shoulder: A long term follow-up. *J Bone Joint Surg* [Am] 1992, 74:738–746.

Restriction of motion was present in 60% of patients at long-term follow-up.

14. Murnaghan JP: Frozen shoulder. In *The Shoulder*. Edited by Rockwood CA Jr., Matsen FA III. Philadelphia: WB Saunders; 1990:837.
15. Ozaki J, Nakagawa Y, Sakurai G, *et al*.: Recalcitrant chronic adhesive capsulitis of the shoulder: Role of contracture of the coracohumeral ligament and rotator interval in pathogenesis and treatment. *J Bone Joint Surg* [Am] 1989, 71:1511–1515.
16. Nobuhara K, Sugiyama D, Ikeda H, *et al*: Contracture of the shoulder. *Clin Orthop* 1990, 254:105–110.
17. Kieras DM, Matsen FA III: Open release in the management of refractory frozen shoulder. *Orthop Trans* 1991, 15:801.
18. Hazleman B: Why is a frozen shoulder frozen? *Br J Rheumatol* 1990, 29:130.
19. Kay N, Slater D: Fibromatosis and diabetes mellitus. *Lancet* 1981, 2:303.
20. • Hannafin JA, DiCarlo EF, Wickiewicz TL: Adhesive capsulitis: Capsular fibroplasia of the glenohumeral joint [abstract]. *J Shoulder Elbow Surg* 1994, 3(suppl):5.

Histologic correlation of the clinical stages (*see* Table 2).

21. Haeri GB, Maitland A: Arthroscopic findings in the frozen shoulder. *J Rheumatol* 1981, 8:149–152.
22. Detrisac DA, Johnson LL: *Arthroscopic shoulder anatomy: Pathological and surgical implications*. Thorofare, NJ: Slack; 1986:111–113.
23. • Uitvlugt G, Detrisac DA, Johnson LL, *et al*.: Arthroscopic observations before and after manipulations of frozen shoulder. *Arthroscopy* 1993, 9:181–185.

Found vascular synovitis. There were no intra-articular adhesions or degenerative changes. An immediate postmanipulation second-look arthroscopy showed there was synovial and capsular hemorrhage indicative of tearing from the manipulation.

24. Neviaser TJ: Arthroscopy of the shoulder. *Orthop Clin North Am* 1987, 18:361–372.
25. Neviaser TJ: Adhesive capsulitis. In *Operative Arthroscopy*. Edited by McGinty. New York: Raven Press; 1991:561–566.
26. Wiley AM: Arthroscopic appearance of frozen shoulder. *Arthroscopy* 1991, 7:138–143.
27. • Esch JC, Baker CL: Frozen shoulder. In *Arthroscopic Surgery. The Shoulder and Elbow*. Philadelphia: JB Lippincott; 1993.

Book chapter on the arthroscopic treatment of the frozen shoulder.

28. Fareed DO, Gallivan WR Jr: Office management of frozen shoulder syndrome: Treatment with hydraulic distention under local anesthesia. *Clin Orthop* 1989, 242:177–183.
29. Andren L, Lundberg BJ: Treatment of rigid shoulders by joint distention during arthrography. *Acta Orthop Scand* 1965, 36:45–53.
30. Parker RD, Froimson AI, Winsberg DD: *et al*.: Frozen shoulder: Part I: chronology, pathogenesis, clinical picture, and treatment. *Orthopedics* 1989, 12:869–873.
31. • Johnson LL: *Diagnostic and surgical arthroscopy of the shoulder*. St. Louis: Mosby-Yearbook; 1992:353–358.

Excellent chapter on author's experience with arthroscopic treatment of the frozen shoulder.

32. Haggart GE, Dignam RJ, Sullivan TS: Management of the "frozen" shoulder. *JAMA* 1956, 161:1219–1222.
33. Ogilvie-Harris DJ, Wiley AM: Arthroscopic surgery of the shoulder: A general appraisal. *J Bone Joint Surg [Br]* 1986, 68:201–207.
34. Hill JJ, Bogumill H: Manipulation in the treatment of frozen shoulder. *Orthopedics* 1988, 11:1255–1260.
35. Parker RD, Froimson AI, Winsberg DD: *et al*. Frozen shoulder, Part II. Treatment by manipulation under anesthesia. *Orthopedics* 1989, 12:989.
36. Bradley JP: Arthroscopic treatment for adhesive capsulitis. *Oper Techn Ortho* 1991, 1:248.

12

CHAPTER

Arthroscopic Stabilization of Acute, Initial Anterior Shoulder Dislocations

ROBERT A. ARCIERO

The traditional treatment of patients with initial anterior shoulder dislocation has been nonoperative, including a period of immobilization followed by supervised rehabilitation and a delay in return to full activity [1–5]. These efforts have been inconsistent in reducing recurrence rates. In fact, the principle prognostic factor for recurrence after the initial dislocation has been the age of the patient [1–3]. For patients less than 20 years of age, recurrence rates have been quoted as high as 94% [3].

At the United States Military Academy, a strenuous physical curriculum is required for graduation. In addition to a Division I intercollegiate athletic program, nonvarsity cadet-students must participate in collision intramural sports such as eight-man tackle football, boxing, wrestling, or rugby. In addition, required military training such as participation in obstacle courses and hand-to-hand combat places great demand on the shoulders. In this environment, shoulder instability is a common orthopedic problem. With these young, active athletes, nonoperative treatment after the initial anterior shoulder dislocation has yielded disappointing results. As arthroscopic stabilization procedures were developed for the treatment of chronic instability, we began to investigate the use of arthroscopy as treatment after the initial event in this high-demand population.

In 1989, Wheeler and coworkers [4] reported a comparison study of nonoperatively treated cadet-athletes with arthroscopic treatment after an acute, initial dislocation. In the nonoperative group, 35 of 38 (92%) patients developed recurrent instability. Nine patients were treated arthroscopically with two recurrences (22%). Subsequently, a prospective study was designed to evaluate the role of arthroscopic treatment for this injury. Arciero and coworkers [5] compared nonoperative treatment with arthroscopic transglenoid suture repair of the Bankart lesion. In the nonoperative group treated with 4 weeks of immobilization, 3 months of rehabilitation, and a delay in return to sports for 4 months, the recurrence rate was still 80%. Arthroscopic suture repair resulted in 18 of 21 patients (86%) with no recurrence at an average follow-up of 33 months.

Both of these initial studies involved cadet-athletes (young, high demand) who sustained an initial anterior shoulder dislocation. All dislocations required a manual reduction and arthroscopy was performed within 10 days. Arthroscopy was done under general anesthesia and in the lateral position. The examination of the shoulder revealed abnormal anterior glenohumeral translation in all cases. Importantly, a hemarthrosis and a capsulolabral avulsion of the inferior glenohumeral ligament (IGHL) from the glenoid (Bankart lesion) was encountered in all 30 initial cases. This pathology is amenable to repair with current arthroscopic techniques.

Encouraged by the early results of arthroscopic treatment for this injury, we sought methods that would minimize morbidity associated with arthroscopic repair.

Starting in December 1991, we began to use interscalene anesthesia. This type of anesthesia provides excellent intraoperative and postoperative analgesia and permits outpatient procedures as well [6]. The arthroscopic technique has been changed to one using the sitting position [7]. This position avoids any traction on the brachial plexus and allows easy conversion to an open procedure. Coupled with interscalene block, this technique allows the patient to assist with positioning. The final significant change in our approach has been the use of a bioabsorbable cannulated fixation device (Suretac; Acufex Microsurgical, Norwood, MA) [8]. This method avoids drilling through the scapular neck and possible suprascapular nerve injury. Also, this fixation repairs the Bankart lesion directly to bone and avoids tying sutures posteriorly over muscle and fascia.

The remainder of this chapter focuses on the specific technique of arthroscopic stabilization of initial anterior shoulder dislocations with a bioabsorbable tack using the sitting position and interscalene anesthesia. Our preliminary results are also described.

TECHNIQUE

We consider arthroscopic stabilization for patients who sustain an anterior shoulder dislocation by using the following criteria: 1) the dislocation was the first instability episode; 2) the dislocation required reduction for initial treatment; 3) the patient was high demand and less than 23 years old; 4) there was no neurologic injury; 5) no history of subluxation or "dead arm" syndrome; and 6) no greater tuberosity fracture.

The patient is initially supine on a standard operating table. A deflated vacuum bean bag is placed beneath the neck, shoulders, and torso of the patient.

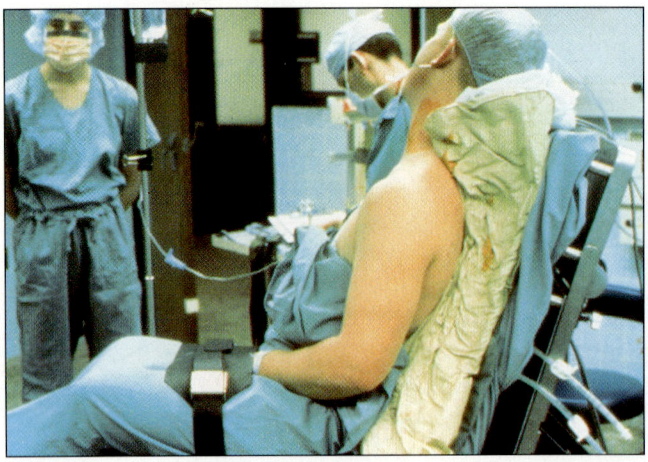

Figure 12-1. Patient in a sitting position with bean bag supporting torso and shoulder projecting from table.

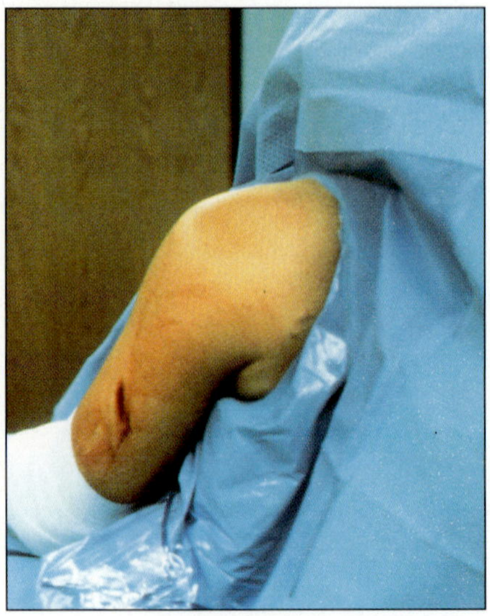

Figure 12-2. Patient in sitting position prepared and draped.

Interscalene anesthesia is administered using a 50/50 mixture of 0.75% bupivacaine and 3.0% chloroprocaine. After satisfactory anesthesia, an examination for anterior, inferior, and posterior glenohumeral translation is performed and recorded. The table is then brought to a sitting position by forward flexing the back of the table and flexing the end or foot of the table. With the patient sitting, the bean bag is bunched along the vertebral border of the scapula of the operative side. The bean bag is cradled about the torso and the neck for support and then inflated (Fig. 12-1). With the bean bag inflated in this position, it can effectively extend the table and allows excellent access to the shoulder. The shoulder is projected laterally over the edge of the table and away from it, maximizing exposure (Fig. 12-2).

Diagnostic arthroscopy is initiated from a posterior portal. A hemarthrosis has always been encountered and an anterior superior portal (ASP) is rapidly established. First, an 18-gauge needle is placed entering the joint just medial to the biceps tendon. From outside this portal it is positioned approximately 1 cm anterior and 1 cm medial to the anterior edge of the acromion (Fig. 12-3). A 5-mm cannula is placed into the ASP. The use of an infusion pump will rapidly clear the hemarthrosis. A probe can be inserted through the ASP and a thorough arthroscopic exam is done. Using the indications mentioned above, a capsulolabral avulsion of the IGHL complex from the glenoid has been encountered in 97% of our cases (Fig. 12-4). A 4-mm motorized shaver is brought through the ASP to remove clot and debris. Abrasion and decortication of the scapular neck follows. This is necessary to provide a suitable healing bed. To improve exposure, the 25° arthroscope is removed and replaced with a 70° arthroscope. This allows good visualization of the anterior glenoid and scapular neck. A 4-mm round burr is used through the ASP to perform the abrasion while viewed posteriorly (Fig. 12-5).

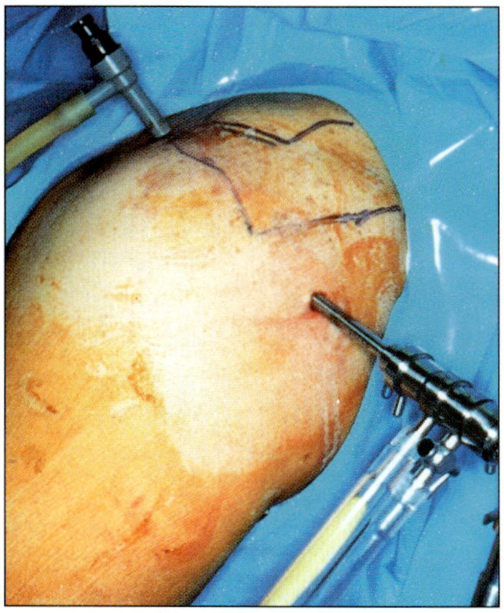

Figure 12-3. Outside views with anterior superior portal placement.

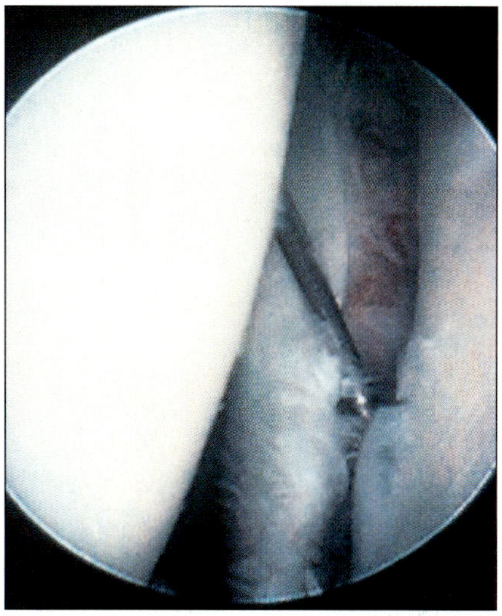

Figure 12-4. An acute Bankart lesion with robust capsulolabral tissue.

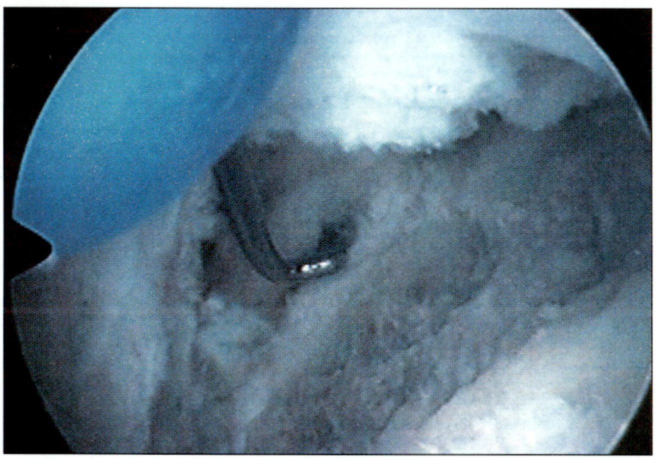

Figure 12-5. Arthroscopic view with 70° arthroscope looking over anterior glenoid rim demonstrating decortication of scapular neck.

After abrasion, a specially designed soft-tissue grasper (Acufex Microsurgical, Norwood, MA) is placed through the ASP, and a trial reduction of the Bankart lesion is performed (Fig. 12-6). This is to insure that the capsulolabral complex can be brought to its anatomic position.

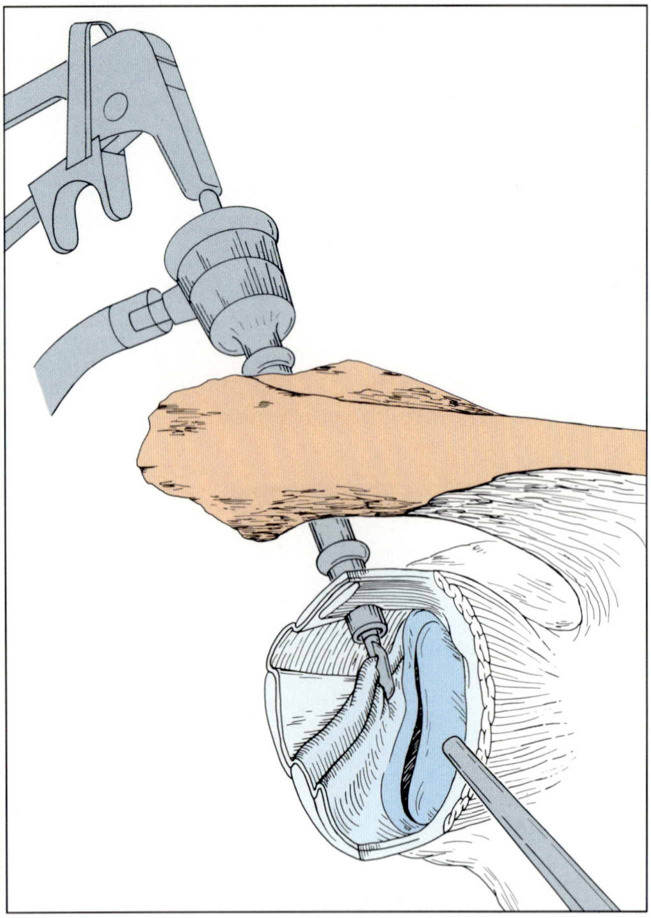

Figure 12-6. Soft-tissue grasper placed through anterosuperior portal and grasping Bankart lesion for trial reduction.

The next step is establishment of the anterior inferior portal (AIP). An 18-gauge spinal needle is used to ensure accurate portal placement. From outside the joint, the needle is started just lateral to the coracoid process (Fig. 12-7). The needle should come into the joint just superior to the superior edge of the subscapularis tendon. Meticulous attention to detail is necessary to guarantee accurate portal placement. The 18-gauge needle is also used to judge the angle of direction as it approaches the glenoid (Fig. 12-8). The bioabsorbable tack fixation system requires drilling into the anterior glenoid. If the AIP is created at too acute an angle to the glenoid, the drill will have a great tendency to "walk" or "skive" off the scapular neck. By coming just superior to the leading edge of the subscapularis tendon, crowding of the two anterior portal cannulas will be minimized. Once satisfied with the position of the needle, the AIP is created with a #11 blade surgical knife, and an 8-mm cannula is positioned (Fig. 12-9).

The bioabsorbable cannulated fixation device used requires initial drilling with a reamer and guidewire. The reamer that is cannulated has a locking nut to secure it to the guidewire. The reamer is placed over the guidewire and secured with the tip of the guidewire protruding 3-mm beyond the reamer (Fig. 12-10). Piercing the Bankart lesion will be easier with the guidewire in this position. A capable assistant provides visualization with the arthroscope and grasps the Bankart lesion with the soft-tissue grasper from the ASP. The assistant reduces the lesion anatomically. The surgeon can then pierce the Bankart lesion inferiorly with the reamer guidewire in preparation for the first tack (Fig. 12-11). Drilling commences at approximately the 8-o'clock position

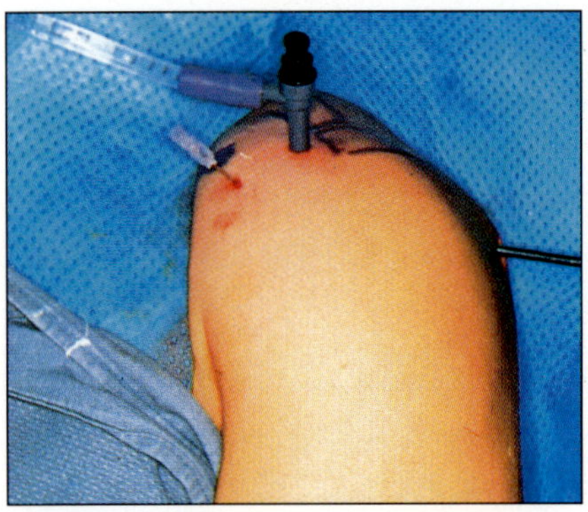

Figure 12-7. Outside view of 18-gauge spinal needle just lateral to coracoid process for creation of an anterior-inferior portal.

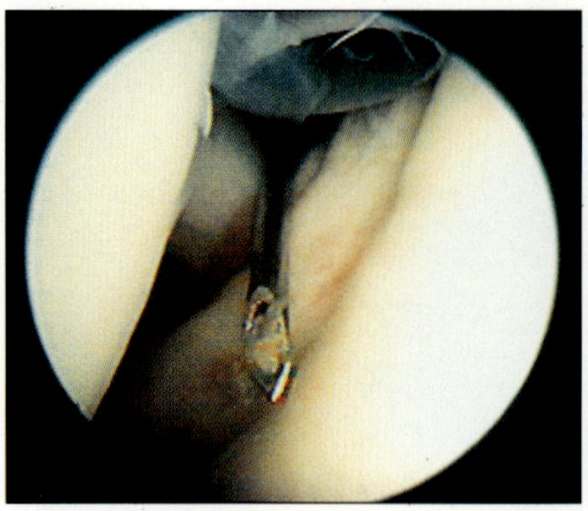

Figure 12-8. View of 18-gauge spinal needle entering the joint just superior to the superior edge of subscapularis and minimizing oblique approach to the glenoid.

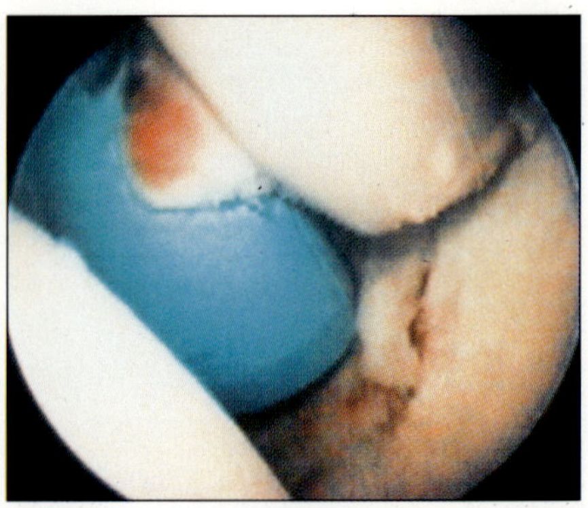

Figure 12-9. Arthroscopic view of antero-inferior cannula (*blue area*) and anterosuperior cannula (*gray area*).

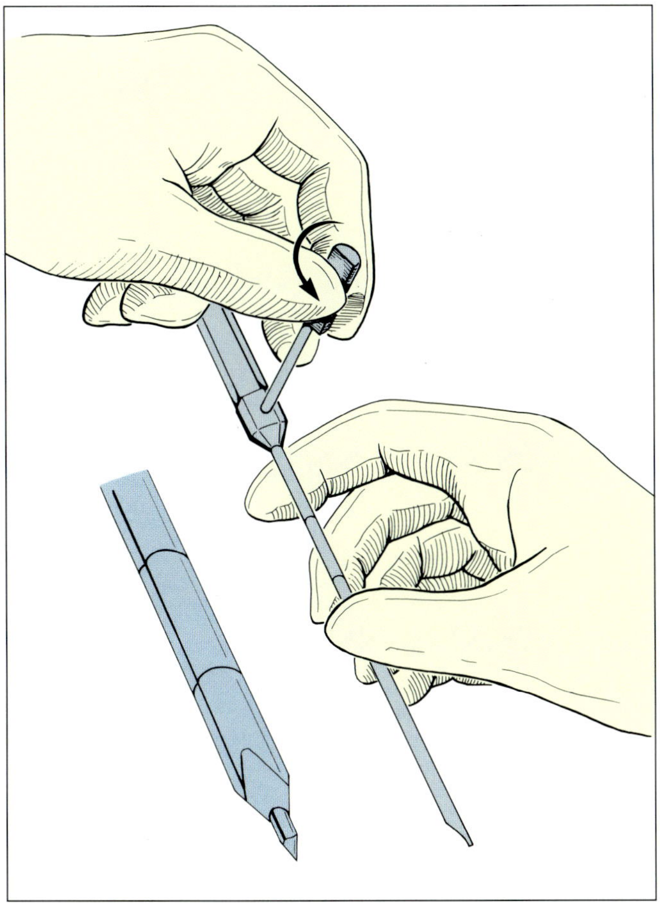

Figure 12-10. Guidewire secured to reamer with 3 mm of tip protruding from end of reamer.

for a left shoulder (4-o'clock on the right shoulder) to a depth of 1.5 cm (Fig. 12-12). The locking nut is loosened and a wire tamp is placed over the guidewire (Fig. 12-13). Several light taps with a mallet will free the guidewire from the reamer. A special black hex handle is secured to the reamer and the reamer is backed out over the guidewire (Fig. 12-14). Constant vigilance is required to prevent extraction of the guidewire when removing the reamer. After the reamer has been removed, an 8-mm cannulated tack is placed over the guidewire (Fig. 12-15). A cannulated impactor facilitates full seating of the tack in its final position (Fig. 12-16). These steps are repeated for an additional tack placed at the 10-o'clock position (2-o'clock for the right) (Fig. 12-17).

The shoulder is immobilized for 4 weeks. A supervised rehabilitation program follows, emphasizing strengthening of the rotator cuff and scapular rotators.

RESULTS

From September 1986 to February 1994, a total of 61 patients were treated with arthroscopy for an acute, initial anterior dislocation of the shoulder. This figure includes nine patients from the initial study of Wheeler and coworkers [4], 21 patients treated with arthroscopic transglenoid suture repair reported by Arciero and coworkers [5], and 31 patients treated with Suretac stabilization as outlined previously.

The average age of the affected patients was 19.5 years (range, 17–23 years). The examination under

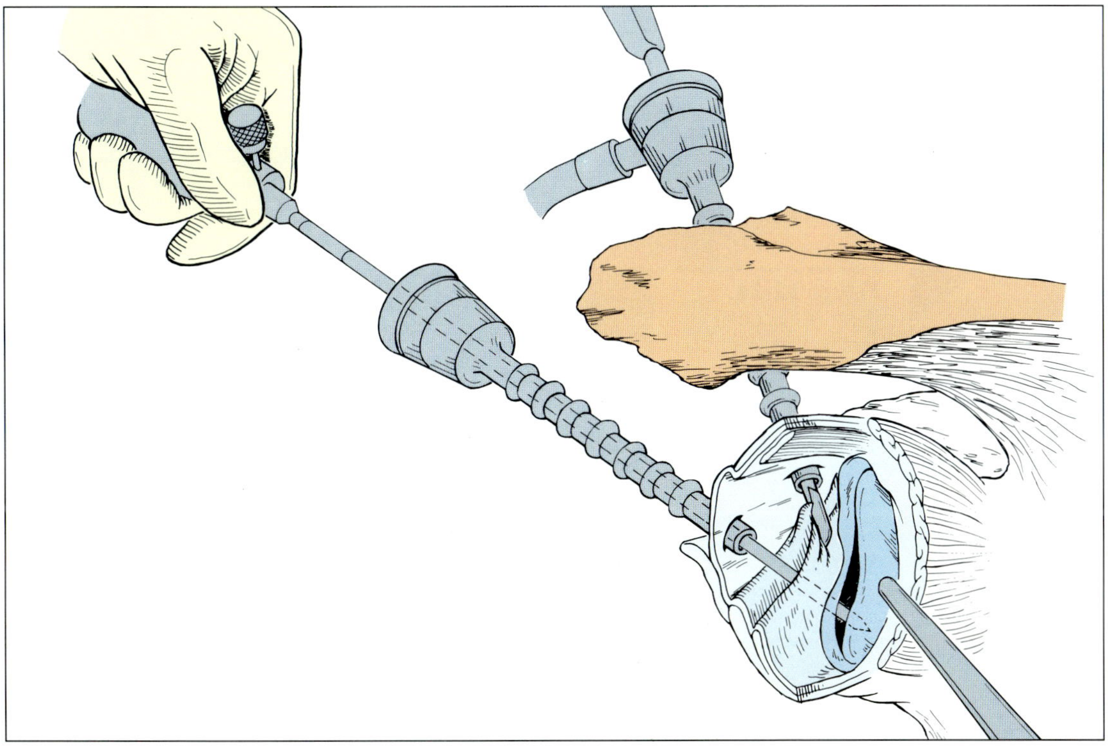

Figure 12-11. Guidewire reamer unit piercing Bankart lesion from anteroinferior portal while assistant maintains reduction of lesion from anterosuperior portal.

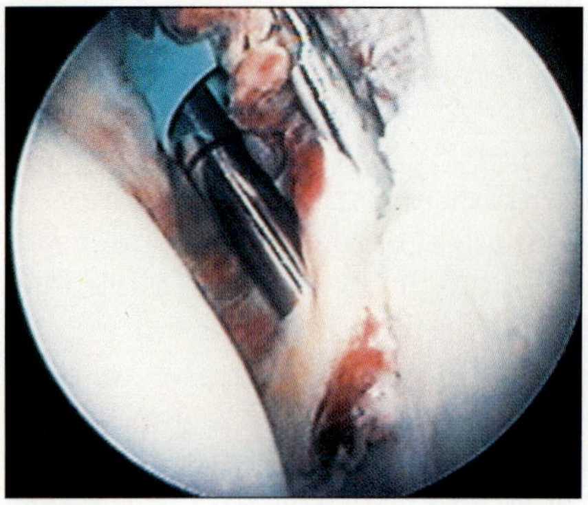

Figure 12-12. Guidewire reamer drilled to proper depth. Assistant maintaining reduction of Bankart lesion with a soft-tissue grasper from the anterosuperior portal.

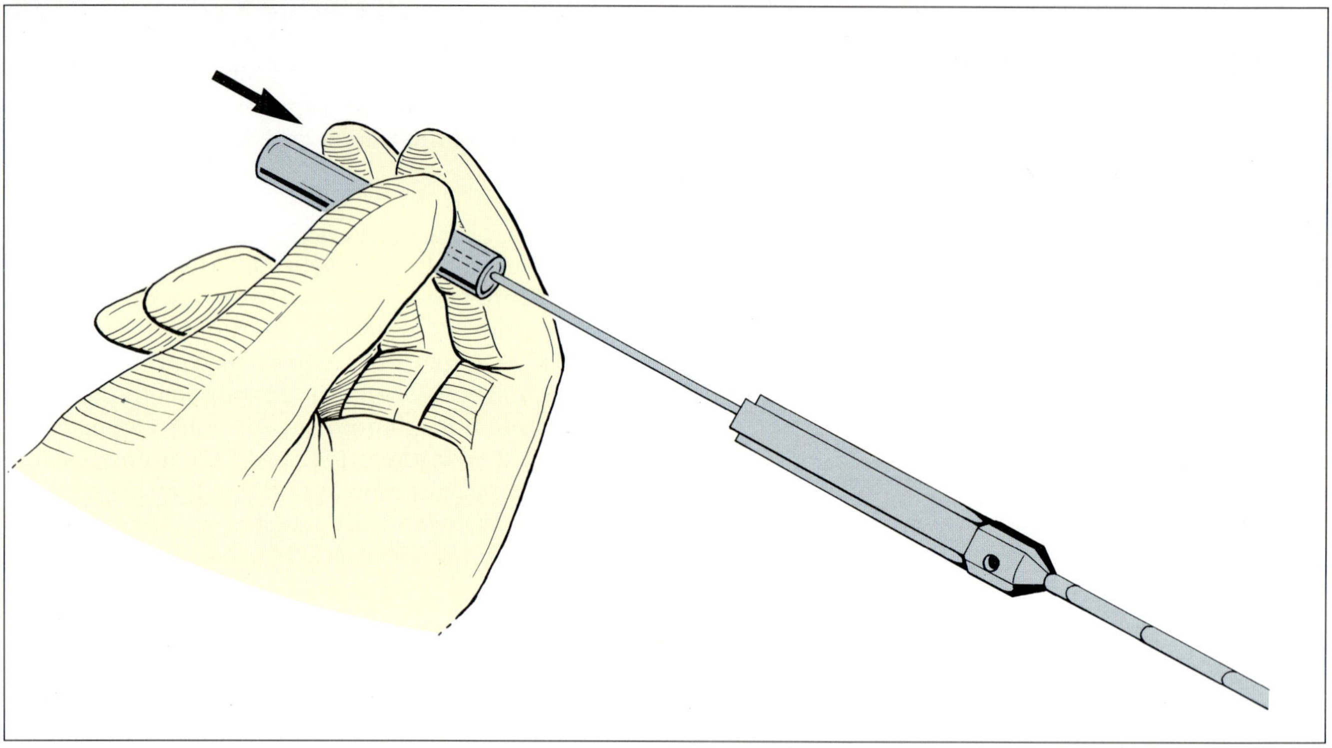

Figure 12-13. Locking nut has been loosened. Several taps of tamp placed over guidewire will free wire from reamer.

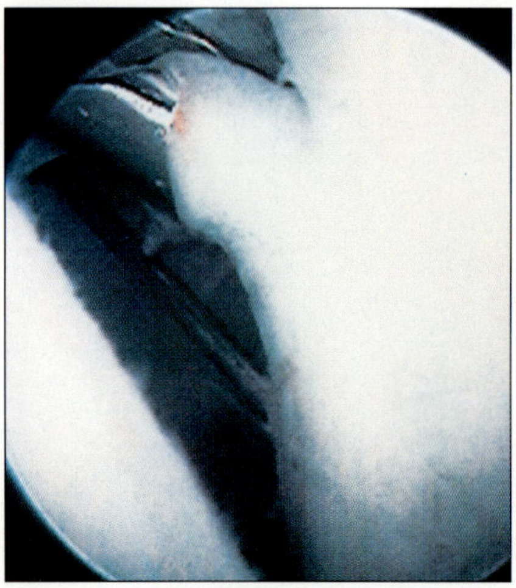

Figure 12-14. Reamer has been removed leaving guidewire in place.

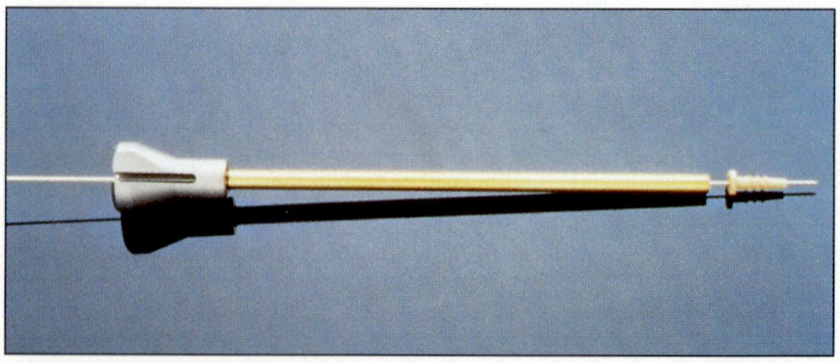

Figure 12-15. Cannulated tack placed over guidewire to be seated with cannulated impactor.

anesthesia revealed abnormal anterior glenohumeral translation in all cases (31 with a laxity grade of 2+; 30 with 3+). Table 12-1 demonstrates the arthroscopic pathology encountered in patients treated with tack fixation.

The remainder of the results will concern the experience with bioabsorbable tack fixation. Since December 1991, 31 patients have been treated with a bioabsorbable cannulated tack. An average of two tacks have been used (one patient with one tack, 28 patients with two tacks, and two patients with three tacks). The average operative time has been 70 min (range, 47–110 min). Twenty patients have been followed for more than 1 year and there has been no recurrence in dislocations, but one patient sustained a single episode of subluxation while boxing. The Rowe shoulder score based on stability, range of motion, and function averaged 95 points (range, 60–100 points). There have been no complications to date.

DISCUSSION

The rationale for considering arthroscopic treatment of an acute dislocation is based on poor results after nonoperative treatment. Our results of 92% and 80% recurrence in two independent studies support the findings of previous authors. In young, active patients who cannot or will not modify their activity, arthroscopic treatment appears to alter the natural history favorably.

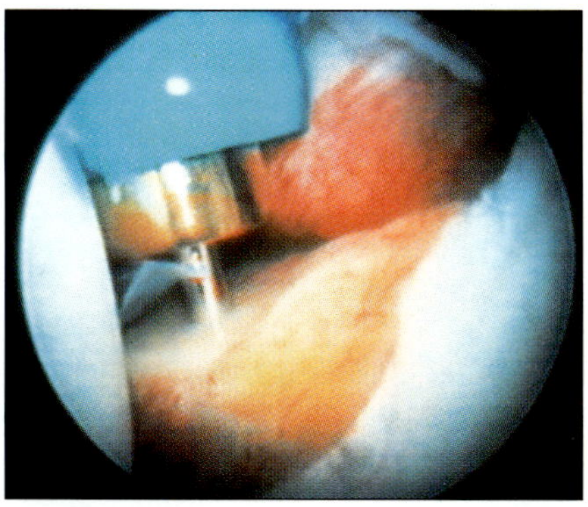

Figure 12-16. Tack in final position over guidewire reapproximating Bankart lesion.

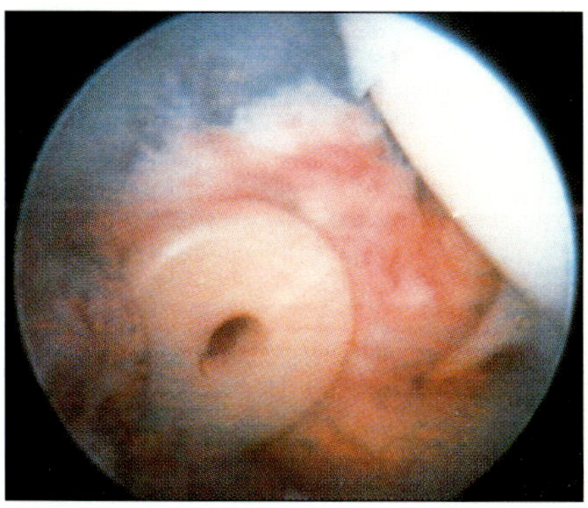

Figure 12-17. Anterior view of left shoulder (from anterior superior portal) demonstrating two tacks reapproximating Bankart lesion.

The principle pathologic entity responsible for recurrence after the initial dislocation has been termed the Bankart or Perthes lesion. An avulsion of the IGHL complex from the glenoid has been cited as the lesion responsible for allowing abnormal glenohumeral translation [9,10]. This has been verified in cadaver studies and supported clinically by the success of open procedures that focus on repair of this lesion in the chronically unstable shoulder [9,10].

In the past decade, arthroscopists have demonstrated the technical ability to repair this lesion arthroscopically for chronic instability [11–14]. However, the results of arthroscopic stabilization compared with open Bankart repair have been less favorable, with recurrence rates after repair quoted as high as 25% [12]. This finding suggests that arthroscopic techniques do not predictably address all components of instability in the chronic situation. Several investigators have implicated the role of capsular injury or redundancy in contributing to instability [15]. In the chronically unstable shoulder, the Bankart lesion, capsular redundancy, a degenerative or absent labrum, the Hill-Sachs lesion, and subscapularis deficiency may all contribute to instability. However, after the acute, initial dislocation a hemarthrosis has been always present. An avulsion of the IGHL as a capsulolabral complex has been observed 97% of the time. Furthermore, if a capsular injury has occurred, no chronic attenuation is present, and the labrum is not degenerated as is frequently observed in chronic instability. We believe this represents the optimum situation for arthroscopic repair.

Baker and coworkers [16] described three types of Bankart lesions present at arthroscopy in a series of 45 patients evaluated after an acute dislocation [16]. Our series deals with a very uniform young age population.

Table 12-1 Arthroscopic pathology in patients with acute, initial anterior shoulder dislocation

Patients, *n*	Pathology
29	Capsulolabral avulsion of inferior glenohumeral ligament from glenoid
1	Lateral detachment of inferior glenohumeral ligament
1	Capsular tear medial to labrum
27	Hill-Sach defects
3	Superior labral anterior to posterior lesions
0	Cuff tears

The indications for arthroscopic intervention were strict. Subsequently, the examination under anesthesia and the arthroscopic findings have been remarkably consistent. This may explain the high incidence of a complete capsulolabral avulsion of the IGHL found at arthroscopy in our patients. The quality of tissue for repair is robust and conducive to tack stabilization.

Our surgical technique has been in evolution. Initially, general anesthesia, the lateral decubitus position, and a metal staple was used. Subsequently, to avoid any problems associated with metallic implants, a transglenoid suture technique was used.

When attempting to develop a new technique, or in this case, use an established technique in a new clinical situation, it is important that potential risks be minimized. The use of the sitting position, interscalene anesthesia, and a bioabsorbable cannulated tack satisfies this prerequisite. In using this technique, general anesthesia is avoided, there is no traction on the brachial plexus, no transglenoid drilling and suturing over posterior soft tissues, and there is no use of metal. This procedure has been reproducible with low morbidity.

Our results have been encouraging but still must be considered preliminary. In our young, active population, the results have been consistently favorable compared with nonoperative treatment with regard to recurrence. Arthroscopic treatment of an acute, initial anterior shoulder dislocation in this population appears to be a reasonable treatment option.

References and Recommended Reading

Papers of interest, published recently, have been highlighted as:
- • Of special interest
- •• Of outstanding interest

1. Hovelius L: Anterior dislocation of the shoulder in teenagers and young adults. *J Bone Joint Surg* 1987, 69A:393–399.
2. Kiviluoto O, Posila M, Jaronia H, *et al.*: Immobilization after primary dislocation of the shoulder. *Acta Orthop Scand* 1980, 51:915–919.
3. McLaughlin HL, MacLellan DI: Recurrent anterior dislocation of the shoulder. *J Trauma* 1967, 7:191–201.
4. Wheeler JH, Ryan JB, Arciero RA, *et al.*: Arthroscopic versus nonoperative treatment of acute shoulder dislocations in young athletes. Arthroscopy 1989, 5:213–217.
5.• Arciero RA, Wheeler JH, Ryan JB, *et al.*: Arthroscopic Bankart repair vs. non-operative treatment for acute, initial, anterior shoulder dislocations. *Am J Sports Med,* 1994, 22:589–594.

Comparative study evaluating arthroscopic Bankart repair with nonoperative treatment after the initial anterior shoulder dislocation. The study, done in a uniform population of young athletes, demonstrated a marked reduction in recurrence rates and the need for secondary open surgery in the arthroscopic-treated group.

6.• Brown AR, Weiss R, Greenberg C, *et al.*: Interscalene block for shoulder arthroscopy: comparison with general anesthesia. *Arthroscopy* 1993, 9:295–300.

A large retrospective study evaluating interscalene regional anesthesia with general anesthesia for shoulder arthroscopy at a medical center practice. Interscalene anesthesia was found to be safe and effective with fewer side effects, fewer hospital admissions, and a shortened hospital stay than with general anesthesia used for shoulder arthroscopy.

7. Skyhar MJ, Altchek DW, Warren RF, *et al.*: Shoulder arthroscopy with the patient in the beach-chair position. *Arthroscopy* 1988, 4:256–259.
8. Warner JP, Warren RF: Arthroscopic Bankart repair using a cannulated, absorbable fixation device. *Operative Techniques in Orthop* 1991, 1:192–198.
9. Turkel SJ, Panie MW, Marshal JL, *et al.*: Stabilizing mechanisms preventing anterior dislocation of the glenohumeral joint. *J Bone Joint Surg* 1981, 63A:1208.
10. O'Brien SJ, Neves MC, Arnoczky SP, *et al.*: The anatomy and histology of the inferior glenohumeral ligament complex of the shoulder. *Am J Sports Med* 1990, 18:449.
11. Morgan CD, Bodenstab AB: Arthroscopic Bankart suture repair: technique and early results. *Arthroscopy* 1987, 3:111–112.
12. Coughlin L, Rubinovich M, Johansson J, *et al.*: Arthroscopic staple capsulorrhaphy for anterior shoulder instability. Am J Sports Med 1992, 20:253–256.
13. Hawkins RB: Arthroscopic stapling repair for shoulder instability. a retrospective study of 50 cases. *J Arthroscopy* 1989, 5:122–128.
14. Matthews LS: Anterior staple capsulorrhaphy for recurrent anterior shoulder instability. *Arthroscopy* 1988, 1:106–111.
15. Ticker JB, Bigliani LU, Soslowsky LJ, *et al.*: Viscoelastic and geometric properties of the inferior glenohumeral ligament. *Orthop Trans* 1992, 16:304–305.
16. Baker CL, Uribe JW, Whitman C: Arthroscopic evaluation of acute initial shoulder dislocations. *Am J Sports Med* 1990, 18:25–28.

13

CHAPTER

Arthroscopic Shoulder Stabilization Using the Bioabsorbable Tack

CLAUDE T. MOORMAN III, KEVIN P. SPEER, RUSSELL F. WARREN

Arthroscopic shoulder stabilization has recently come of age as an alternative to more extensive open procedures [1–4]. Advantages of the arthroscopic approach include 1) decreased postoperative pain or morbidity, 2) less anatomic distortion, and 3) decreased operative time. Because of the diminished perioperative morbidity of the surgery, patients can often be stabilized on an outpatient basis. Recently, a bioabsorbable tack (Suretac; Acufex Microsurgical, Norwood MA) has been developed at our institution for use in arthroscopic shoulder stabilization [5–7••]. This device affords the advantages of a biodegradable implant and obviates the need for drilling through the scapular neck or typing sutures over posterior soft tissue. In this chapter, we review the physical and degradation properties of this tack, discuss indications for its use and insertion technique, and outline postoperative management.

THE BIOABSORBABLE TACK

The bioabsorbable tack was developed in response to problems with first and second generation techniques for arthroscopic stabilization. Johnson [8] advocated the use of metallic staples for anterior capsulorrhaphy in the early 1980s. Unfortunately, the rate of recurrence and dangers of hardware extrusion with subsequent joint destruction have been unacceptably high with this technique [9,10]. Transosseous suture placement has been developed as an effective alternative to anterior hardware, although it adds the hazards of suturing over the posterior soft tissue and drilling through the scapula [11]. The tack system was designed to circumvent these shortcomings and provide for secure fixation of the capsulolabral complex to the anterior glenoid. Because the tack is inserted anteriorly, no transosseous drilling or posterior soft-tissue compromise is necessary. Because the device is bioabsorbable, there are no problems with hardware extrusion.

The biodegradable tack used at our institution is constructed from polygluconate, a synthetic copolymer similar to that used in bioabsorbable suture materials. It is pressure-molded into shape in 6- and 8-mm sizes, with a flat head and ribbed shank to increase surface area and maximize soft-tissue holding power (Fig. 13-1). For purposes of shoulder reconstruction, we use the 8-mm tack; the guidewire is larger and serves as a more effective "joy-stick" to mobilize the tissue superiorly without bending. This device is cannulated for ease of insertion over a guidewire. Pull-out strength is about 100 N at the time of insertion. The tack has a biodegradation profile that allows for about 4 weeks of gradually decreasing fixation strength (Fig. 13-2). Soft-tissue healing to an appropriately prepared glenoid surface has been shown to reliably occur during this time frame [12]. Degradation is accomplished by passive hydrolysis alone [7]. Should the device inadvertently extrude into the joint, it would be dissolved by the joint fluid rapidly, minimizing damage to the articular surface. Although this mechanism is advantageous in terms of degradation, it does require airtight packaging of the device to avoid unintentional degradation by the moisture in room air.

INDICATIONS

The most important variable in the success of stabilization using the bioabsorbable tack system is patient selection. In the review of the first 52 patients treated with this technique, 79% had excellent stability at follow-up (2 to 5 years). Of the 11 failures, four patients sustained reinjuries in violent contact sports. The remaining seven patients experienced dislocations (four patients) or subluxations (three patients) with minor trauma. Eight of the 11 patients required subsequent open anterior stabilization. All eight demonstrated excellent healing of the repaired labrum to the glenoid but gross laxity of the capsular envelope.

Our review suggests that patients with gross laxity, poor-quality anterior tissue, or multidirectional instability (particularly of an atraumatic onset) are poorly suited for tack stabilization. We feel that candidates for tack fixation must meet three essential criteria: 1) the lesion should be traumatic in etiology, 2) the patient must have a discrete Bankart lesion with good tissue quality, and 3) the patient must demonstrate no evidence of multidirectional instability (negative sulcus sign). Furthermore, it would appear that the chances for success are increased if repair is performed early (after the initial dislocation) when the plastic deformation of the capsulolabral envelope is less than after multiple dislocations or subluxations. Based on information from the preliminary study and the results since, an algorithm has been conceived to assist with the process of patient selection (Fig. 13-3).

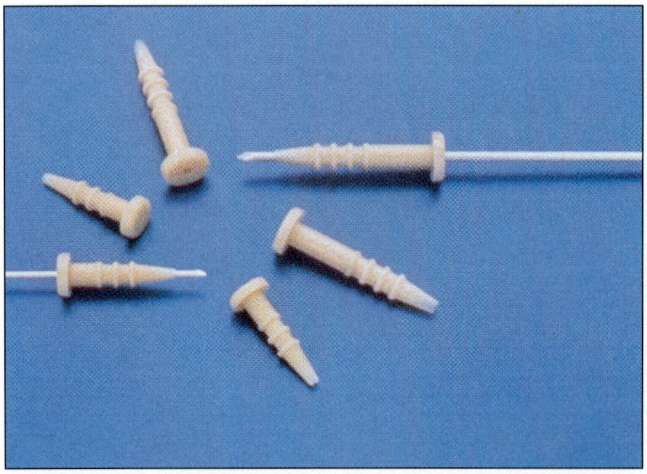

Figure 13-1. Cannulated bioabsorbable tack anchors; both 6- and 8-mm sizes are available. The 8-mm tack is used most often for shoulder stabilization. (*From* Speer and Warren [13]; with permission.)

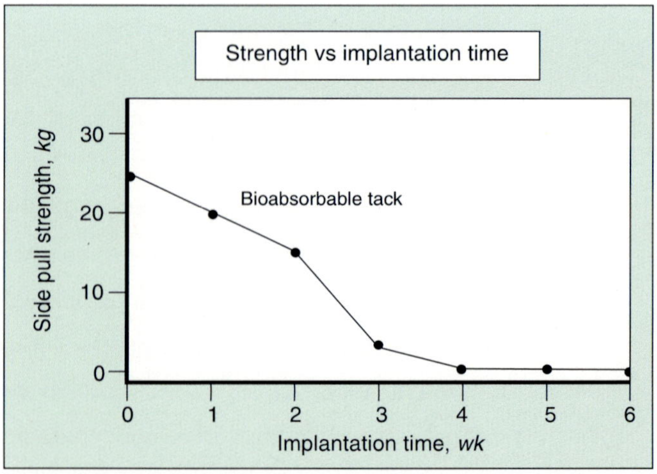

Figure 13-2. Biodegradation profile of the tack. Note that fixation strength gradually decreases over a 4-week period. (*From* Speer and Warren [13]; with permission.)

More recently, we have expanded the indications for tack stabilization to include labral injury superiorly as in the biceps anchor (superior labral anterior to posterior) lesion. The type 2 or 4 variety with detachment of the biceps anchor leads to increased anterior translation and may cause instability symptoms or aggravate instability secondary to more inferior labral injury (Bankart lesion). Repair of the biceps anchor lesion is performed by rasping the bony attachment site superiorly from the 11-o'clock position to the 2-o'clock position. Tacks are placed at the biceps anchor insertion through a high medial portal.

TECHNIQUE OF TACK STABILIZATION

Positioning

We perform arthroscopic tack stabilization in the beach-chair position with the patient seated upright under an interscalene anesthetic (Fig. 13-4). This position provides several advantages over the lateral decubitus position: 1) no traction or suspension apparatus necessary for the arm, 2) simpler conversion to an open procedure, 3) better access to the anterior shoulder, and 4) improved patient tolerance under regional anesthetic.

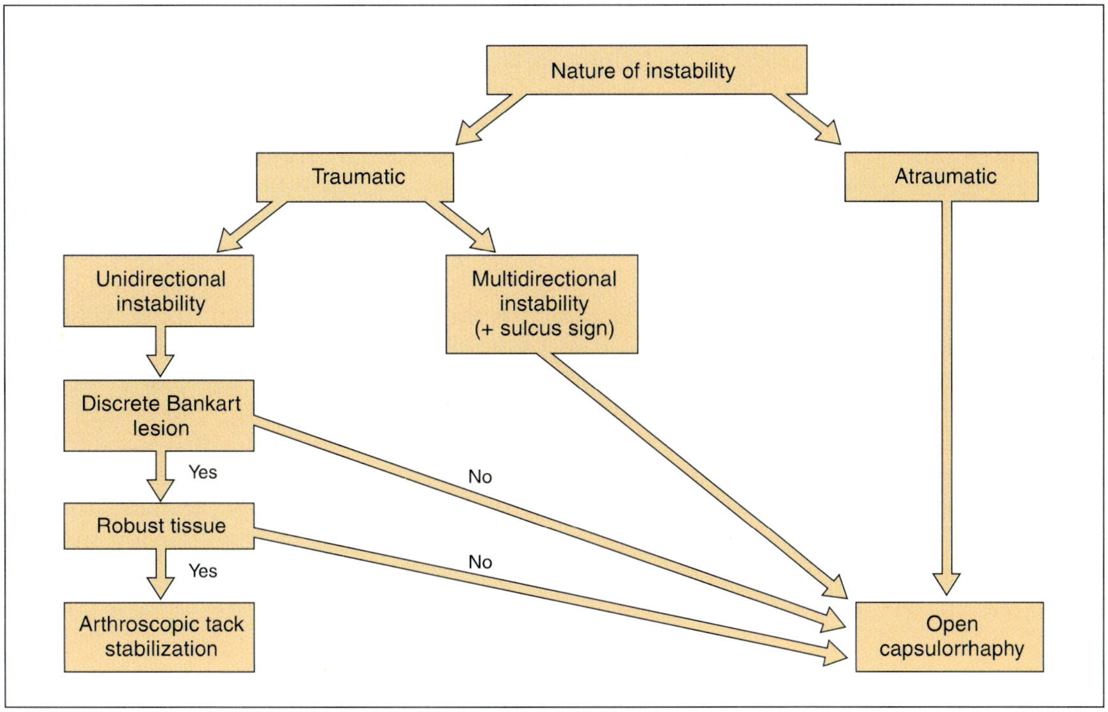

Figure 13-3. Patient selection algorithm for shoulder stabilization.

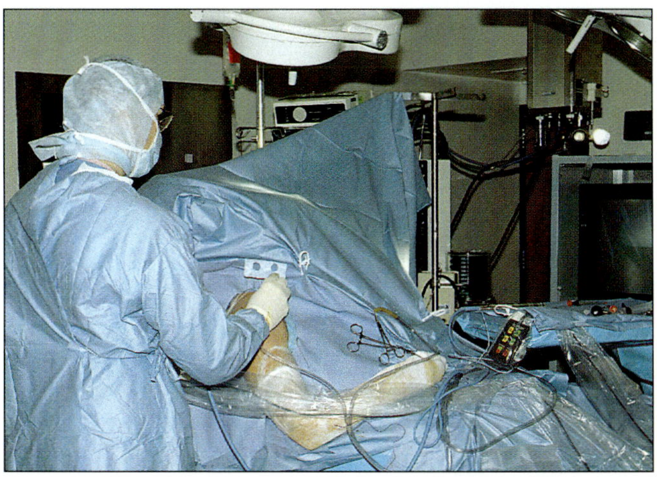

Figure 13-4. Beach-chair position for shoulder arthroscopy under an interscalene block anesthetic.

Examination Under Anesthesia

With the patient appropriately positioned and anesthetized, the shoulder is carefully examined. This stability examination focuses on evaluation of inferior and anteroposterior (AP) stability. Inferior stability is assessed using the sulcus test, applying inferior force to the humeral diaphysis with the glenohumeral joint adducted (arm at the side). Assessment is made of inferior translation of the humeral head relative to the undersurface at the acromion. Normal translation is 30% to 50% of the glenoid height (approximately 1 cm). Grading is 1+, 2+, and 3+ for translations of 1 cm, 2 cm, or > 2 cm, respectively; a grade of 2+ or greater on the sulcus test is diagnostic of inferior instability (Fig. 13-5).

Anteroposterior translation is evaluated at 45° of abduction with the shoulder in the plane of the scapula (slightly flexed) and in neutral rotation. Axial force is applied with one examining hand through the elbow (to the shoulder joint proximally) to center the head (Fig. 13-6). The other hand is used to apply AP force to the humeral diaphysis and to evaluate translation. Normal translation of the humeral head is 50% of the width of the glenoid surface (approximately 1 cm) anteriorly and posteriorly. Grading is as follows: 1+, translation of glenoid rim; 2+, head subluxes over rim but reduces when force is released; and 3+, head dislocates (locks out without return when force is released). A combination of 2+ or greater AP instability with a sulcus test of 2+ or greater is diagnostic of multidirectional instability. These patients are best suited for open stabilization. Patients with 2+ unidirectional instability and a negative sulcus test are considered for tack stabilization (Fig. 13-3).

Arthroscopic Set-up

The arthroscope is inserted through a standard posterior portal (Fig. 13-7). Two anterior portals are required for tack stabilization. The first is placed superiorly in the rotator interval, just anterior to the biceps tendon, and used both to prepare the glenoid and to grasp the labral tissue. The labrum is fully detached anteriorly down to the 6-o'clock position using a knife-rasp (Fig. 13-8). The rasp is then used to freshen the anterior glenoid in preparation for the tacks. The 4.5 mm full-radius intra-articular shaver is often helpful as an accessory for this process. A grasper, or alternatively, a suture passer is used to capture the tissue complex for superior mobilization. A second inferior portal is placed anteriorly. This portal is positioned by using a spinal needle for localization and oriented to be as low as possible while still clearing the intra-articular portion of the subscapularis tendon. More recently, we have placed a cannula through the subscapularis muscle, staying lateral to the conjoined tendon (45° anterior angle). The portal is placed slightly lateral to the joint line to allow for a lateral to medial inclination (for drilling purposes). The guidewire drill complex is loaded with approximately 4 to 5 mm of the sharp guidepin protruding through the tip of the drill and passed into the joint through the inferior portal (Fig. 13-9). The labrum inferior glenohumeral ligament complex (IGHLC) tissue is advanced through the superior portal 5- to 15 mm as

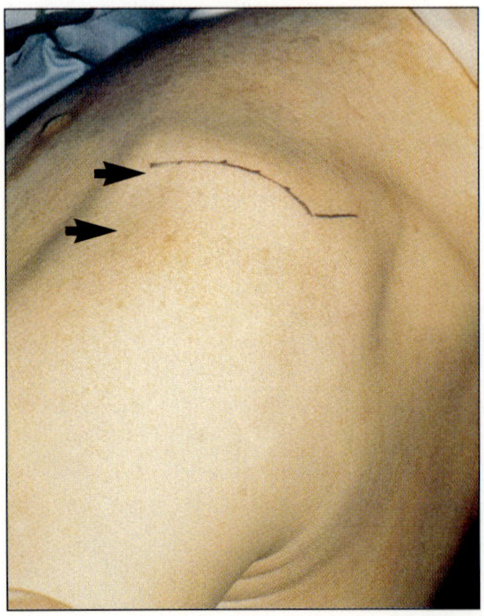

Figure 13-5. Positive sulcus sign. Note that inferior translation of humeral head is greater than 1 cm relative to the acromion.

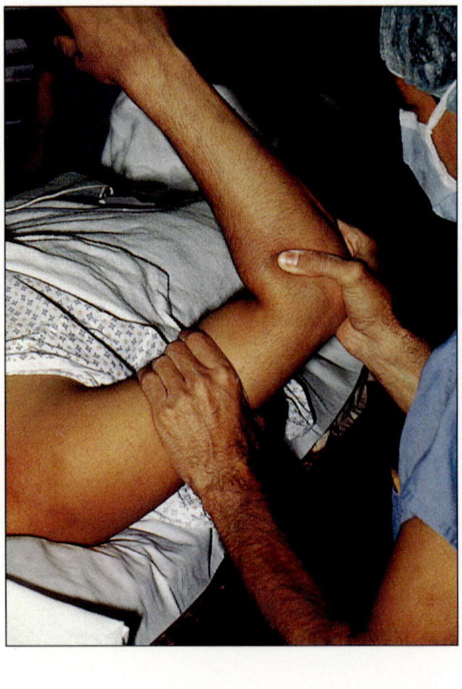

Figure 13-6. Position for evaluation of anteroposterior shoulder stability. The examiner's right hand (left for opposite shoulder) is used to control position and apply axial load to center the humeral head in the glenoid. Maximal translation will be appreciated in the scapular plane (slight flexion), 45° abduction, and neutral rotation. The left hand supplies anteroposterior force and senses translation.

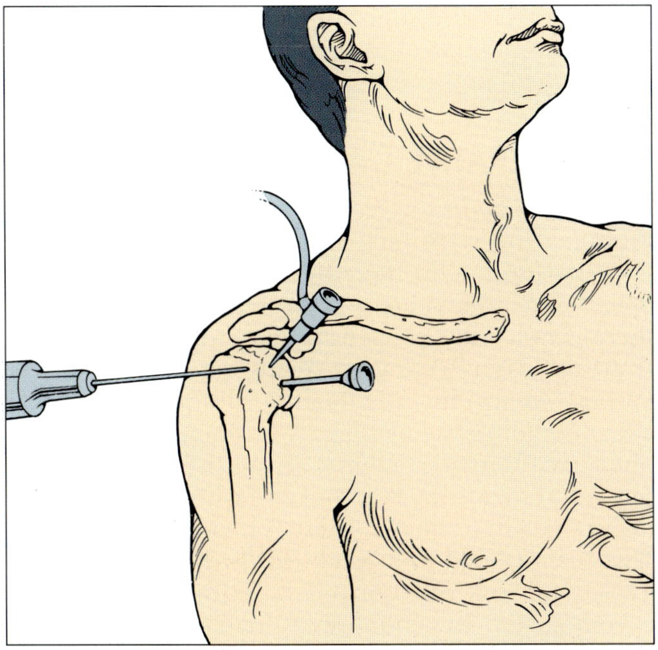

Figure 13-7. Overview of portal placement for tack stabilization. A standard posterior arthroscope portal is used for visualization. Twin anterior instrument portals are required for tissue mobilization and tack insertion.

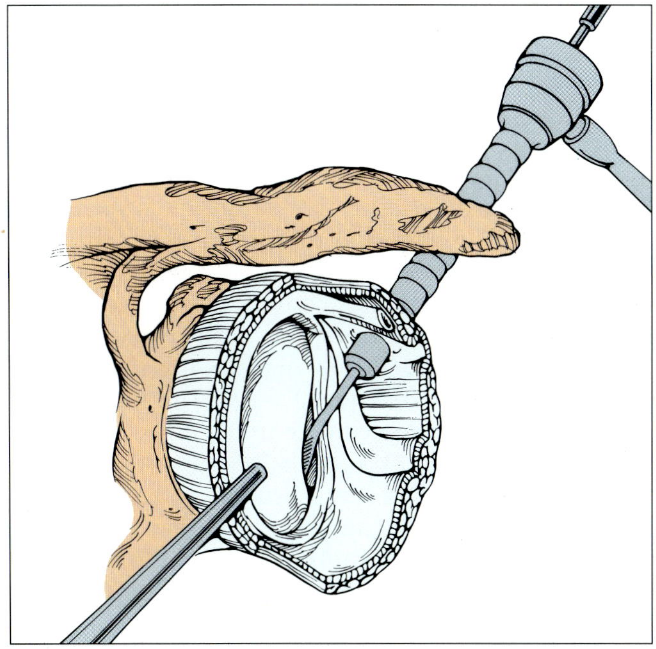

Figure 13-8. The anterosuperior portal is placed as high as possible in the rotator interval, just anterior to the biceps tendon. The knife-rasp is used to fully detach the labrum anteriorly and freshen the anterior surface of the glenoid in preparation for tack placement.

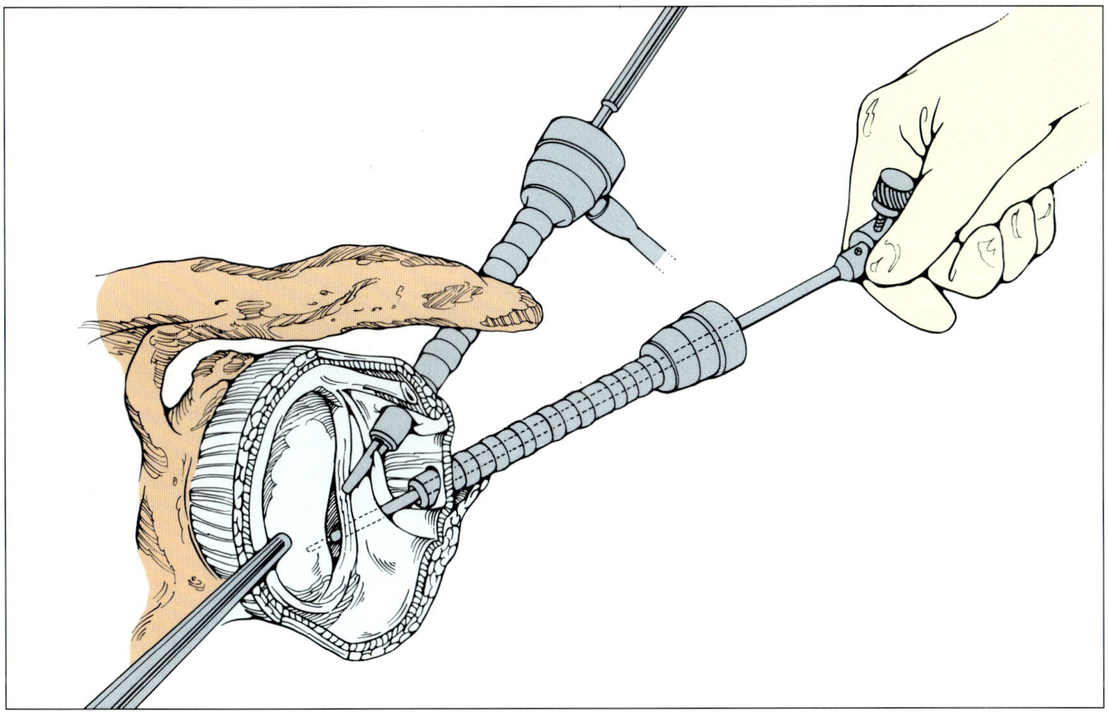

Figure 13-9. The anteroinferior portal is placed as low as possible while still clearing the subscapularis tendon. The portal is placed lateral to the joint line to provide for a slight lateral to medial inclination for the guide-wire-drill apparatus. The guidewire-drill apparatus is placed through the inferior portal by hand, used to pierce the tissue, and then used to place the capsulolabral tissue at the articular margin at the 4:30 position (right shoulder) on the glenoid.

the soft tissue allows. With the labrum-IGHLC mobilized superiorly, the guidewire is used to impale the tissue and secure it to the glenoid at the 4:30 (right shoulder) or 7:30 (left shoulder) position (Fig. 13-10). Power is used to advance the drill bit to a depth of 12 mm (Fig. 13-11). The thumb screw is loosened at the base of the drill bit and the guidepin, now freely mobile, is tapped about 2 to 3 mm further into the bone. Hand power is used with a gentle back and forth rotational torque to remove the drill, leaving the guidepin in place (Fig. 13-9). A tack is placed on the guidewire and tapped into place using the slotted impactor and a mallet (Fig. 13-12). The tack enters the joint and the prepared hole under direct visualization with the arthroscope. With the inferior tack securing the IGHLC, a second superior tack is placed in the 2-o'clock (right shoulder) or 10-o'clock (left shoulder) position to mobilize the middle glenohumeral complex superiorly and supplement the fixation of the first tack (Fig. 13-13). Although two tacks provide sufficient holding power, often we are able to get three tacks into the tissue depending on the size of the glenoid and the fixation requirements for the soft-tissue envelope. If a third tack is used, the second tack is placed at the 3-o'clock position (9-o'clock left shoulder) and the superior tack at the 1:30 position (10:30 left shoulder) to provide adequate separation (about 1 cm) of the drill holes.

Postoperative Care

We tend to be less aggressive in initial postoperative mobilization with tack-stabilization patients than with patients who have been stabilized using the open technique. There are two reasons for this. First, there is much less propensity for anterior scarring, so there is less urgency in regaining early motion. Second, we feel that the fixation, although more than adequate for tissue healing, is less immediately postoperative with the tack than with techniques for open stabilization. For these reasons, patients are maintained in a sling in internal rotation for 4 weeks. This is shortened to 3 weeks in throwing athletes to avoid the loss of external rotation. Patients are encouraged to do pendulum exercises, elbow range of motion work, and hand-wrist strengthening for this immobilization period. At the end of the immobilization period, patients are instructed in pulley exercises and allowed assisted flexion to 90° and external rotation to 0° with the arm at the side. Isometric

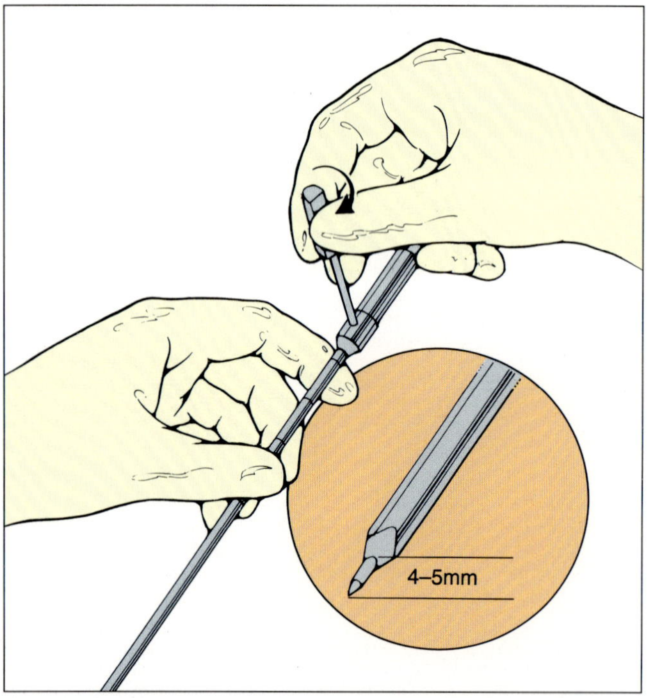

Figure 13-10. Guidewire-drill apparatus. A hex-head screw in the handle stabilizes the drill bit to the guidewire. The guidewire is set to protrude through the tip of the drill bit approximately 4 to 5 mm. The hex-screw is loosened following drilling to allow for selective removal of the drill bit, leaving the guidewire in the bone for tack insertion. (*From* Pagnani and Warren [6••]; with permission.)

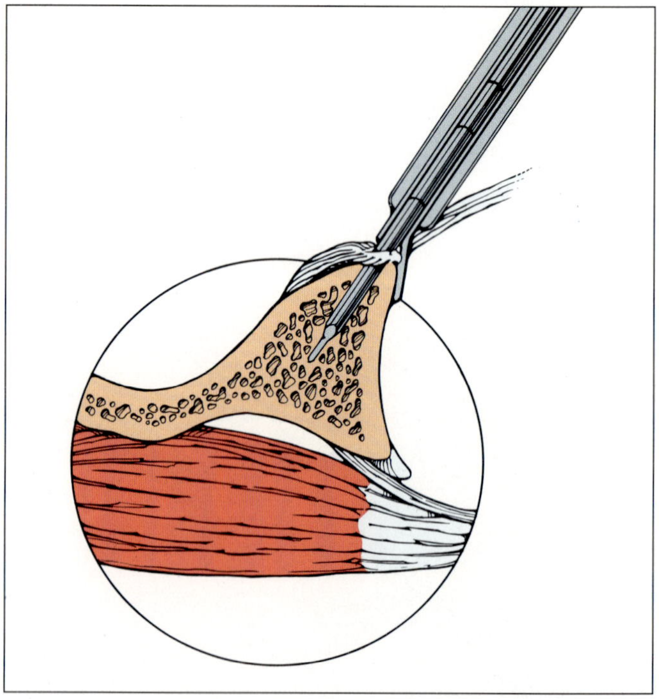

Figure 13-11. Axial view of the guidewire-drill apparatus inserted approximately 12 to 14 mm into the bone. The optional glenoid guide is depicted.

strengthening of the deltoid, biceps, and triceps are initiated at this time. At 8 weeks, motion is advanced and elastic tubing exercises are instituted for internal and external rotator strengthening. Our goal is restoration of full motion by the 12-week mark. Weights are added for strengthening at 12 weeks. Patients are allowed to return to contact sports at 5 to 6 months if rehabilitation has progressed smoothly. Throwers are returned to light overhand activity at 5 months and advanced to full-speed throwing over a 6 to 8 week period with a goal of return to sport by 7 months.

COMPLICATIONS

Complications with tack stabilization have been infrequent, generally minor, and related to the learning curve. The most common complication, as with other arthroscopic stabilization techniques, is recurrent instability. We feel this relates more to patient selection than to failure of the technique. Tack stabilization is not designed to treat patients with multidirectional instability or with grossly lax patulous capsular tissue. The algorithm (Fig. 13-3) we currently use for patient selection has drastically reduced this complication.

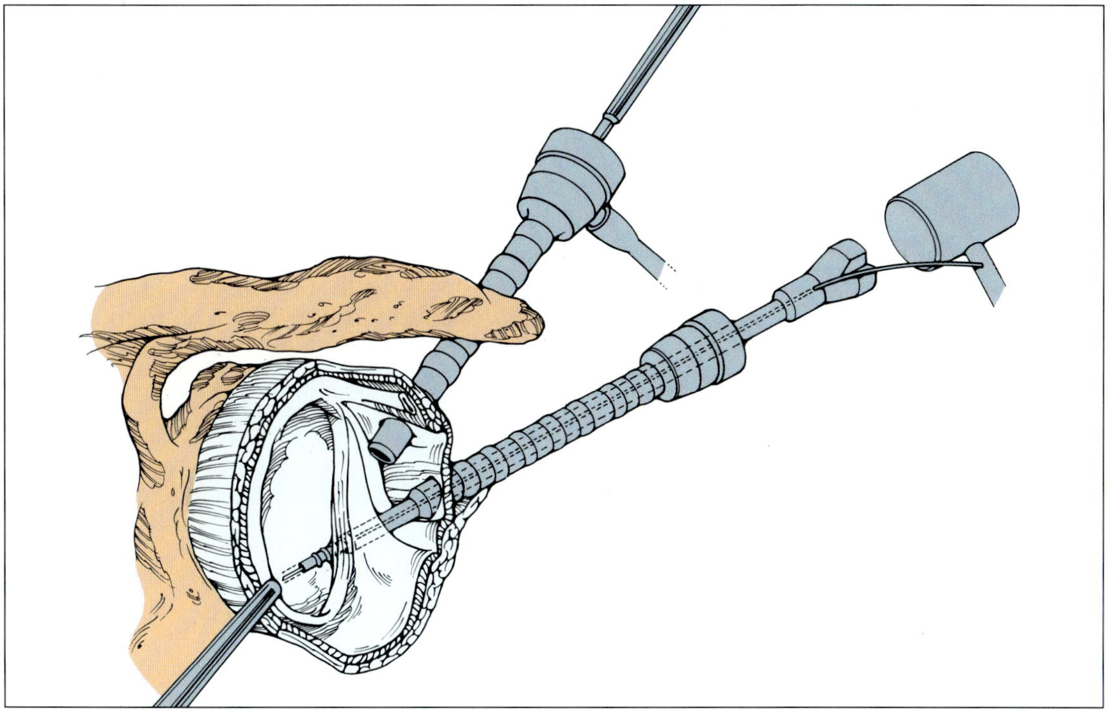

Figure13-12. Placement of the cannulated inferior tack over the guidewire. The tack is tapped into position using the cannulated impactor.

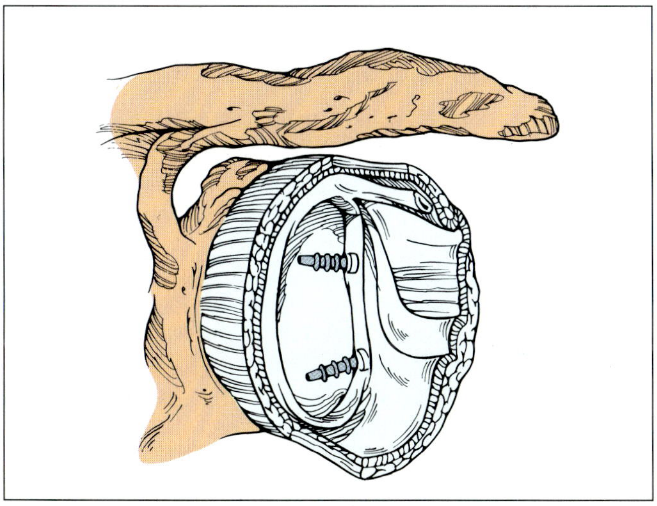

Figure 13-13. The superior tack is placed at the 2-o'clock position to finish the stabilization construct.

Failure of the tack device itself is generally due to one of two problems. First, the head can slip through the hole in the capsule with a consequent loss of purchase on the soft-tissue sleeve. This results when the tissue is of poor quality, or a technical error is made in not impaling enough of the soft-tissue wad to acquire holding strength. Loss of tack fixation in the bone has not been a problem. Second, eccentric tapping on the tack during insertion can shear off the anchoring head. This generally occurs when the guidewire is removed and the surgeon tries to give the tack a few free-hand blows for good measure. In this case, a new tack is inserted directly adjacent to the sheared one.

Discomfort at 6 to 8 weeks has been noted on occasion following tack stabilization. This transient phenomena may represent head separation, loosening of the tines, or synovitis. We have managed these conditions with anti-inflammatory agents and decreased activity over the 1- to 2-week period. No long-term sequelae has been noted.

The majority of other problems with tack stabilization relate to portal placement. If the top anterior portal is placed too low, it is difficult to mobilize the tissue properly. If the inferior portal is placed too high, it will be difficult to get the inferior tack low enough. If the inferior portal is placed too medial, it is difficult to angle the drill medial enough to avoid "mole-hilling" the articular surface of the glenoid. If the drill is bent or toggled during insertion, the hole may be grossly enlarged, compromising fixation. For these reasons, attention to detail of portal placement is imperative.

SUMMARY

The bioabsorbable tack is quite effective in repairing Bankart and biceps anchor lesions when the tissue is of good quality. It has eliminated the need for metallic fixation devices and has obviated the necessity for suturing over posterior soft-tissue structures. The device has suitable initial holding strength and is degraded by hydrolysis over a 4-week period. The technique for insertion is straightforward provided a few key principles are observed. Success relates to patient selection, a process facilitated by the presented algorithm. The postoperative course has been standardized and allows return to most activities by 6 months. The bioabsorbable tack provides the surgeon with an additional option that has been used successfully in well-selected patients with shoulder instability.

REFERENCES AND RECOMMENDED READING

Papers of interest, published recently, have been highlighted as:
- • Of interest
- •• Of outstanding interest

1. Hawkins R: Arthroscopic stapling repair for shoulder instability: a retrospective study of 50 cases. *Arthroscopy* 1989, 5:122–128.

2. Morgan C, Bodenstab A: Arthroscopic bankart suture repair: technique and early results. *Arthroscopy* 1987, 3:111–122.

3. Wiley A: Arthroscopy for shoulder instability and a technique for arthroscopic repair. *Arthroscopy* 1988, 4:25–30.

4. Yahiro M, Matthews L: Arthroscopic stabilization procedures for recurrent anterior shoulder instability. *Orthop Rev* 1989, 11:1161–1168.

5.•• Pagnani M, Galiant B, Warren RF: Glenohumeral instability. In *Orthopaedic Sports Medicine: Principles and Practice.* Edited by J Delee and D Drez. Philadelphia, WB Saunders: 1994: 580–622.

A comprehensive review of the pathophysiology, etiology and treatment of all forms of glenohumeral instability. This reference provides excellent indications and technique sections for both open and arthroscopic stabilization.

6.•• Pagnani M, Warren RF: Arthroscopic shoulder stabilization. *Operative Techniques in Sports Med* 1993, 1:276–284.

An excellent treatise demonstrating the technical pearls of bioabsorbable tack application.

7.•• Speer K, Warren R, Pagnani M: Arthroscopic stabilization of the shoulder using a bioabsorbable tac: a 2–5 year follow-up study. *J Bone Joint Surg* 1994, in press.

The first long-term follow-up study of the bioabsorbable tack.

8. Johnson L: Shoulder arthroscopy. In *Arthroscopic Shoulder Surgery: Principles and Practice,* Edited by L. Johnson. St. Louis: Mosby; 1986:180.

9. Small N: Complications of arthroscopy: the knee and other joints. *Arthroscopy* 1986, 2:253–258.

10. Zuckerman J, Matsen F: Complications about the glenohumeral joint related to the use of screws and staples. *J Bone Joint Surg* 1984, 66A:175–180.

11. Caspari R, Savoie F: Arthroscopic reconstruction of the shoulder: the bankart repair. In *Operative Arthroscopy,* Edited by J. McGinty. New York: Raven Press; 1991:507–516.

12. Rodeo S, Arnoczky S, Torzilli P, *et al.*: Tendon-healing in a bone tunnel. A biomechanical and histological study in the dog. *J Bone and Joint Surg* 1993, 75:1795–1803.

13. Speer KP, Warren RI: Arthroscopic shoulder stabilizaiton: a role for biodegradable materials. *Clin Orthop* 1993, 291:67–74.

14

CHAPTER

Technique of Capsulorrhaphy (Caspari Technique)

FELIX H. SAVOIE III
CHRISTOPHER D. MILLER

Traumatic anterior instability was initially described by Perthes [1] and then several years later by Bankart [2,3]. Both described a lesion in which the anterior labrum is detached from the glenoid. The key lesion was later shown by Turkel and coworkers [4] to be a detachment of the anterior inferior glenohumeral ligament (anterior band of the inferior glenohumeral ligament). In traumatic anterior instability, this structure must be reconstructed to restore anterior stability to the shoulder.

A variety of repairs have been described for the treatment of traumatic anterior instability of the shoulder and have been classified by Rowe [5] into six groups of reconstructive procedures (Table 14-1). Most current procedures primarily deal with repairing the torn labrum or capsule back to the glenoid rim (Bankart lesion). Several techniques of repair have been described, including the use of multiple sutures [2,3,6,7•], use of a suture attached to the capsulolabral structures which is then pulled through drill holes to the back of the shoulder [8,9], or by staple or screw fixation of the capsule and labrum to the glenoid neck (Warren, Paper presented at the AAOS 55th Annual Meeting, Las Vegas, 1989) [10].

As shoulder arthroscopy has developed, it has contributed greatly to our understanding of the anatomy and pathophysiology of instability of the shoulder [11]. Subsequently, there has been a large interest in the development of arthroscopic techniques for treatment. Arthroscopic procedures, through the use of small puncture wounds instead of a surgical dissection, have the advantages of reduced discomfort, minimal complications, and improved motion and strength of the shoulder during the early postoperative period. However, these procedures should have results equal to or better than those currently available with open techniques to be acceptable.

Arthroscopic Techniques

Most arthroscopic techniques are modifications of previously reported open operations and fall into three basic procedural groups. The Gallie [12] procedure utilizes fascia lata allograft to recreate an anterior inferior sling and has been successfully adapted by Caspari [13••] for an arthroscopically assisted procedure. Caspari initially reported 80% satisfactory results in 51 patients.

Most arthroscopic techniques attempt to repair the labrum by a modification of the Bankart procedure. Caspari [7•] has utilized multiple sutures with 96% satisfactory results in 49 patients, similar to the results obtained by Rowe [6] in the open version of the procedure.

Johnson [14], Maki (Paper presented at the AAOS 55th Annual Meeting, Las Vegas, 1989), and Matthews [15] have reported on arthroscopic modifications of the Dutoit staple, repair with success rates ranging from 66% to 85%. Warren has further modified the Dutoit technique by utilizing a screw instead of a staple (Warren, 1989). Most recently, Wolf has reported on his technique utilizing a suture anchor (Wolf, Paper presented at AANA Specialty Day, AAOS New Orleans, 1994).

Pathology of Anterior Instability

Each of the previously described procedures attempts to address the primary lesion of traumatic anterior shoulder instability—a detachment or midsubstance tear of the anterior inferior glenohumeral ligament (AIGHL) [4]. In the normal shoulder, the labrum functions to deepen and widen the bony glenoid and also serves as an attachment for the capsuloligamentous stabilizing structures of the shoulder. In traumatic anterior dislocation, the AIGHL can be torn near its labral attachment, in midsubstance, or may be avulsed with the labrum (Figs. 14-1 and 14-2). Tom Neviaser [16•] has recently described an avulsion of the labrum with the underlying periosteal sleeve that causes a medial displacement and inferior rotation of the labrum (the anterior labroligamentous periosteal sleeve avulsion lesion). Even though this lesion heals, the displacement results in incompetence of the AIGHL and subsequent anterior instability. McGlynn and Caspari [11] have conducted an arthroscopic study of the function of the labrum in which he reproduced the findings of Turkel and coworkers [4]. Avulsion of the labrum with the AIGHL resulted in anterior instability of the shoulder, whereas injury to the labrum without detachment of the AIGHL did not result in anterior instability.

The results of these studies indicate that injury to the AIGHL is the primary lesion resulting in traumatic anterior instability of the shoulder. Other lesions that have been described as associated with anterior instability (attenuation of the anterior capsular structures, Hill-Sachs lesion, chondromalacia of the anterior

Table 14-1 Reconstructive procedures for anterior instability

I	Capsulolabral complex repair
II	Subscapularis shortening
III	Muscle-tendon sling procedures
IV	Bone block procedures
V	Osteotomies
VI	Muscle transfers

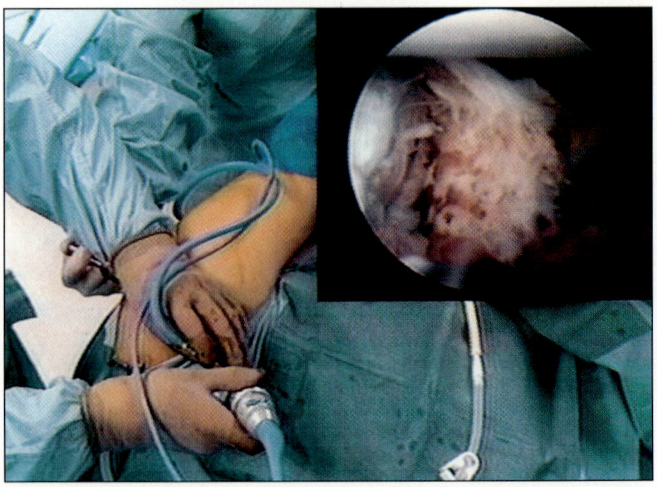

Figure 14-1. View through anterior portal of detached labrum–anterior inferior glenohumeral ligament complex.

glenoid, or flattening of the anterior rim) occur as secondary changes due to the repetitive excess anterior translation. Nevaiser and coworkers [17] have also reported on the association of rotator cuff tears with traumatic anterior dislocation in those patients who sustained their initial dislocation at greater than 50 years of age.

ARTHROSCOPIC CAPSULORRHAPHY

Indications

The primary indication for arthroscopic capsulorrhaphy is recurrent anterior instability in a patient in whom a supervised attempt at nonoperative treatment, including rehabilitation or bracing, has failed. Other indications include traumatic or atraumatic anterior subluxation, such as in the throwing athlete, or previously failed anterior reconstructive procedures, depending on the pathology found at the previous operation and the procedure that was performed (Caspari, Paper presented at the 55th Annual Meeting of the American Academy of Orthopaedic Surgery, Las Vegas, 1989) [3,7•,13••,14].

Contraindications

Contraindications to anterior capsulorrhaphy include those patients with voluntary or multidirectional instability, generalized hyperelasticity, or those patients unable to follow the postoperative rehabilitation requirements. In addition, the operating surgeon should be thoroughly familiar with the arthroscopic technique as well as alternative arthroscopic and open reconstructive techniques should the suture punch capsulorrhaphy prove unsatisfactory.

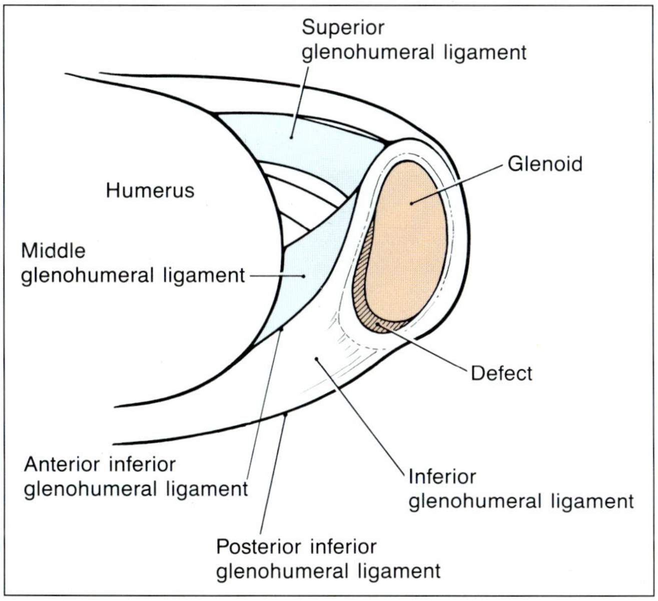

Figure 14-2. The key lesion of anterior instability. The anterior inferior glenohumeral ligament–labral complex is illustrated detached from the anterior-inferior glenoid.

Patient Positioning and Set-up

All reconstructions are performed with the patient under general anesthesia. An examination under anesthesia is done to confirm the diagnosis. This examination is normally done laterally because it allows easier compression of the humeral head into the glenoid. It is also important at this time to check for posterior or multidirectional instability, because this may alter the reconstruction that is required. Comparison should be made with the normal contralateral shoulder.

The patient is then placed in the lateral decubitus position on a bean bag and rolled back 30° to provide adequate access to the anterior aspect of the shoulder. The arm is placed sterilelly in a traction apparatus that allows removal and replacement of the arm in traction without compromising the sterile field. The shoulder should be in a position of 30° to 45° of abduction and 15° of frontal flexion. Ten to 15 lbs of weight is normally used to suspend the shoulder and maintain distraction during the procedure.

A standard posterior visualization portal is established 2 cm inferior and 2 cm medial to the posterolateral corner of the acromion in the mid-equatorial line of the glenohumeral joint. The arthroscopic sheath should be essentially level with the surface of the glenoid and entered directly at the posterior joint line. The portal passes through the interval between the infraspinatus and teres minor to limit damage to either of these musculotendinous structures. The inflow through the arthroscopic sheath is initially utilized. Initial inspection of the joint can be accomplished at this time to confirm the diagnosis and need for reconstruction. After confirming diagnosis, an anterior instrument portal may be established. A superior inflow portal may also be established or a fluid management (pump) system may be used if reconstruction is planned but is not necessary for less extensive procedures.

Several points are key to the success of arthroscopic capsulorrhaphy. These include 1) establishment of the anterior portal at the proper placement from outside to in; 2) rotation of the suture punch when placing the sutures; 3) cornering the drill hole for the transglenoid beath pin; and 4) using a passing suture to pull the sutures through the posterior aspect of the shoulder (Fig. 14-3).

Precise placement of the anterior portal is critical to the success of the procedure. As little as 1 to 2 mm of variation may cause considerable difficulty in adequately placing the sutures or in drilling across the glenoid, while proper placement will insure an easy procedure. This should be accomplished by testing with a spinal needle. The external landmark for placement of this portal is just lateral to the coracoid process, while the intra-articular location is in the rotation interval in a triangular area lateral to the middle glenohumeral ligament, superior to the subscapularis tendon, and inferior to the superior glenohumeral ligament (Fig. 14-4). As the spinal needle enters the joint, the tip should be able to reach the neck of the glenoid at the 1:30 to 2-o'clock position 3 mm or more medial to the edge of the articular surface of the glenoid. It should also be angled so that a projected line through the glenoid neck will exit the infraspinatus fossa posteriorly, 5 cm or more medial to the posterior arthroscopic portal. The needle should also be able to reach the entire anterior labral ligamentous complex from the 12-o'clock to the 6-o'clock positions. When proper placement is confirmed, the anterior portal is established.

Arthroscopic Findings in the Unstable Shoulder

A complete arthroscopic examination of the shoulder should be performed at this time. Findings will include detachment of the AIGHL with or without the labral complex. This will almost always involve the 3-o'clock to 6-o'clock positions of the anterior glenoid, but may extend superiorly up to the biceps tendon and inferiorly to the edge of the posterior inferior glenohumeral ligament. Secondary changes may include a patulous anterior capsule, partial or full-thickness rotator cuff tears, chondromalacia of the anterior glenoid, a superficial or deep Hill-Sachs lesion, or degenerative tears of the anterior labrum.

Arthroscopic Capsulorrhaphy

The area of detachment of the AIGHL-labral complex is noted and then degenerative fraying of the labrum and scar tissue are debrided. This allows for ease of visualization during reconstruction and the preparation of fresh surfaces for healing. Chondromalacic areas of the anterior glenoid can be debrided or abraded as necessary at this time. If the AIGHL-labral complex is intact, but the anterior capsule is incompetent, then an arthroscopic Bankart lesion is created by detaching the capsule from the anterior neck of the glenoid. An estimation of the amount of capsule that will need to be removed is made by mentally projecting a line forward from the plane of the glenoid to where it intersects the anterior capsule. This usually requires resection of no more than 5 to 10 mm of anterior capsule. If the anterior capsuloligamentous structures are very thin or absent, or if the capsular tear is lateral, then the patient is not a candidate for this type of repair.

Another key point of this procedure is adequate abrasion of the anterior glenoid neck. This creates a bleeding surface to allow adequate healing of the capsuloligamentous reconstruction. The abrasion should extend from the superior-most extent of the tear down to the 6-o'clock position on the glenoid. Although this would be difficult to accomplish in a stable shoulder, the anterior instability allows distrac-

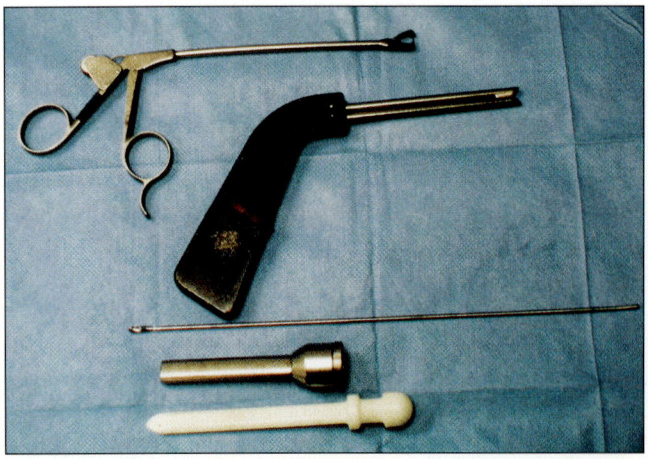

Figure 14-3. Equipment used during capsulorrhaphy. *Top* to *bottom*, suture punch, drill guide, transglenoid beath pin, suture punch cannula with dull trocar.

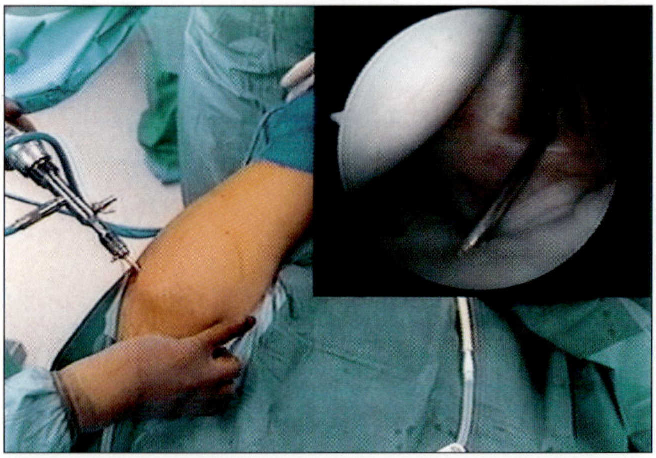

Figure 14-4. Position for establishment of anterior portal.

tion of the humerus, which can be easily accomplished by an assistant, thus affording access to the entire anterior aspect of the glenoid (Fig. 14-5). Adequate abrasion can be assured by checking visually utilizing the 70° arthroscope though the posterior portal, or a standard 30° arthroscope through the anterior portal (Fig. 14-6).

The anterior cannula is then replaced with a suture punch cannula and the suture punch utilized to place six to 10 sutures into the detached labrum-AIGHL complex, depending on the size of the tear. The initial suture is placed at the "V" of the split where the ligament has been torn off (Figs. 14-7 and 14-8). The suture punch is placed into the joint and then rotated into the tear. A size 0 polydioxanone (PDS) suture is usually used at this point and the adequacy of the bite can be tested by pulling on the suture punch. After insuring proper placement, the suture is then fed into the joint. The suture punch is then disengaged from the tissues, rotated back into the joint, and then removed through the suture punch cannula. As it is slowly withdrawn, it is important to keep the suture punch from closing and to continue threading the suture, otherwise breakage will occur. By placing traction on the initial suture, the inferior capsule can be pulled upward, allowing improved access to the infe-

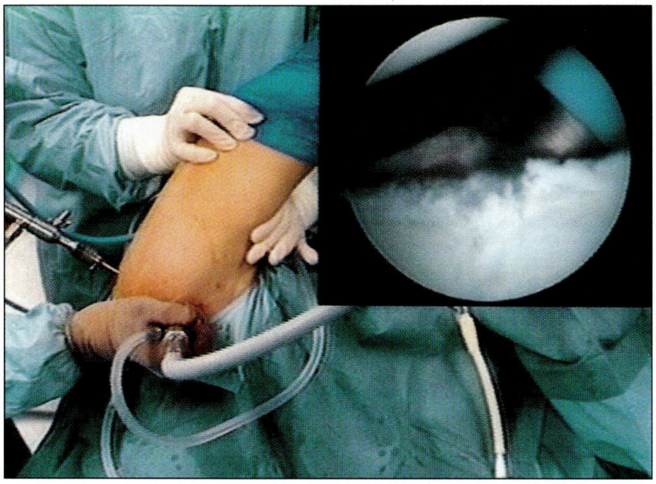

Figure 14-5. The shoulder may be distracted by an assistant during debridement and abrasion of the anterior inferior glenoid neck.

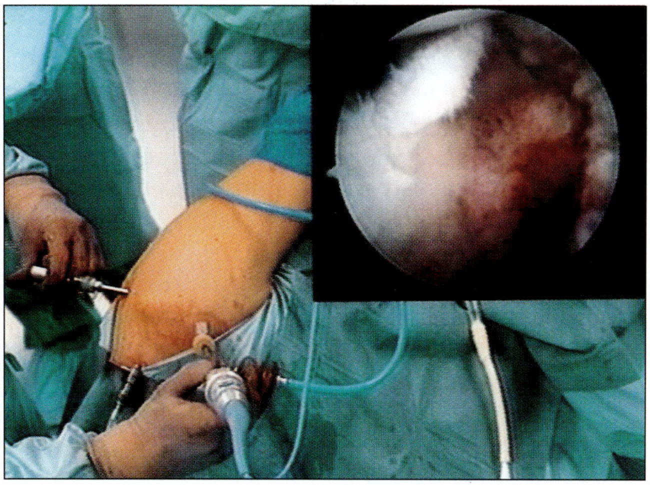

Figure 14-6. View through anterior portal showing abrasion of the anterior-inferior glenoid neck down to bleeding bone.

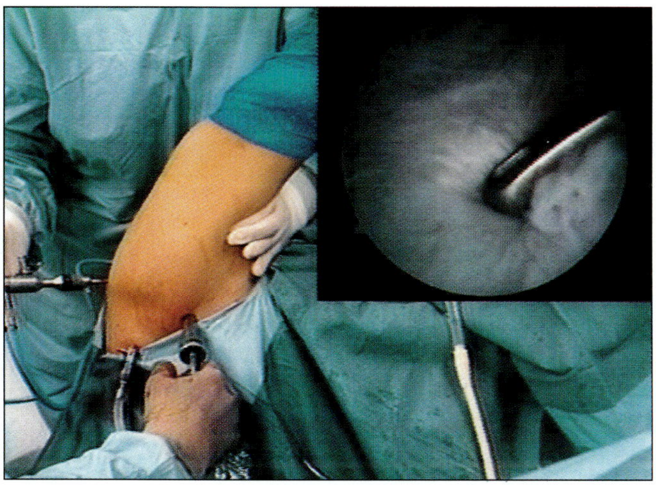

Figure 14-7. Initial suture placement.

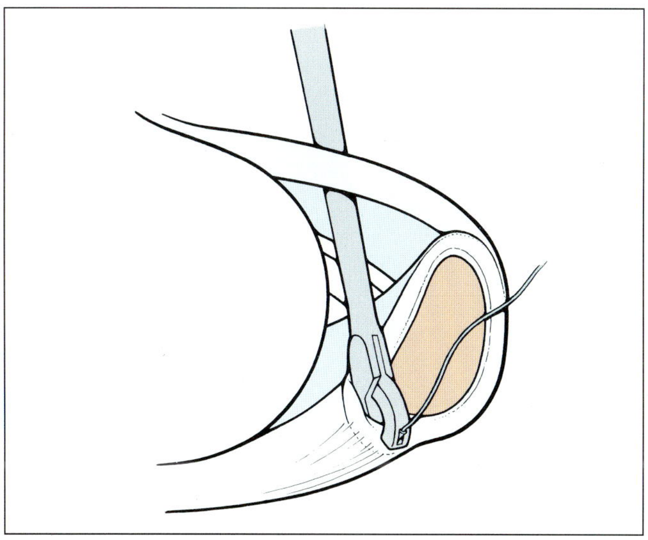

Figure 14-8. Schematic drawing of initial suture placement. A size 0 polydioxanone suture is placed into the "V" of the defect.

rior-most aspect of the capsule and placement of a second 0 PDS suture. These two inferior-most sutures allow improved shifting of the anterior-inferior capsule, thus enhancing the stability of the reconstruction by removing any excess inferior capsular laxity. Two 0 PDS sutures are then placed in sequential fashion approximately 5 mm apart in the anterior capsuloligamentous structures, and all are retracted through the anterior portal. While a simple stitch is often adequate, the anterior capsule can be plicated by placement of a mattress suture. This can be accomplished by taking an initial bite with the suture punch farther into the anterior capsule, then rotating it and punching through the capsule a second time before threading the suture, thus effectively closing the gap.

Once all of the sutures have been positioned, the drill guide is used through the cannula to direct a 3/16-in drill–suture-passer though the glenoid neck from anterior to posterior and out through the infraspinatus fossa. There are two holes on the drill guide. Originally, it was used for allograft reconstruction, and the medial hole was recommended. The lateral hole is now used so that the drill hole can be cornered on the face of the glenoid, allowing the sutures to be advanced upward and anteriorly to more accurately recreate the capsulolabral complex. The starting point is located near the 1:30 to 2-o'clock position on the glenoid face (Figs. 14-9 and 14-10). As the pin is observed to exit posteriorly, a small incision is made to allow it to exit the skin. A #2 passing suture is then tied to the eyelet at the end of the pin, and the reconstructive sutures are then placed through this passing suture. By pulling on the beath pin, the passing suture and subsequent reconstructive sutures are pulled through the glenoid and out through the posterior incision. As traction is applied to the sutures, the superior shift of the capsule is visualized, and satisfactory reduction and stability can be confirmed (Figs. 14-11 and 14-12). The AIGHL-labral complex is seen to be reconstituted as it is advanced superiorly and medially against the abraded glenoid neck. The arm is then removed from traction and adducted and internally rotated to remove the stress on the anterior capsule. The sutures are pulled tightly to approximate the repaired ligament to the glenoid neck. The sutures are then divided into two bundles by individually tensioning each suture. After proper tensioning is accomplished, one or both bundles of suture are passed through the infraspinatus fascia before tying (Fig. 14-13).

If further arthroscopic procedures are to be performed, the sutures are passed posteriorly, but not tensioned before proceeding with subacromial arthroscopy or other required procedures. After all procedures have been completed and the posterior suture is tied, the anterior and posterior incisions are sutured and a dressing and shoulder immobilizer are applied. This procedure can easily be accomplished in an outpatient setting and the patient can return home within 2 to 4 hours following the procedure.

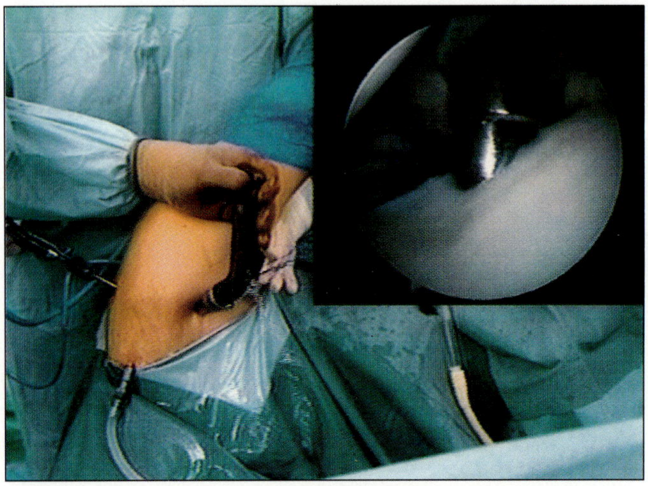

Figure 14-9. Placement of drill guide for the transglenoid beath pin.

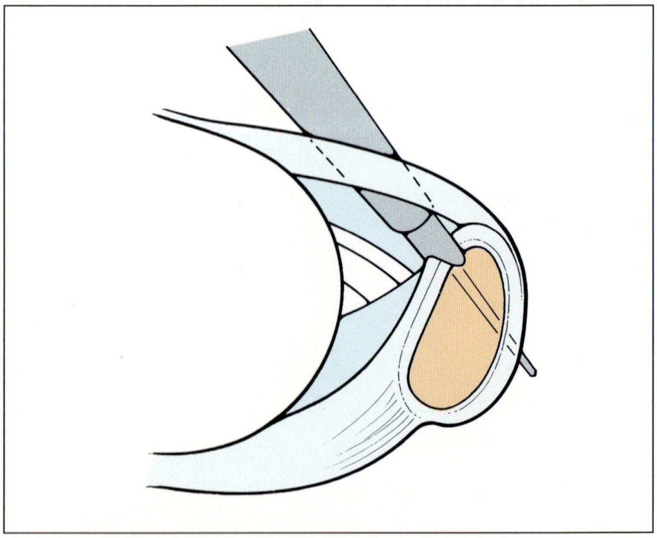

Figure 14-10. Schematic drawing of placement of the drill guide for the transglenoid pin. The drill guide should be placed at approximately the 10:30 position in a left shoulder and at the 1:30 position in a right shoulder.

Postoperative Regimen

The arm is maintained in an immobilizer and the patient is instructed to leave it on until the first postoperative visit, usually at 7 to 10 days following surgery. Patients are also instructed in routine wound management, which consists of removal of the dressing at 48 hours and replacement with band-aids. After the first postoperative visit, the patient is allowed to wear a sling during the day. Depending on the age and confidence in his or her compliance, the patient may begin a gentle range of motion. This consists of gentle active-assisted exercises in frontal flexion and external rotation to neutral. It is strongly emphasized to the patient that these exercises are to be done within the limits of comfort and should not produce pain. At 4 weeks following surgery, the sling is discontinued but may be intermittently used for an additional 2 weeks. The immobilizer is maintained while sleeping until 6 weeks following the procedure. Physical therapy is begun at 4 weeks emphasizing range of motion exercises but avoidance of a position of abduction and external rotation. Range of motion and strengthening is advanced at the tolerance of the patient. By 6 weeks postoperatively, all immobilization is discontinued and the patient is begun on a more aggressive range of motion and strengthening program. Full range of motion should be achieved by 8 to 12 weeks. Functional rehabilitation of athletes is also begun at this time and may continue for as long as 6 months postoperatively. Noncontact athletes may begin competition at 3 months, but strenuous contact athletes, such as football players, should avoid participation for a minimum of 6 months postoperatively.

RESULTS

In our patient series, to determine the efficacy of the Caspari technique, we dealt with 163 patients with traumatic anterior instability during a 3-year period

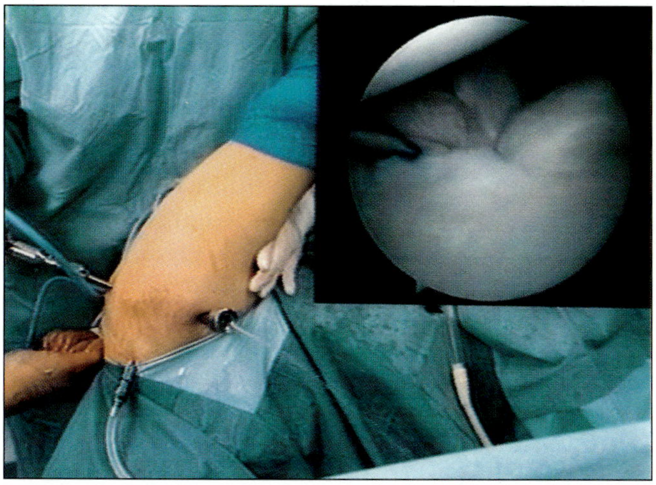

Figure 14-11. Tensioning of sutures, showing shift of capsule and reduction of humerus head.

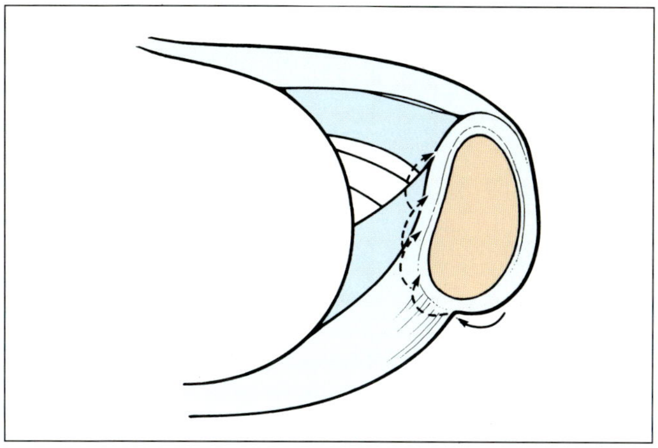

Figure 14-12. Illustration of the capsuloligamentous shift that is created by reconstruction.

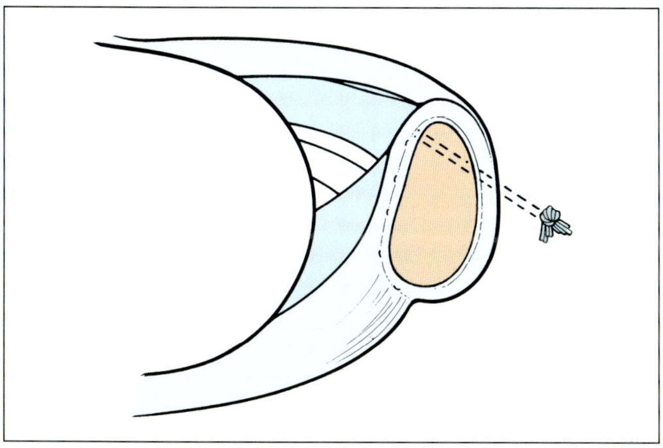

Figure 14-13. The sutures are tied posteriorly over the infraspinatus fascia.

(Savoie, Paper presented at Arthroscopy Specialty Day, AAOS, New Orleans, 1994). One hundred sixty-one of these patients were re-examined with a minimum of 2 years follow-up. Repair was satisfactory in 91% of these patients. Outcome in 14 patients was classified as failure, which was defined as any reported episode of subluxation or dislocation. All throwing athletes were able to return to their sport at or above their previous level of competition. These results were quite favorable when compared with other reports of arthroscopic procedures. Caspari [7•] published a 96% success rate using the suture punch technique in the first 50 patients in his series. Morgan [9] has reported a 100% success rate in a limited number of patients operated on under very strict guidelines. However, Grana and coworkers [18•] found only a 54% success rate in his series of patients utilizing the Caspari technique.

In our current study, there was a clear association between age and the failure rate of this procedure. Younger age was clearly associated with an increased incidence of failure. In those patients aged 22 years or older a 98% satisfactory rate was noted but in those patients 16 years of age or younger the success rate was only 76%. Simply by excluding these patients, the success rate for the remaining patients (age ≥ 17) is 94%.

Reeves [19] has noted that the attachment of the ligaments and labrum to the glenoid does not fully mature until the latter half of the midteens, indicating that failure in the younger age group may not be a failure of the procedure, but rather a failure of the healed structures to maintain adequate strength.

Complications

Of the 14 failed outcomes in our series, three of the patients had a single episode of subluxation, underwent rehabilitation, and had no further symptoms. Three patients had a single episode of a dislocation that reduced spontaneously. None of these patients have yet required reconstruction. Eight patients had multiple recurrences of dislocation. Six of these patients underwent an open reconstructive procedure. A seventh patient had a reconstructive procedure performed by another surgeon that failed and is planning a third reconstructive procedure. No other complications were noted in this series.

Two complications were reported in the series by Caspari [7•]. One patient who received reconstruction with a nonabsorbable suture tied posteriorly over a button outside the skin developed a synovial fistula through the glenoid neck to the posterior incision. Open debridement of the posterior incision and removal of the suture eradicated the fistula with no apparent sequelae. One additional patient with a combined instability and rotator cuff debridement had persistent weakness and required open rotator cuff repair one year following reconstruction, at which time the labral repair was noted to have healed.

CONCLUSIONS

Arthroscopic capsulorrhaphy of anterior instability provides results similar to those reported by Rowe with the open Bankart procedure. The procedure can be accomplished on an outpatient basis through minimal incisions and puncture wounds. Complications are low. Patient morbidity is greatly reduced without compromising long-term results. In our patient series, satisfactory results were achieved in 91% of the patients. There appears to be an age-related association with failure of the procedure. In those patients who were age 17 and older, 94% satisfactory results were noted but only 76% satisfactory results were seen in those patients 16 years and under. We feel this technique may have limited indications in those individuals aged 16 years or under.

REFERENCES AND RECOMMENDED READING

Papers of particular interest, published recently, have been highlighted as

- • Of special interest
- •• Of outstanding interest

1. Perthes G: Uber Operationen der habituellen Schulterluxation. *DTZ Chir* 1906, 85:199.

2. Bankart ASB: Recurrent or habitual dislocation of the shoulder. *Br Med J* 1923, 2:1132.

3. Bankart ASB: The pathology and treatment of the recurrent dislocations of the shoulder joint. *Br J Surg* 1938, 23–29.

4. Turkel SJ, Panio MW, Marshall JL, *et al.*: Stabilizing mechanisms preventing anterior dislocation of the glenohumeral joint. *J Bone Joint Surg* 1981, 63A:1208–1217.

5. Rowe CR: Dislocations of the shoulder. In *The Shoulder*. Edited by Rowe CR. New York: Churchill Livingstone; 1988:165.

6. Rowe CR, Patel D, Southmayd WW: The Bankart procedure. A long term end result study. *J Bone Joint Surg* 1978, 60A:1–16.

7.• Caspari RB, Savoie FH, Myers JF, *et al.*: Arthroscopic reconstruction of anterior shoulder instability. In *Surgery of the Shoulder*. Edited by Post M, Morrey BF, Hawkins RJ. Chicago: Mosby-Yearbook; 1990.

A description of the early results of the Caspari technique for shoulder instability.

8. Eyre-Brook AL: Recurrent dislocation of the shoulder. Lesions discovered in seventeen cases, surgery employed and immediate report of results. *J Bone Joint Surg* 1948, 30B:39.

9. Morgan CD, Bodenstab AB: Arthroscopic Bankart suture repair: technique and early results. *Arthroscopy* 1987, 3:111.

10. Dutoit GT, Roux D: Recurrent dislocation of the shoulder. A 24 year study of the Johannesburg stapling operation. *J Bone Joint Surg* 1956, 38A:1–12.

11. McGlynn FJ, Caspari RB: Arthroscopic findings in the subluxating shoulder. *Clin Orthop* 1984, 183:173.

12. Gallie WE, Lemesurier AB: Recurring dislocation of the shoulder. *J Bone Joint Surg* 1948, 30B:9

13.•• Caspari RB, Savoie FH: Arthroscopic reconstruction of the shoulder: the Bankart repair (suture technique) In *Operative Arthroscopy*. edn 2. Edited by McGinty JB, Caspari RB, Jackson RW, Poehling GG. New York: Raven Press; 1995.

A comprehensive description of the technique of arthroscopic suture reconstruction with an excellent historical overview.

14. Johnson LL: Shoulder arthroscopy. In *Arthroscopic Surgery: Principles and Practice*. Edited by Johnson LL. St. Louis: Mosby-Yearbook; 1986:1301–1445.

15. Matthews LS, Vetter WL, Oweida SJ, *et al.*: Arthroscopic staple capsulorrhaphy for recurrent anterior shoulder instability. *Arthroscopy* 1988, 4:106–111.

16.• Neviaser TJ: The anterior labroligamentous periosteal sleeve avulsion lesion: A cause of anterior instability of the shoulder. *Arthroscopy* 1993, 9:17–21.

A superb description of a seldom recognized pathologic variant of which all surgeons must be aware.

17. Neviaser RJ, Neviaser TJ, Nevaiser JS: Concurrent rupture of the rotator cuff and anterior dislocation of the shoulder in the older patient. *J Bone Joint Surg* 1988, 70A:1308–1311.

18.• Grana WA, Buckley PD, Yates CK: Arthroscopic Bankart suture repair. *Am J Sports Med* 1993, 21:348.

This article details the problems that may be encountered during the "learning curve" of arthroscopic reconstruction.

19. Reeves B: Experiments on the tensile strength of the anterior capsular structures of the shoulder in man. *J Bone Joint Surg* 1968, 50B:858–865.

15

CHAPTER

Shoulder Capsulorrhaphy Using Suture Anchors and Nonabsorbable Sutures

STEPHEN J. SNYDER AND JOHN P. BELZER

Nearly a century has passed since Perthes described the essential lesion in the shoulder following a traumatic anterior shoulder dislocation [1]. In his two publications, Bankart further highlighted this pathology, which now bears his name [2,3]. More than 100 techniques for surgical stabilization of traumatic shoulder instability have since been described. These include capsular repair procedures, such as the Bankart repair, subscapularis advancing procedures, such as the Magnusson-Stack, and bony procedures, such as the Bristow-Laterjet. Although all of these techniques have been shown to be relatively successful, the Bankart repair remains the standard of surgical treatment with which all other methods are compared.

Rowe [4], in a clinical series of long-term follow-up of Bankart repairs, reported a 96% success rate. Rowe [5] later stated that "it is timely that surgery of the shoulder advance to careful atraumatic technique preserving the viability, motion, and function of shoulder tissues so that the patient obtains a free, unrestrained, strong, and coordinated shoulder."

With the advent of arthroscopic technology, the concept of atraumatic shoulder surgery has reached a higher level while maintaining a successful clinical outcome. Arthroscopic surgery affords the surgeon the opportunity to directly visualize the glenohumeral pathology, and in conjunction with physical findings and imaging studies, tailor treatment appropriately. Arthroscopic capsulorrhaphy using suture anchors is a versatile and effective method of treating anterior shoulder instability by adhering to these atraumatic principles [6,7]. In addition, Green and Cristensen [8••] reported a significant reduction in operative time, perioperative complications, days of hospitalization, and other important parameters following arthroscopic stabilization when compared with a similar open procedure.

PATHOPHYSIOLOGY

Several reports in the literature support the role of the subscapularis in providing anterior shoulder stability [8••,9]. However, the majority of both the basic science and clinical literature implicate the anterior capsulolabral structures, specifically the inferior glenohumeral ligament anterior labral complex, as the stabilizing factors with the arm in a position of 90° of abduction [10–12,13•,14,15] (Fig. 15-1).

Turkel and coworkers [11], using selective cutting techniques in a cadaveric model, demonstrated the stabilizing role of the inferior glenohumeral ligament with the arm in the position of risk, greater than 90° abduction, and external rotation. When this ligament was left intact while all other structures were cut, the shoulder remained stable. O'Brien [12] similarly demonstrated the importance of the posterior inferior glenohumeral ligament in preventing posterior instability with the arm in internal rotation.

Reeves [16] reported on the tensile strength of the anterior capsulolabral ligaments and their injury pattern following anterior dislocation. He noted in a cadaveric study that the force needed to avulse the labrum from the anterior glenoid increased from 15 kg in infancy to 64 kg at 25 years of age. Anterior dislocation was found to avulse the labrum from the glenoid in shoulders of patients under 45 years of age, whereas capsular rupture and subscapularis injury occurred in shoulders of patients over 45 years. He concluded that acute anterior dislocation of the shoulder occurs with failure of the weakest anterior shoulder structures, and it is this weakest point that influences recurrent instability.

It is the labral avulsion pattern of injury—and thus the younger patient population—that appears to be more prone to recurrent instability. Rowe [4] reported in his clinical series of Bankart repairs that approxi-

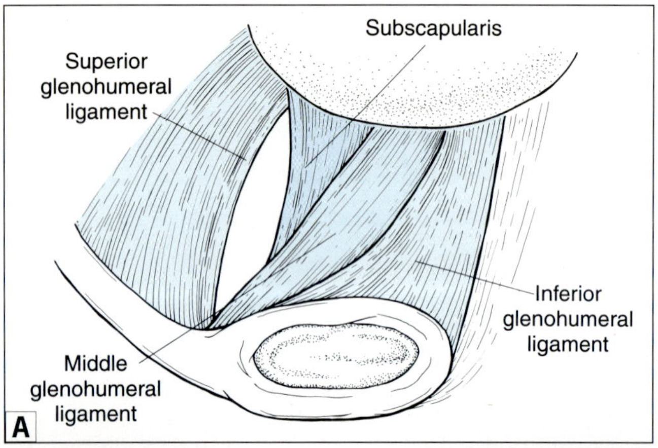

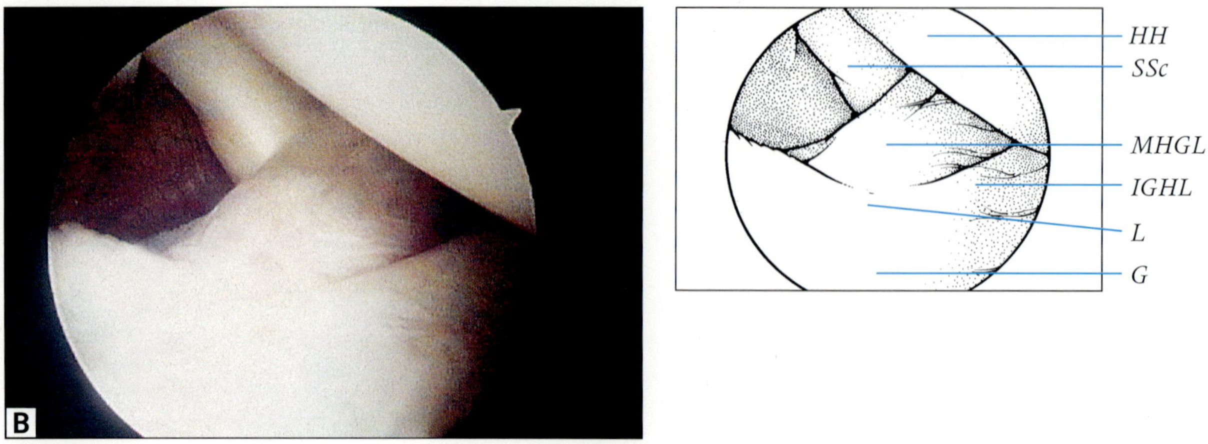

Figure 15-1. Classic ligament pattern of normal shoulder anatomy. **A**, graphic depiction, **B**, arthroscopic view. G—glenoid; HH—humeral head; IGHL—inferior glenohumeral ligament; L—labrum; MGHL—middle glenohumeral ligament; SSc—subscapularis tendon.

mately 85% of patients with recurrent anterior instability had an avulsion of the labrum from the anterior glenoid noted at the time of reconstructive surgery. Of the 15% of patients without a Bankart lesion, over half were patients with atraumatic instability. Less than 1% of his patients were noted at the time of surgery to have a deficient subscapularis. Similarly, in other clinical studies, abnormalities of the labrum were noted arthroscopically in all patients with subluxating shoulders [15] and in the majority of patients with dislocating shoulders [13•].

HISTORY

Arthroscopic techniques for the treatment of traumatic anterior instability have been derived from previously described open techniques. These include transglenoid suturing techniques, stapling techniques, and more recently, methods using suture anchors. The transglenoid technique has had good clinical success [8••,17,18]. However, this technique requires significant technical skill to avoid complications such as penetration of the articular surface of the glenoid and damage to the suprascapular nerve during passage of the suture pin [7]. In addition, the sutures passed in this technique are tied over the infraspinatus fascia, which is often distended with extravasated fluid. This may result in loosening of the repair over a short period with reabsorption of this fluid [6]. The arthroscopic stapling technique has not been as successful in long-term clinical follow-up [19], and the use of staples has been associated with complications due to loosening and migration of the implants [20].

Among instruments designed or modified for arthroscopic surgery, suture anchors have been adapted for arthroscopic use and have proven to be a viable alternative to the techniques previously described [7]. The use of suture anchors provides the arthroscopic surgeon with a versatile system in which the labral structures can be repaired anatomically to the anterior glenoid. Additionally, capsular tissue can be mobilized and if necessary advanced or plicated to address associated laxity of these anterior structures that may have developed with multiple subluxations or dislocations.

SURGICAL INDICATIONS

Arthroscopic shoulder stabilization procedures continue to be modified and improved. Patients with an *A*traumatic, *M*ultidirectional, *B*ilateral, responding to *R*ehabilitation and—if surgery is necessary—*I*nferior capsular shift should be performed (AMBRI) type of shoulder instability infrequently have traumatic structural abnormalities [21]. Patients with an AMBRI shoulder disability should be treated with exercise programs that strengthen the rotator cuff and learn to avoid positions of risk [22]. If these patients do not respond to a rehabilitation program, we sometimes perform an arthroscopic capsular plication technique (Snyder, personal communication) or an open capsular shift surgery [23] which does not require the use of suture anchors.

Patients with a *T*raumatic, *U*nidirectional, with *B*ankart lesion, responding to *S*urgery (TUBS) type of shoulder instability, in contradistinction, have been noted to have a Bankart lesion in 85% of the cases [4]. When presenting the surgeon with recurrent instability, TUBS patients represent the ideal candidate for arthroscopic repair with suture anchors. In addition, Rowe [4] reported that in patients under 20 years of age, the redislocation rate in patients presenting traumatic instability was more than 90%. Other studies have reported similarly high redislocation rates [24]. Because of the high recurrence rate in this age group, particularly in athletes [25], we recommend counseling these patients and their parents regarding the likelihood of recurrent dislocation and presenting the patients with the option of undergoing arthroscopic repair following the first dislocation.

TECHNIQUE

Equipment

There are many variations on the suture anchor. The suture anchor design must fulfill two criteria. First, the anchor should fixate into the bone tunnel firmly and have a pull-out strength approaching or ideally surpassing the tensile strength of the suture being used. Second, the suture anchor must have an eyelet that allows for sliding of the selected suture, which facilitates knot tying. The anchors we prefer allow for passage of a #2 braided nonabsorbable suture.

We are currently using the Mini Revo (Linvatec Corp., Largo, FL) and the Mitek GII (Mitek Surgical Products, Westwood, MA) suture anchor for the majority of our capsulorrhaphies (Fig. 15-2A). The Mitek anchor consists of a titanium core with two wire arcs. These arcs flex with insertion of the anchor, and following insertion, the arcs re-expand to seat the anchor firmly in the glenoid, preventing potential dislodging. The pull-out strength of the Mitek GII anchor is approximately equal to the tensile strength of a #2 braided suture [26]. The disadvantage of the Mitek anchor is that it is a permanent implant. If complications occur such as knot locking prior to tightening, suture breakage, or inadvertent unloading of the suture of an implanted anchor, the anchor is not retrievable and remains imbedded in bone, functionless.

For this reason, we have used two other devices, the Mini Revo and the absorbable Bio Anchor (Linvatec Corp., Largo, FL), the latter on an investigational basis (Figs. 15-2B and 15-2C). The Mini-Revo is a threaded anchor that is screwed into bone. This anchor offers the benefit of being easily retrievable should suture failure occur intraoperatively or if repeat surgery is necessary at a future date. The Bio Anchor is a bioabsorbable implant that is impacted into a bone tunnel. It is made of a polylactide polymer that maintains its strength for over 6 months. This allows adequate time for the repaired anterior structures to heal before subsequent reabsorption of the implant. The Bio Anchor is not retrievable but may be drilled out should a complication occur.

Prior to implantation, the suture anchors are each loaded with a #2 braided nonabsorbable suture. The authors feel that a nonabsorbable suture is preferable to an absorbable suture, because it ensures that the labral repair is firmly held in proper position for an adequate period of time to allow for healing. This gives added security against premature suture breakage in the young, active population. The absorbable suture has been shown to lose some of its tensile strength within a few weeks, potentially before complete healing of labrum to bone has occurred [27].

The use of a nonabsorbable braided suture has become feasible with the advent of the Shuttle Relay (Linvatec Corp., Largo, FL) (Fig. 15-3A). The Shuttle is a nylon-coated, multistrand wire measuring 30 inches in length. At the midpoint of the Shuttle, the wire is exposed and strands are separated, forming an eyelet for passage of the suture. The Shuttle is passed through labral or ligament tissue by using instruments such as a modified suture punch (Fig. 15-3B), a suture hook device (Fig. 15-3C), or a 17-gauge epidural needle (Fig. 15-3D). It can then be used to "shuttle" the strong, flexible, braided suture through these tissues in either an anterograde or retrograde fashion to form a simple stitch, figure-of-eight stitch, or mattress stitch.

The loop-handled knot pusher is a 10-cm rod with an eyelet on one end and thumb loop on the other (Fig. 15-3E). One strand of the suture is passed through the eyelet of the knot pusher, allowing for the throws of the knots to be made extra-articularly and then advanced down a cannula intra-articularly to secure the desired structures.

Operating Room Set-up

A complete discussion of operating room set-up for arthroscopy of the shoulder is beyond the scope of this chapter. Here we describe our basic techniques and highlight points that we feel are essential in performing a successful capsulorrhaphy with suture anchors.

Prior to arriving in the operating room, the patient may choose to undergo an interscalene block. The advantages of this procedure are excellent postoperative analgesia and motor block, which help to prevent the patient from injuring the shoulder in the immediate postoperative period. Once in the operating room, the patient is given a general anesthetic and supported in the lateral decubitus position with a vacuum bean bag. The surgical table is rotated 45° to allow the surgeon easy access to both anterior and posterior shoulder portals.

The involved shoulder is examined thoroughly for range of motion and stability. Attention is paid to the direction and magnitude of any laxity observed.

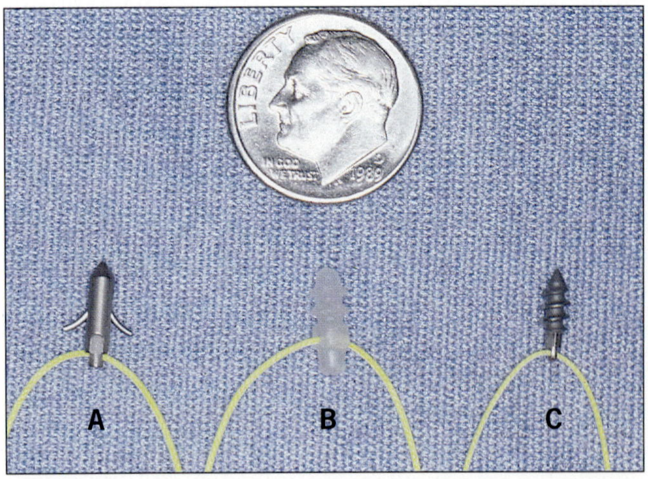

Figure 15-2. Suture anchors used in arthroscopic stabilization, **A**, Mini Revo (Linvatec Corp., Largo, FL), **B**, Bio Anchor (Linvatec Corp., Largo, FL), **C**, Mitek GII (Mitek Surgical Products, Westwood, MA).

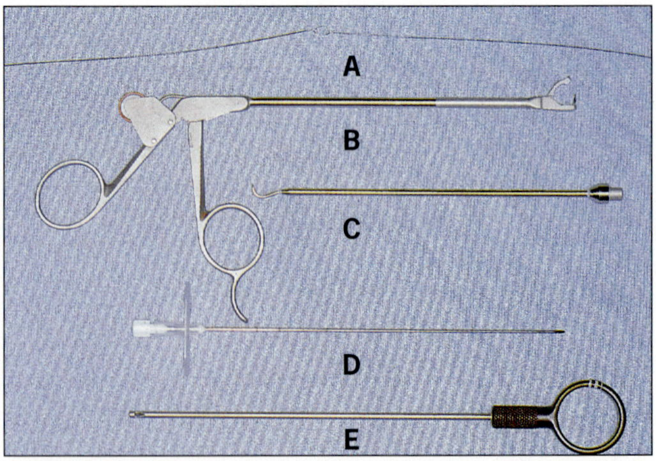

Figure 15-3. Equipment used for suture anchor capsulorrhaphy. **A**, Shuttle Relay (Linvatec Corp., Largo, FL), **B**, modified Caspari suture punch (Linvatec Corp., Largo, FL), **C**, suture hook (Linvatec Corp., Largo, FL), **D**, 17-gauge epidural needle, and, **E**, loop-handled knot pusher.

The shoulder and arm are then cleansed with an antimicrobial solution and a surgical drape is applied. We prefer a specialty drape that includes a collection bag to minimize arthroscopic fluid spillage on the patient's head and neck and to help keep the floor dry. The arm is placed in a sterile foam shoulder traction and rotation sleeve (STaR; Arthrex, Naples, FL), which is subsequently attached to the Arthrex shoulder traction apparatus (Arthrex, Naples, FL). These two items are designed to work together (Fig. 15-4A). The Arthrex shoulder holder allows for easy and rapid positioning of the arm in both the glenohumeral and bursal arthroscopy positions. The upper bar is an adjustable telescopic arm. When extended, it allows for use of a sterile lateral traction strap to apply direct lateral traction and rotation of the shoulder (Fig. 15-4B). The use of the lateral traction strap is necessary to distract the humerus away from the glenoid and internally rotate the extremity, reducing tension of the anterior structures during surgical repair.

For all shoulder arthroscopic procedures, we use an arthroscopic fluid pump system and a 30° video arthroscope. The pump supplies a variable flow of fluid to maintain a set intra-articular pressure. This helps minimize bleeding and maintains a desired joint distention during the procedure.

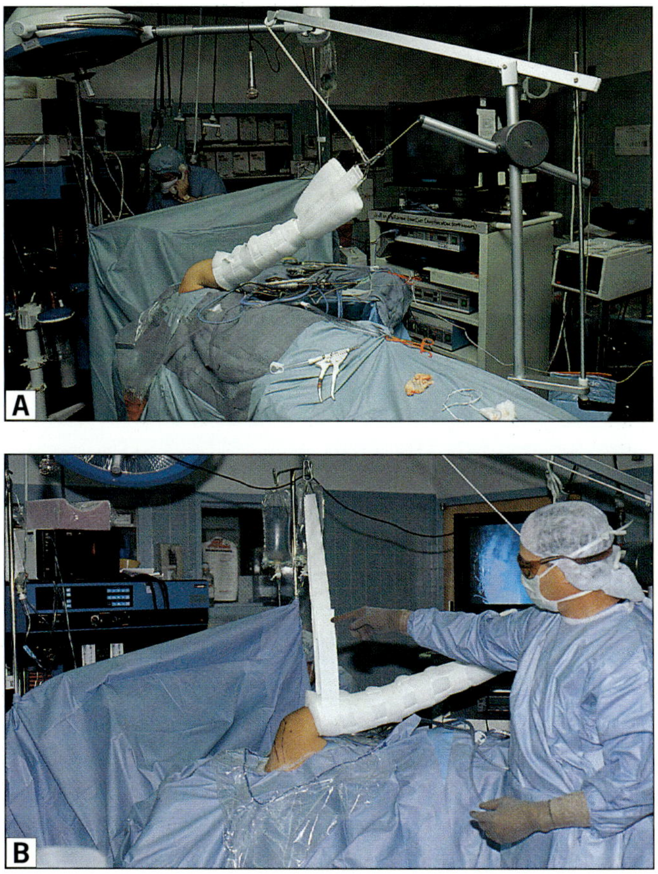

Figure 15-4. **A**, STaR sleeve (Arthrex, Naples, FL) and Arthrex shoulder traction apparatus (Arthrex, Naples, FL) in position for diagnostic arthroscopy. **B**, Lateral traction strap applied to proximal aspect of STaR sleeve for appropriate arm position for arthroscopic anterior capsulorrhaphy.

SURGICAL TECHNIQUE

Portals

Standard arthroscopy portals previously described by Wolf [28] are used for this technique with a few variations. A posterior portal is created 2 to 3 cm medial and 4 to 5 cm caudal to the posterolateral corner of the acromion. This portal is used for visualization during the procedure.

Two anterior portals are established. The anterosuperior portal is created after the posterior portal by passing the arthroscope, under visual control, just superior to the biceps tendon in the rotator interval. Once in this position, the arthroscope is removed from the sheath and a switching stick is inserted and advanced anteriorly through the capsule and into a subcutaneous position 2 cm inferior to the anterior acromial edge. A superficial skin incision is made and a second cannula is advanced over the switching stick into the joint in a retrograde fashion.

Using these two portals, the diagnostic portion of the procedure is performed. The anterior midglenoid portal is created prior to performing the Bankart repair. This is performed only after the arm has been placed in two-point traction as described by Gross [29]. The portal is created using an outside-in technique. A 5-mm superficial skin incision is made approximately 4 cm inferior and 2 cm lateral from the anterosuperior portal, well lateral to the tip of the coracoid process. A 6-mm operating cannula with a blunt obturator is passed through the anterior structures and penetrates the joint at the superior margin of the subscapularis tendon, approximately 3 cm lateral to the glenoid. By creating the two anterior portals at the opposite borders of the rotator interval, the distance between the two anterior cannulae is maximized to facilitate concomitant instrumentation from the anterior portals.

Diagnostic Arthroscopy

The shoulder is initially held in 70° of abduction and 10° of flexion with approximately 10 lbs of suspension for diagnostic arthroscopy. A 15-step diagnostic technique previously described by the senior author [30], which includes arthroscopic evaluation of the entire glenohumeral joint from both anterior and posterior portals, is used. This method assures that a thorough examination of the anterior capsuloligamentous and labral structures is performed, and that other pathologic entities, such as the Hill-Sachs lesion or rotator cuff pathology, are documented.

It is imperative that the surgeon be familiar with normal arthroscopic anatomy of the shoulder. The misdiagnosis of such entities as a sublabral hole, a meniscoid labrum, or a Buford complex such as pathologic lesions may lead to inappropriate treatment and result in a poor outcome due to stiffness or pain (Fig. 15-5 A–C).

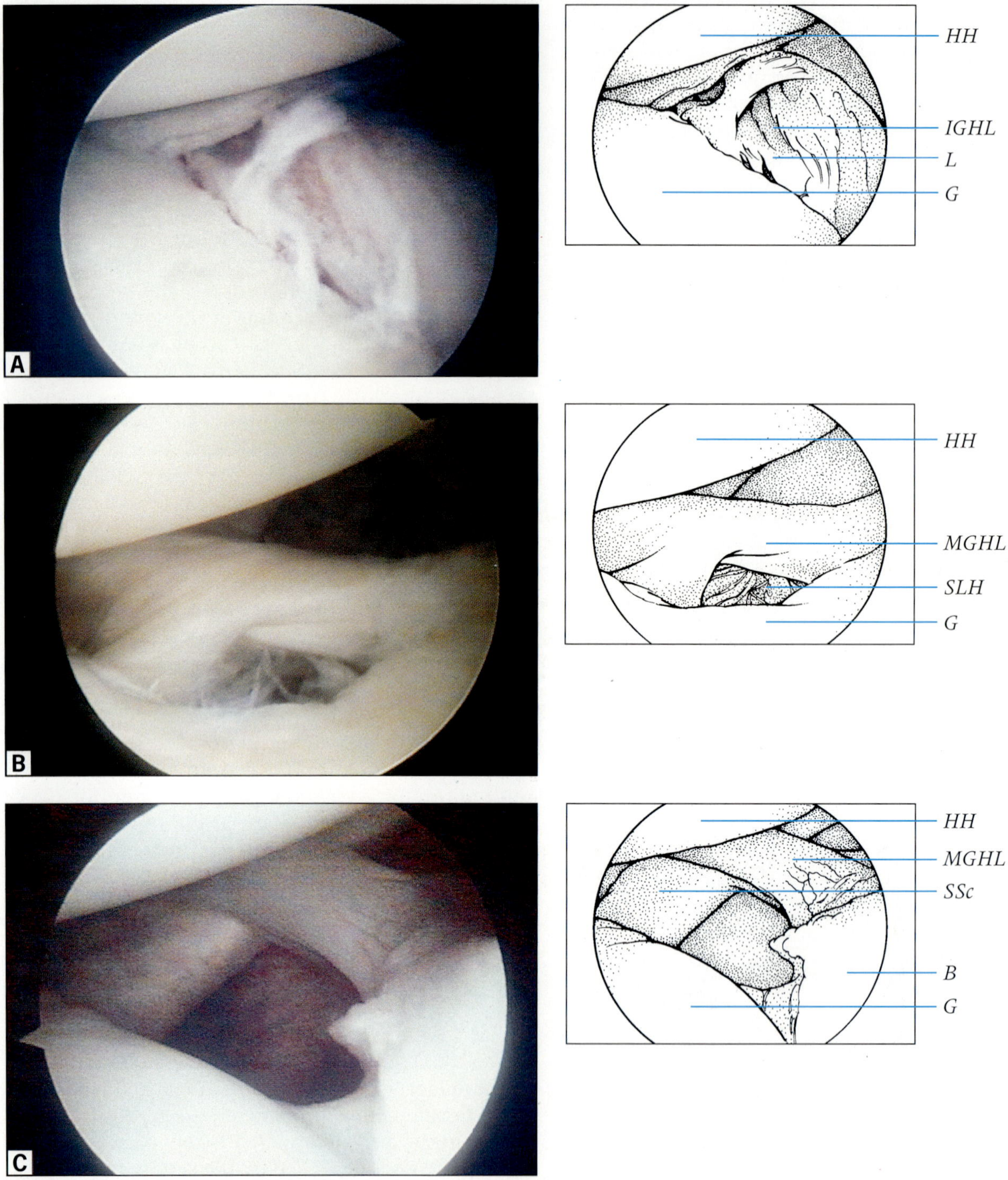

Figure 15-5. Arthroscopic view of pathologic and normal variants of anterior shoulder structures. **A,** Arthroscopic view of Bankart lesion. **B,** Arthroscopic view of sublabral hole, normal variant. **C,** Arthroscopic view of Buford Complex, normal variant. B—biceps tendon; G—glenoid; HH—humeral head; IGHL—inferior glenohumeral ligament; L—labrum; MGHL—middle glenohumeral ligament; SLH—sublabral hole.

Surgical Technique for Anterior Stabilization

Arm Position

Once the diagnostic portion of the arthroscopy is complete and a Bankart lesion has been documented, the surgeon may proceed with the anterior stabilization. The shoulder is placed in two-point traction with the arm in approximately 30° abduction and slight forward flexion. Five lbs of weight are used for distal traction in line with the arm. The 2-in wide lateral traction strap is applied to the most proximal aspect of the STaR sleeve, and 10 to 15 lbs of lateral traction is applied only as long as needed. The arm is held internally rotated by the lateral traction strap to relax the anterior structures. The anterior midglenoid portal is then created.

Glenoid Rim Preparation

With the arthroscope in the anterior superior (AS) portal, a shaver is used through the anterior midglenoid (AMG) portal to debride fibrous tissue from the anterior glenoid rim. Debridement is carried out over the extent of the labral detachment. If the capsulolabral structures are chronically medially retracted and require advancement, an arthroscopic Liberator (Linvatec Corp., Largo, FL) elevator is used to mobilize these tissues from the anterior scapular neck (Fig. 15-6A).

Next, a 4-mm round burr is used to remove a superficial layer of the anterior glenoid bone over the entire region of soft-tissue avulsion from the articular cartilage edge down the glenoid neck medially (Fig. 15-6B). This procedure promotes a fibroblastic healing response. A suction punch is helpful to trim loose articular cartilage and soft tissue from the glenoid edge. This is important because it allows for direct visualization of the subchondral bone of the anterior glenoid rim for accurate placement of the suture anchors.

Imprudent use of the motorized shaver or burr in this part of the procedure can result in damage to the anterior soft-tissue structures, scalloping, or excessive bone excision. To avoid these complications, the burr may be used with the suction closed to avoid winding up of labral tissue. Damage to the anterior soft tissue can limit the surgeon's ability to repair the ligaments adequately to bone. Excessive bone excision from the

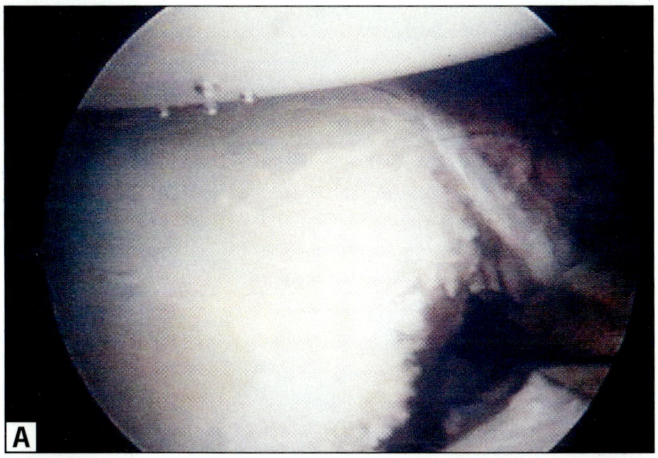

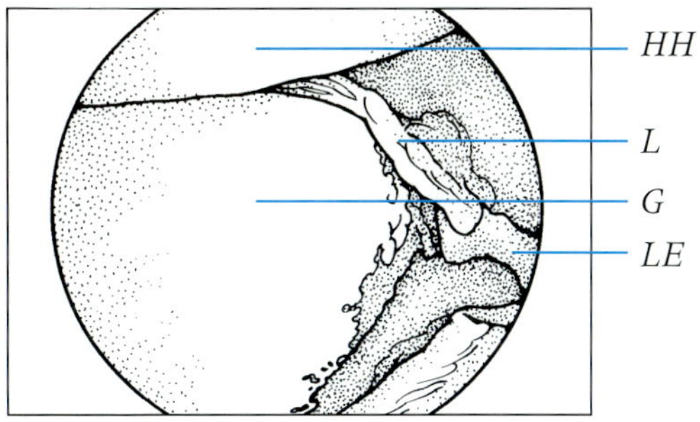

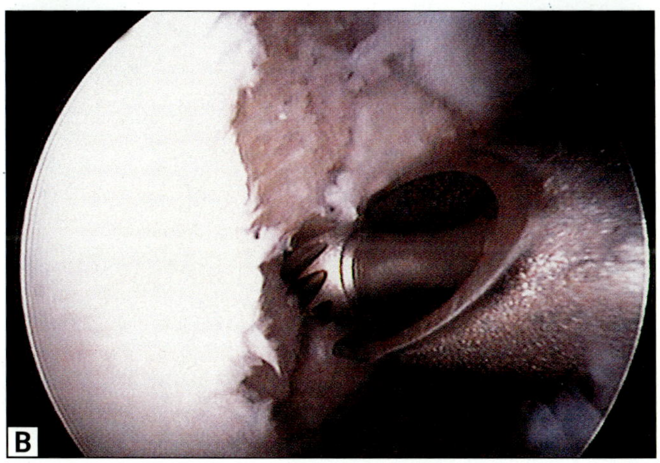

Figure 15-6. A, The Liberator (Linvatec Corp., Largo, FL) elevator in use to elevate and mobilize medially retracted labral and ligamentous structures. G—glenoid; HH—humeral head; L—labrum; LE—Liberator elevator. **B**, Burr removing superficial layer of bone to promote fibroblastic healing response.

anterior glenoid decreases the anteroposterior dimension of the glenoid, which may increase the possibility of redislocation.

Drill Hole Placement

Pilot drill holes are made at the edge of the glenoid (Figs. 15-7A and 15-7B). It is imperative that the drill holes are placed at the corner of the glenoid, slightly on the articular surface. Placement of the holes further medially will result in an inadequate labral repair and possible recurrent instability. Two to four drill holes are made between the 2-o'clock position and the 5-o'clock position. In most cases, three anchors are adequate. We do not use a drill guide, but prefer to place the tip of the drill above the chosen sites and carefully advance into the bone while supporting the spinning shaft with the surgeon's fingers. A small basket punch is used to remove debris from the drill holes so that clear visualization is achieved.

Once the anterior edge of the glenoid has been adequately prepared, it is necessary to exchange the

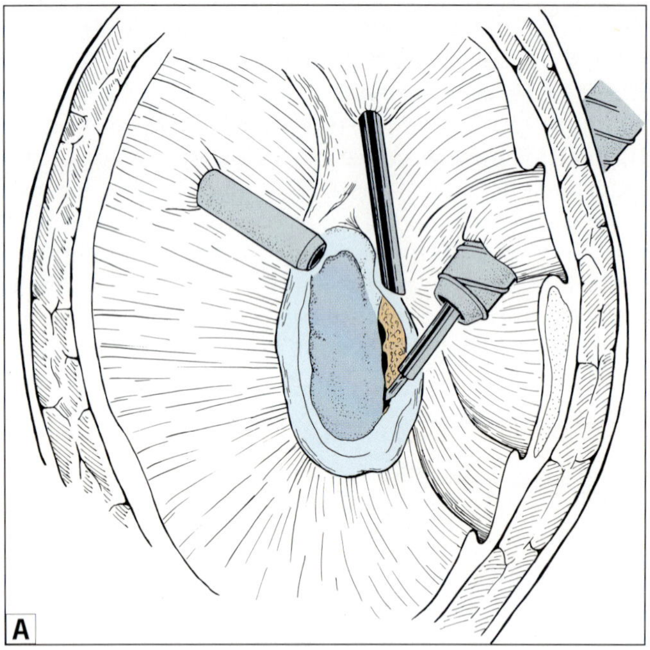

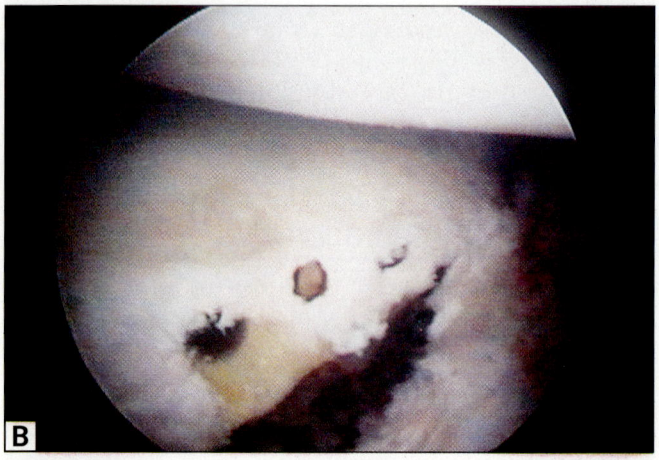

Figure 15-7. Proper placement of suture anchor pilot drill holes on the anterior edge of the articular surface of the glenoid. **A**, Graphic depiction. **B**, Arthroscopic view.

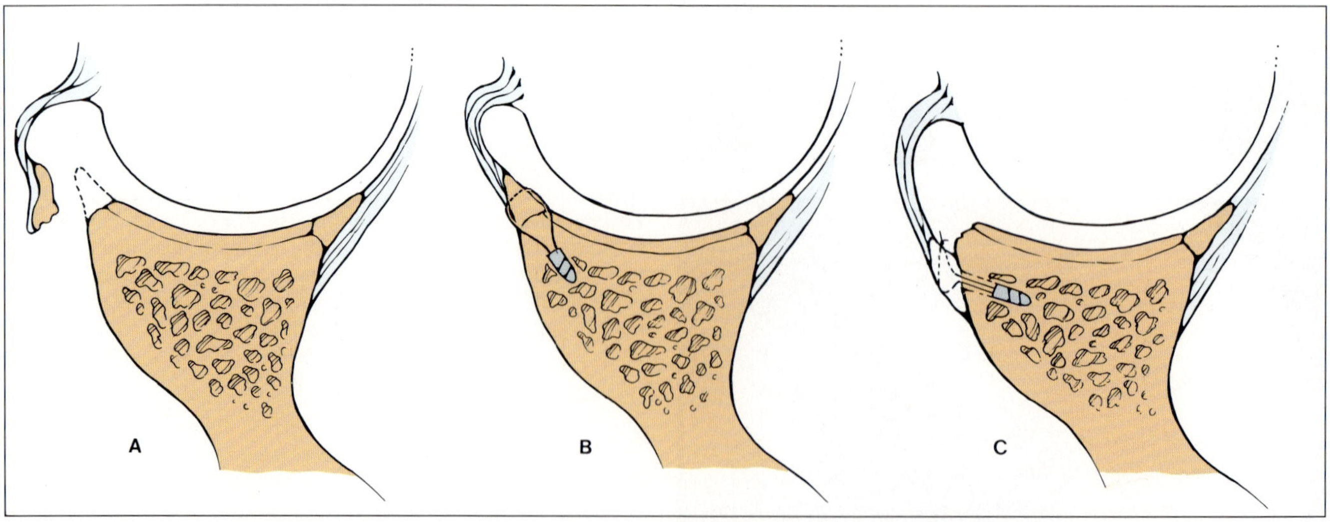

Figure 15-8. **A**, Traumatic anterior shoulder instability usually results in a labral avulsion from the anterior glenoid (Bankart lesion). **B**, Appropriate placement of suture anchors at the edge of the articular surface of the glenoid restores the anatomic attachment of the glenohumeral ligament in addition to recreating normal labral height to improve shoulder instability. **C**, Placement of anchors medially on the neck of the glenoid fail to restore the concavity of the glenoid and may have a less satisfactory result.

AMG operating cannula for an 8.4-mm screw-in operating cannula. This larger cannula is required for the use of the larger capsulorrhaphy instruments. This exchange is easily performed by first enlarging the AMG portal incision slightly and then switching the AMG cannulae over a guiderod.

If the anchor pilot drill holes are made too far medially on the scapular neck, the capsulolabral complex is not advanced to its anatomic position (Fig. 15-8). This fails to reconstitute the normal height of the labrum, a stabilizing mechanism of the glenohumeral joint [31]. It may also result in residual laxity of the ligamentous structures. The surgeon should clear the drill holes of debris; if this is not performed, it may be difficult to locate these holes later at the time of anchor insertion.

Anchor Placement

While viewing through the AS portal, the first anchor is placed through the AMG cannula and inserted into the inferior-most drill hole (Figs. 15-9A and 15-10A). The anchor is then fully seated, either by tapping the inserter with a mallet, in the case of the Mitek or Bio

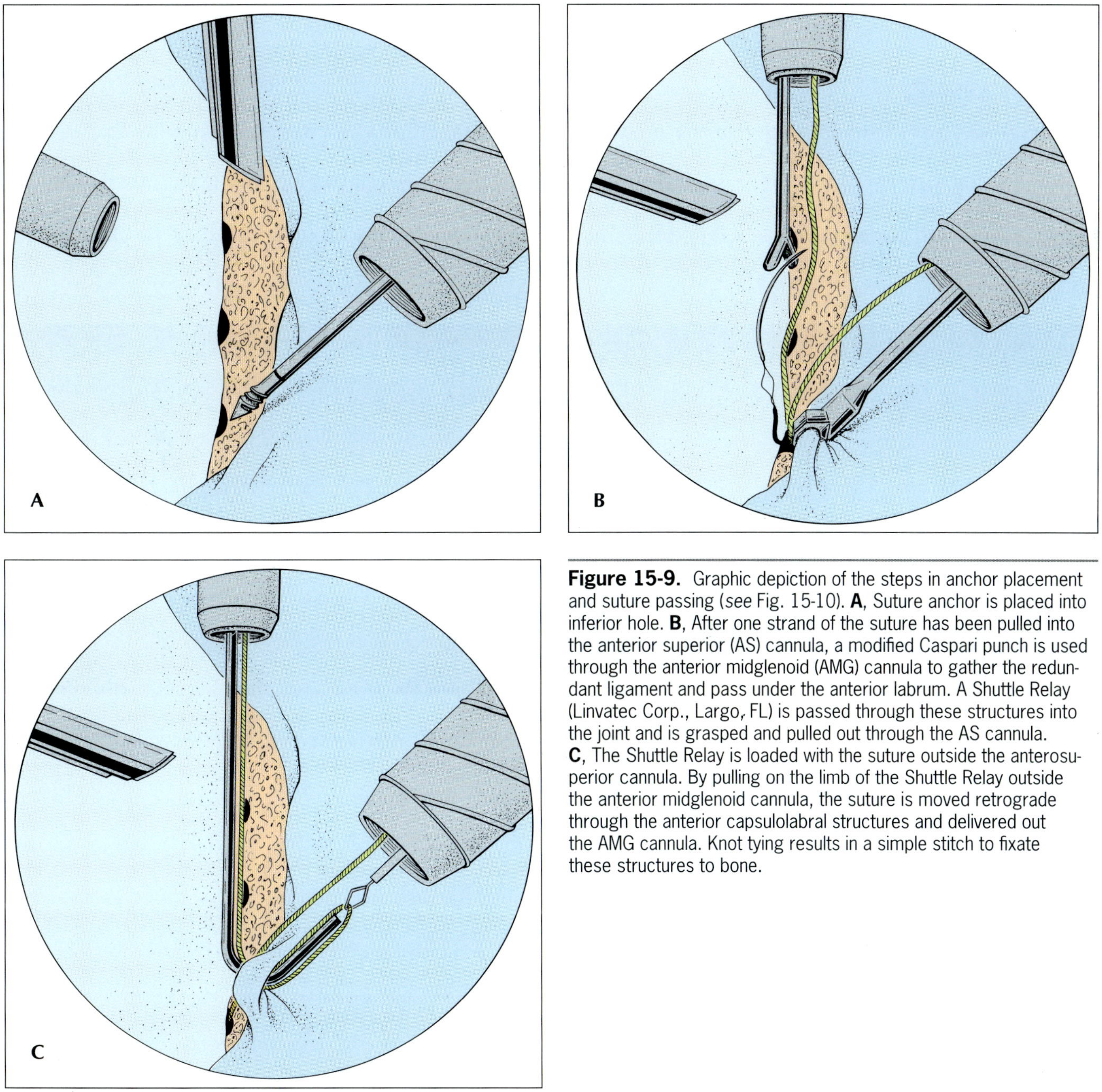

Figure 15-9. Graphic depiction of the steps in anchor placement and suture passing (*see* Fig. 15-10). **A**, Suture anchor is placed into inferior hole. **B**, After one strand of the suture has been pulled into the anterior superior (AS) cannula, a modified Caspari punch is used through the anterior midglenoid (AMG) cannula to gather the redundant ligament and pass under the anterior labrum. A Shuttle Relay (Linvatec Corp., Largo, FL) is passed through these structures into the joint and is grasped and pulled out through the AS cannula. **C**, The Shuttle Relay is loaded with the suture outside the anterosuperior cannula. By pulling on the limb of the Shuttle Relay outside the anterior midglenoid cannula, the suture is moved retrograde through the anterior capsulolabral structures and delivered out the AMG cannula. Knot tying results in a simple stitch to fixate these structures to bone.

Anchor, or by screwing in the implant, in the case of the Mini Revo. The inserter is then removed carefully by retro tapping the handle so as not to pull the sliding suture through the eyelet of the anchor. Once the anchor is seated, tension is placed firmly on the suture to confirm adequate fixation of the anchor in glenoid bone.

The surgeon and operating personnel should confirm that the anchor is firmly attached to the inserter. If the anchor is dislodged from the end of the inserter intra-articularly, it must be removed. The anchor should not be seated any deeper than the stop mark on the seating tool. The risk of penetrating the inferior glenoid may occur if the anchors are inserted too deeply.

Suture Passing

The arthroscope is then changed to the posterior portal for viewing. One strand of the suture is captured using a crochet hook and retrieved through the AS portal. Using either a suture hook or a modified Caspari suture punch (Linvatec Corp., Largo, FL), the anterior labrum and a portion of the inferior glenohumeral ligament are penetrated and a Shuttle Relay (Linvatec Corp., Largo, FL) is advanced through them into the joint. The suture needle should pass below and medial to the labrum so that when tied, the suture holds the labrum up on the edge of the glenoid (Figs. 15-9B and 15-10B). The amount of anterior capsulolabral structures imbricated is dependent on the laxity of these structures. In an extremely lax shoulder, the stitcher is passed 2 to 3 cm inferior and lateral to the anchor so that a capsular tuck is advanced proximally, restoring tension to the tissue.

The end of the Shuttle Relay is then grasped with an arthroscopic clamp and pulled out the AS cannula until the eyelet is visible. The Shuttle eyelet is loaded with the braided suture in the AS portal. The limb of the Shuttle exiting through the AMG portal is pulled, carrying the suture through the anterior structures and out the AMG cannula (Figs. 15-9C and 15-10C). This step results in a simple stitch for fixating the anterior structures to bone. We have been pleased with the simple suture because it bolsters the labrum and rolls it up over the edge of the anterior glenoid, thus increasing the effective depth of the glenoid with a subsequent increase in stability [31]. However, this

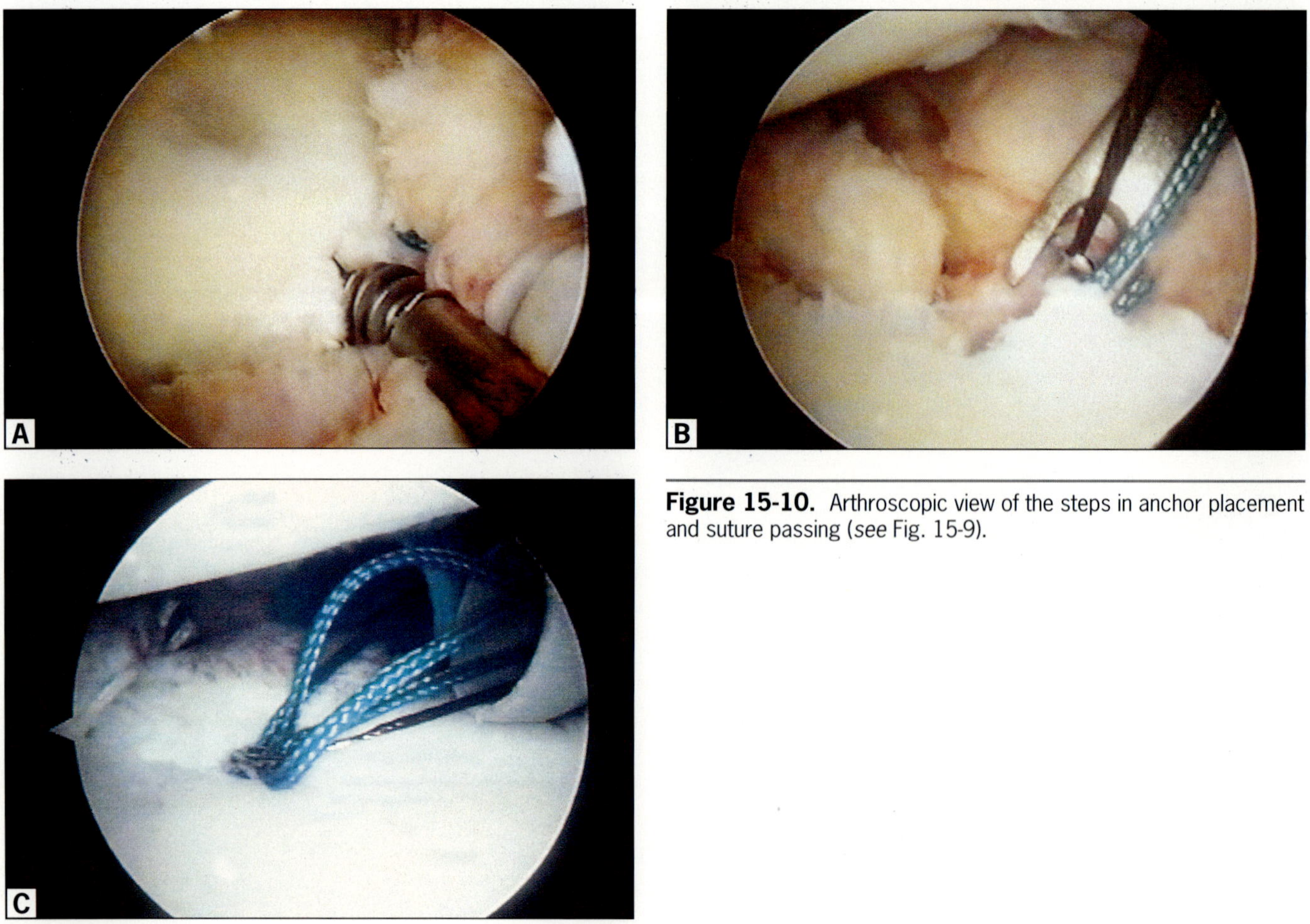

Figure 15-10. Arthroscopic view of the steps in anchor placement and suture passing (*see* Fig. 15-9).

step may be repeated with the other strand of the suture to create a horizontal mattress stitch if desired.

A simple mistake that can be easily avoided is pulling the suture out of the eyelet of the anchor after the anchor has been seated in bone. This is a nuisance with the Mini Revo, because it requires that the anchor be removed, reloaded with suture, and replaced. It is a more significant problem with the Mitek or the Bio Anchor because these anchors are not retrievable and remain in the glenoid without serving a function (Fig. 15-11). We avoid this complication by keeping a clamp on the loose ends of the suture. In addition, close attention is paid to the suture when the crochet hook is used to deliver it from the AMG cannular into the AS cannula. If the suture is seen to be pulling through the eyelet, it must be stabilized by clamping the AMG suture.

Knot Tying

Knot tying can present one of the more demanding aspects of this procedure. The surgeon has only one attempt to perform this task correctly, because a loose stitch is functionless and must be replaced. When using the Mitek, which is not retrievable, a failed knot necessitates placement of an additional anchor. Thus, although seemingly tedious, knot tying must be practiced to perfection using a model prior to attempting it intraoperatively. We have used many knots for this task; the knot we are currently using is the Revo knot. The slip knot we previously used has resulted in several episodes of the knot locking prior to tightening of the suture and thus has been abandoned.

The initial step in tying the Revo knot is to pass the knot pusher down the strand of the suture that was pulled through the AMG cannula by the Shuttle Relay. Any twists or soft tissue on the strands of the suture must be cleared prior to proceeding.

The knot consists of two alternating half-hitches tied around one post, followed by two additional half-hitches, with the second suture strand acting as the post. A fifth half-hitch on the initial post is often used for security.

The first "under" half-hitch is formed outside the cannula and advanced down the post with the knot pusher. Slack in the suture strands is taken up by tensioning the right and left strands in an alternating fashion. This is not a slip knot and the two limbs of the suture remain the same length (Fig. 15-12A).

Once the first half-hitch is snug, a second opposite or "over" half-hitch is placed while tension is continued on the post strand (Fig. 15-12B). Again, the knot pusher is advanced down the strand with the slack in the nonpost strand being taken up with light tension.

Once the first two half-hitches are placed, tension is released on both suture strands, allowing the knot to set. The knot pusher is changed to the opposite suture strand, which now becomes the second post. An "under" half-hitch is thrown around the second post and advanced gently by the knot pusher with mild alternating tension on both sutures (Fig. 15-12C).

Care should be taken not to put significant tension on the second post strand, because this may cause release of the previously set half hitches and loosening of the knot against the capsulolabral tissues. Each of the last two throws of this knot should be tightened by "past pointing" of the knot pusher once the throw has been advanced down to the knot (Fig. 15-12D). This helps to firmly set these final two locking knots. The fourth "over" half-hitch is placed on the second post, again in an opposite direction. This half-hitch is

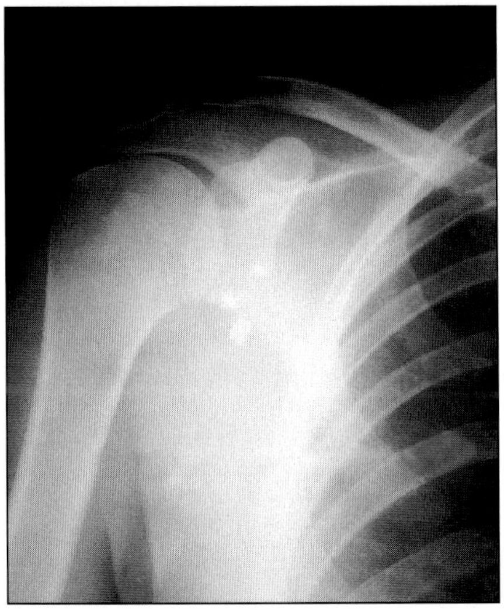

Figure 15-11. Radiograph of completed arthroscopic anterior reconstruction. Note that there are three anchors in the axillary recess. This was the result of inadvertent unloading of the Mitek GII (Mitek Surgical Products, Westwood, MA) after implanting the anchor in bone. The second and third anchors were subsequently inserted in the same pilot hole, forcing the initial anchors out of the inferior glenoid. If a retrievable Mini Revo (Linvatec Corp., Largo, FL) anchor had been used, it could have been removed and reloaded.

gently advanced with light tension on both strands (Fig. 15-12E). A fifth "under" half-hitch is often used on the first post for added security. The tails of the suture are cut using a basket punch or other cutting device, leaving approximately 3-mm ends (Fig. 15-12F).

The most common complication in knot tying is the knot locking prior to snug seating down against the capsulolabral structures. This can be avoided by making sure the post strand of the first two throws is held taut and that excess slack is taken up frequently with light pulls on the nonpost strand of suture. Once these first two strands are set, it is imperative that tension be released on both the nonpost and post strands and that no significant tension be placed on either strand while the second two locking throws are placed. This should allow for firm seating without loosening of the knot occurring and therefore should eliminate this complication. The second most common complication is suture breakage. This can be avoided by using a strong #2 braided suture and firm tension only, not overtensioning the suture strands.

A second and (if desired) a third anchor is placed in the glenoid and the procedure previously outlined is repeated. Once all sutures have been tied, the final repair is visualized and probed to assure firm fixation of the anterior capsulolabral structures to bone (Fig. 15-13A and 15-13B).

POSTOPERATIVE CARE AND REHABILITATION

Many surgeons advocate immediate motion following open Bankart repairs [4]. However, reports have attributed early failures of arthroscopic techniques to the use of a more aggressive postoperative regimen [18,32]. It is likely that this is due to the patient's minimal postoperative symptoms, allowing the patient to utilize his operative extremity much more readily and forcefully than he would following an open procedure, which places the repair at risk.

In light of this, we have used a more conservative postoperative routine. The patient's arm is maintained in a shoulder support for 3 weeks postoperatively. An ideal shoulder support for postoperative immobilization is the DonJoy UltraSling (Smith & Nephew DonJoy, Carlsbad, CA) (Fig. 15-14). This sling maintains the upper extremity in neutral rotation, as opposed to internal rotation that occurs with traditional shoulder immobilizers. It also allows for easier release of the forearm so the patient may begin hand,

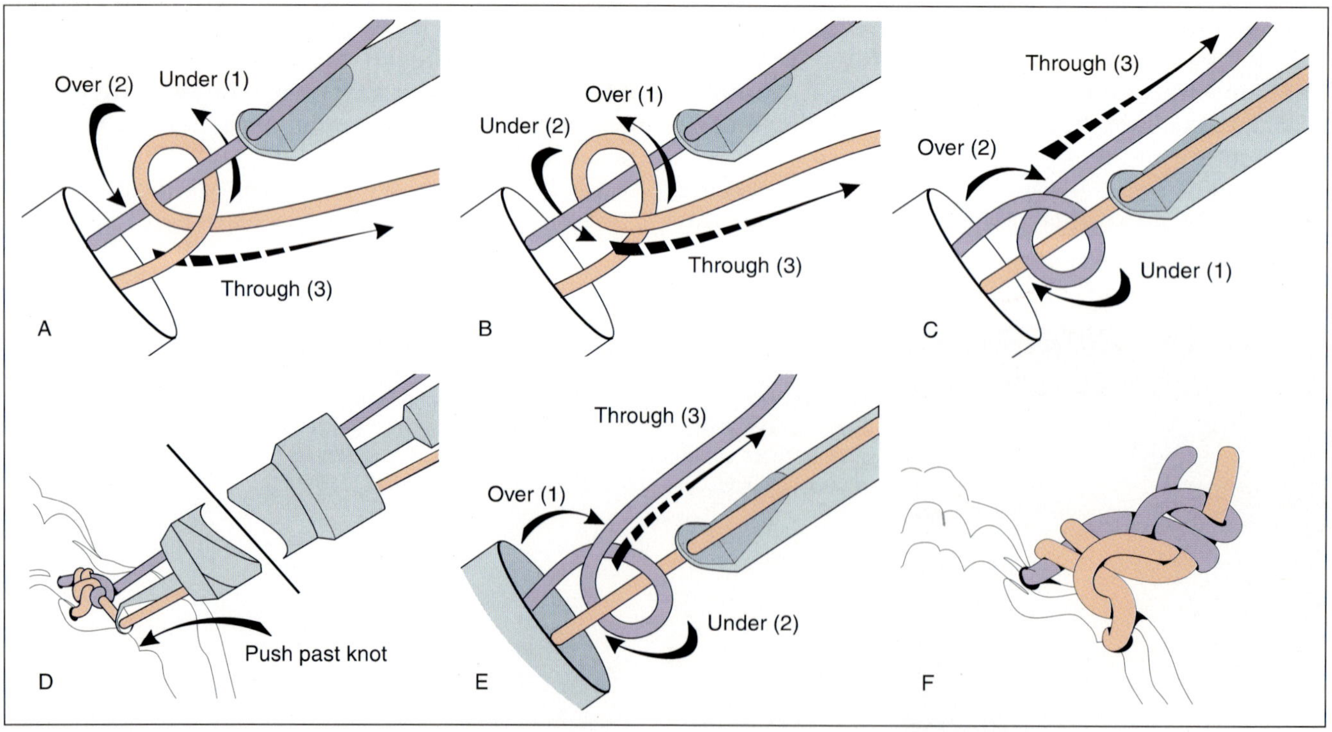

Figure 15-12. Technique for tying the arthroscopic Revo knot, **A**, Underhand half-hitch on the primary post, **B**, overhand half-hitch on the primary post, **C**, underhand half-hitch on the secondary post, **D**, "past pointing" to lock third half-hitch, **E**, fourth half-hitch overhand on the secondary post, **F**, completed Revo knot (a fifth half-hitch is often added on the primary post).

wrist, and elbow motion exercises immediately during postoperative care. In addition to the range of motion exercises of distal upper extremity joints, external rotation of the shoulder is allowed for 20° in the immediate postoperative period.

At 10 days, the patient is taught gentle pendulum exercises. At 3 weeks, subscapularis strengthening exercises are begun, and at 6 weeks, the patient begins active-assisted range of motion exercises. At 10 weeks, full activity is allowed except for forceful exercise in external rotation and abduction. We discourage this for approximately 6 months. At that time, patients may go back to their normal exercise routines, including throwing sports.

As we have become more experienced and comfortable with our methods for anterior stabilization, we have liberalized our postoperative therapy to allow earlier motion of the arm. However, we still prohibit stressful external rotation and abduction exercises as well as a return to sports for 5 to 6 months.

SOUTHERN CALIFORNIA ORTHOPEDIC INSTITUTE RESULTS

At the Southern California Orthopedic Institute, 37 patients undergoing arthroscopic capsulorrhaphy have been followed-up for more than 1 year, with an average follow-up of 22 months. Thirty-three of these patients have been satisfied with the results and have returned to their usual work and sports.

Four patients subsequently developed a recurrent instability postoperatively, each from significant trauma. The first patient suffered a redislocation when

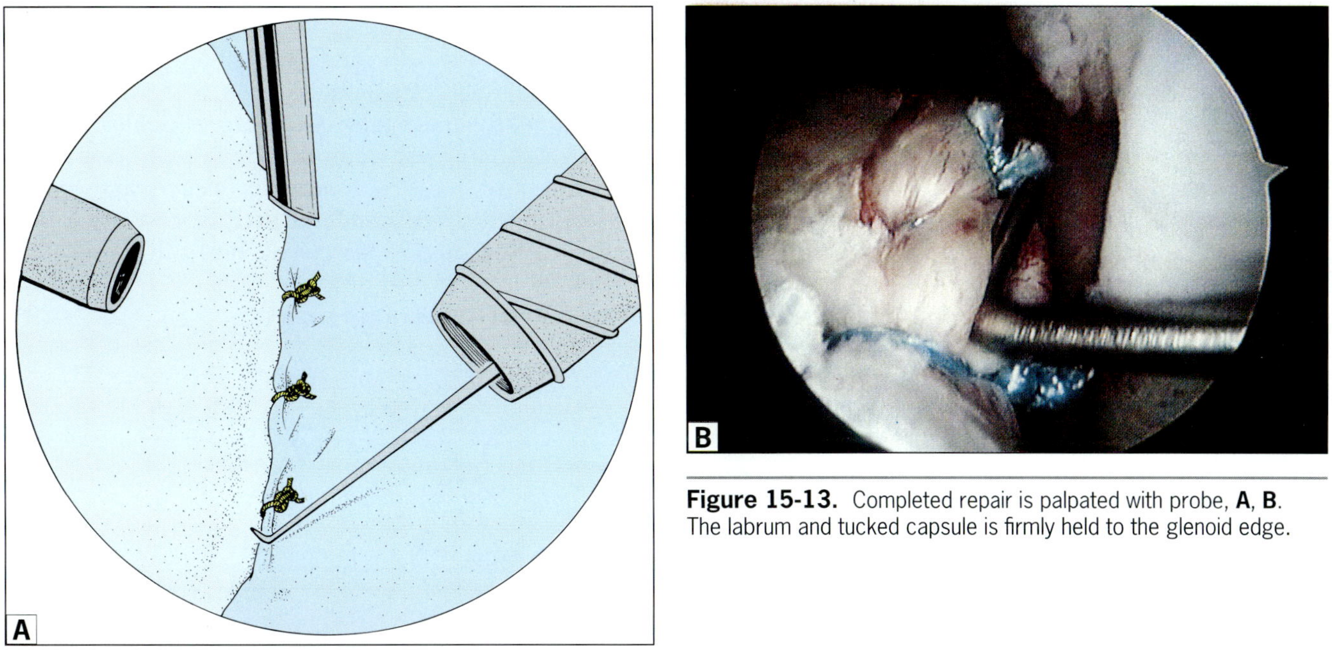

Figure 15-13. Completed repair is palpated with probe, **A**, **B**. The labrum and tucked capsule is firmly held to the glenoid edge.

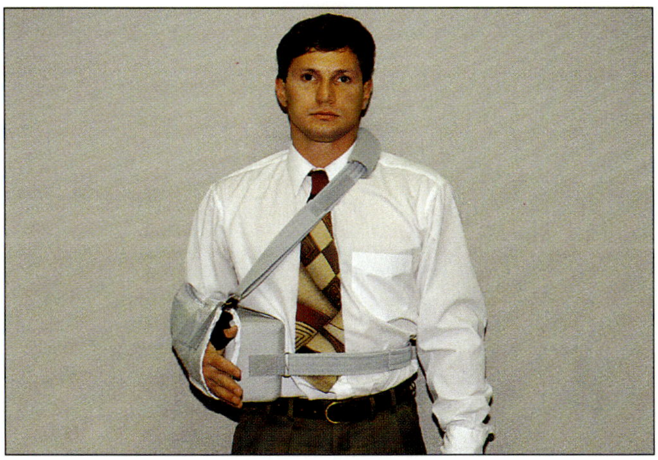

Figure 15-14. The arm is supported postoperatively in an Ultra Sling (Smith & Nephew DonJoy, Carlsbad, CA) in neutral rotation.

he was struck by an automobile and thrown approximately 10 feet. The second patient redislocated during a motocross motorcycle riding accident. A third patient had his arm stressed in extreme hyperabduction and external rotation while rebounding in a pickup basketball game. The final patient redislocated his shoulder during a rock climbing accident. At the time of his redislocation, his arm was in 90° of abduction and 90° of external rotation.

The first two patients underwent revision stabilization procedures. The first patient, due to insurance changes, underwent his revision procedure elsewhere. In the operative summary, the surgeon noted "the capsule had stayed tight down onto the glenoid." A capsular reefing procedure was done because the capsule was suspected of being patulous anteriorly.

The second patient underwent a revision stabilization procedure at Southern California Orthopedic Institute. At the time of surgery, the patient was noted to have a humeral avulsion of the glenohumeral ligaments (Fig. 15-15). In fact, his Bankart repair was solidly healed. A capsular shift was performed on this patient.

Functional subjective scores on all patients in terms of activities of daily living and return to work were all excellent in the patients who did not have complications of redislocation. In addition, this group of patients was noted objectively to have minimal limitations of shoulder range of motion, with the average loss of external rotation being 5° with no evidence of loss of internal rotation.

Radiographs that were performed on 28 patients, including the four patients with recurrent instability, revealed that there was no evidence of degenerative changes, nor were there any instances of hardware loosening or migration. Four patients had extraosseous Mitek GII anchors that had been pushed through the glenoid in an attempt to stack anchors when the suture failed intraoperatively (Fig. 15-11).

CONCLUSION

Arthroscopic techniques for anterior stabilization of the shoulder continue to improve. The use of suture anchors and nonabsorbable sutures effectively allows the Bankart repair to be performed arthroscopically without unnecessary iatrogenic surgical injury. The results of this procedure have been excellent with failures only attributable to severe trauma. Longer follow-up will determine whether this treatment modality will withstand the test of time and replace the Bankart repair as the standard for treatment of the traumatically unstable shoulder. It is our hope that when these and other arthroscopic stabilization procedures have been proven effective, they will be available to treat young athletes after the first dislocation, thereby avoiding the pain, cost, disability, and joint damage from recurrent dislocation that so often follows the traditional conservative approach.

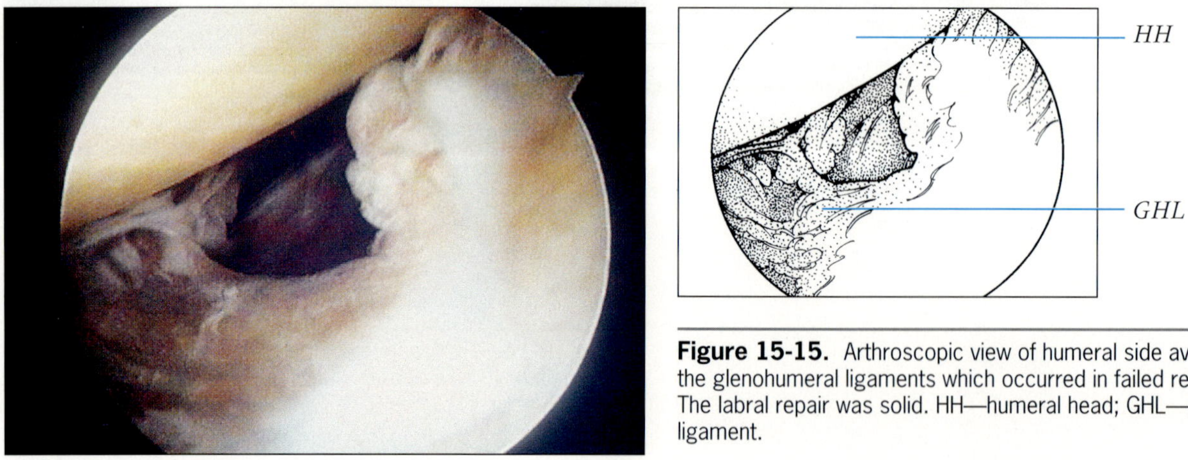

Figure 15-15. Arthroscopic view of humeral side avulsion of the glenohumeral ligaments which occurred in failed reconstruction. The labral repair was solid. HH—humeral head; GHL—glenohumeral ligament.

REFERENCES AND RECOMMENDED READING

Papers of interest, published recently, have been highlighted as:
- • Of interest
- •• Of outstanding interest

1. Perthes G: Über operationen bei habitueller schulterluxation. *Ztscher Chir* 1906, 85:199–227.

2. Bankart ASB: Recurrent or habitual dislocation of the shoulder joint. *Br Med J* 1923, 2:1132–1133.

3. Bankart ASB: The pathology and treatment of recurrent dislocations of the shoulder joint. *Br J Surg* 1938, 26:23–29.

4. Rowe CR, Patel D, Southmayd WW: The Bankart procedure: A long-term end-result study. *J Bone Joint Surg* [Am] 1978, 60:1–16.

5. Rowe CR: Acute and recurrent anterior dislocations of the shoulder. *Orthop Clin North Am* 1980, 11:253–270.

6. Wolf EM, Wilk RM, Richmond JC: Arthroscopic Bankart repair using suture anchors. *Operative Tech Orthop* 1991, 1:184–191.

7. Snyder SJ, Strafford BB: Arthroscopic management of instability of the shoulder. *Orthopedics* 1993, 16:993–1002.

8.•• Green MR, Christensen KP: Arthroscopic versus open Bankart procedures: a comparison of early morbidity and complications. *Arthroscopy* 1993, 9:371–374.

This study demonstrated a statistically significant reduction in operative time, estimated blood loss, postoperative narcotic use, postoperative fever, postoperative days of hospitalization, and time absent from work when comparing arthroscopic Bankart repairs to those performed using the open technique. Arthroscopic Bankart repair offers significant clinical advantages compared with the open technique, with additional economic advantages due to decreased operative time, hospitalization, and earlier return to work.

9. Symondesis PP: The significance of the subscapularis muscle in the pathogenesis of recurrent anterior dislocation of the shoulder. *J Bone Joint Surg* [Br] 1972, 54:476–483.

10. O'Connell PW, Nuber GW, Mileski RA, *et al.*: The contribution of the glenohumeral ligaments to anterior stability of the shoulder. *Am J Sports Med* 1990, 18:579–584.

11. Turkel SJ, Panio MW, Marshall JL, *et al.*: Stabilizing mechanisms preventing anterior dislocation of the glenohumeral joint. *J Bone Joint Surg* [Am] 1981, 63:1208–1217.

12. O'Brien SJ, Neves MC, Arnoczky SP, *et al.*: The anatomy and histology of the inferior glenohumeral ligament complex of the shoulder. *Am J Sports Med* 1990, 18:449–456.

13.• Baker CL, Uribe JW, Whitman C: Arthroscopic evaluation of acute initial anterior shoulder dislocations. *Am J Sports Med* 1990, 18:25–28.

This study noted three types of lesions following anterior shoulder dislocations. Group III patients, who represented 62% of the study group, had a labral detachment and were grossly unstable when examined under anesthesia. The authors conclude that the intact traumatic lesion in addition to other factors predispose the shoulder to recurrent dislocation.

14. Zarins B McMahon MS, Rowe CR: Diagnosis and treatment of traumatic anterior instability of the shoulder. *Clin Orthop* 1993, 291:75–84.

15. McGlynn FJ, Caspari RB: Arthroscopic findings in the subluxating shoulder. *Clin Orthop* 1984, 183:173–178.

16. Reeves B: Experiments on the tensile strength of the anterior capsular structures of the shoulder in man. *J Bone Joint Surg* [Br] 1968, 50:858–865.

17. Benedetto KP, Glötzer W: Arthroscopic Bankart procedure by suture technique: Indications, technique and results. *Arthroscopy* 1992, 8:111–115.

18. Morgan CD, Bodenstab AB: Arthroscopic Bankart suture repair: Technique and early results. *Arthroscopy* 1987, 3:111–122.

19. Coughlin L, Rubinovich M, Johansson J, *et al.*: Arthroscopic staple capsulorrhaphy for anterior shoulder instability. *Am J Sports Med* 1992, 20:253–256.

20. Zuckerman JD, Matsen FA: Complications about the glenohumeral joint related to the use of screws and staples. *J Bone Joint Surg* [Am] 1984, 66:175–180.

21. Matsen FA III, Thomas SC, Rockwood CA: Anterior glenohumeral instability. In *The Shoulder*. Edited by Rockwood CA, Matsen FA. Philadelphia: WB Saunders Co.; 1990:526.

22. Burkhead WZ, Rockwood CA: Treatment of instability of the shoulder with an exercise program. *J Bone Joint Surg* [Am] 1992, 74:890–896.

23. Neer CS, Foster CR: Inferior capsular shift for involuntary inferior and multidirectional instability of the shoulder. *J Bone Joint Surg* [Am] 1980, 62:897–908.

24. Wheeler JH, Ryan JB, Arciero RA, Molinari RN: Arthroscopic versus nonoperative treatment of acute shoulder dislocations in young athletes. *Arthroscopy* 1989, 5:213–217.

25. Simonet WT, Cofield RH: Prognosis in anterior shoulder dislocation. *Am J Sports Med* 1984, 12:19–24.

26. Barber FA, Cawley P, Prudich JF: Suture anchor failure strength: an *in vivo* study. *Arthroscopy* 1993, 9:647–652.

27. Barber FA, Click JN: The effect of inflammatory fluid on the breaking strength of new "long lasting" absorbable sutures. *Arthroscopy* 1992, 8:437–441.

28. Wolf EM: Anterior portals in shoulder arthroscopy. *Arthroscopy* 1989, 5:201–208.

29. Gross RM: Arthroscopic shoulder capsulorrhaphy: Does it work? *Am J Sports Med* 1989, 17:495–500.

30. Snyder SJ: A complete system for arthroscopy and bursoscopy of the shoulder. *Surg Rounds Orthop* 1989, 57–65.

31. Lippitt S, Matsen F: Mechanisms of glenohumeral joint instability. *Clin Orthop* 1993, 291:20–28.

32. Grana WA, Buckley PD, Yates CK: Arthroscopic Bankart suture repair. *Am J Sports Med* 1993, 21:348–353.

16
CHAPTER

Arthroscopic Transglenoid Suture Capsulorrhaphy for Anterior Shoulder Instability

DONALD J. ROSE

Over the past several years, an increased understanding of the anatomy and pathophysiology of anterior and anteroinferior shoulder instability has occurred. Turkel and coworkers found that as the shoulder approaches 90° of abduction, the inferior glenohumeral ligament, with its attachment to the anteroinferior glenoid labrum, is primarily responsible for maintaining shoulder stability during external rotation [1].

On those shoulders operated on for recurrent anterior shoulder instability, Rowe and coworkers [2,3] found a high incidence of Bankart lesions, defined as an avulsion of the anteroinferior glenohumeral ligament labral complex from the anterior glenoid rim and scapular neck. Excessive anteroinferior capsular laxity was noted to be present in approximately 70% of the initial procedures for anterior shoulder instability and in 83% of failed primary surgeries.

Speer and coworkers (paper presented at the Annual Meeting of American Shoulder and Elbow Surgeons, San Francisco, 1993) concluded, based on biomechanical studies, that the Bankart lesion alone is not accountable for anterior shoulder dislocation, and hypothesized that additional plastic deformation of the inferior glenohumeral ligament must occur. This pathology (Bankart lesion, capsular laxity, or both) results in a loss of the normal static buttress effect (Fig. 16-1).

Although open techniques of anterior shoulder reconstruction have been successful in preventing recurrent dislocations [2,4–6], arthroscopic stabilization procedures offer several potential advantages, including reduced postoperative morbidity and hospitalization time, improved assessment of associated intra-articular pathology, decreased loss of range of motion, and improved cosmesis [7,8].

The following technique of arthroscopic suture capsulorrhaphy corrects, if present, both the Bankart lesion and excessive anteroinferior capsular laxity, thus restoring the buttress effect. The advantages of an arthroscopic procedure are maintained while many of the potential complications associated with the use of arthroscopic staples or other hardware [9–11] are avoided. The procedure takes its historical origins from earlier open transglenoid procedures described by Luckey [12] and Reider and Inglis [13].

SURGICAL TECHNIQUE

Positioning

Following induction of general endotracheal anesthesia, both shoulders are examined. The patient is placed in a lateral decubitus position with the operative shoulder suspended overhead in approximately 40° of abduction (Fig. 16-2). The scapular blade is left exposed during prepping and draping. Double traction [14] is helpful in providing increased arthroscopic exposure anteroinferiorly.

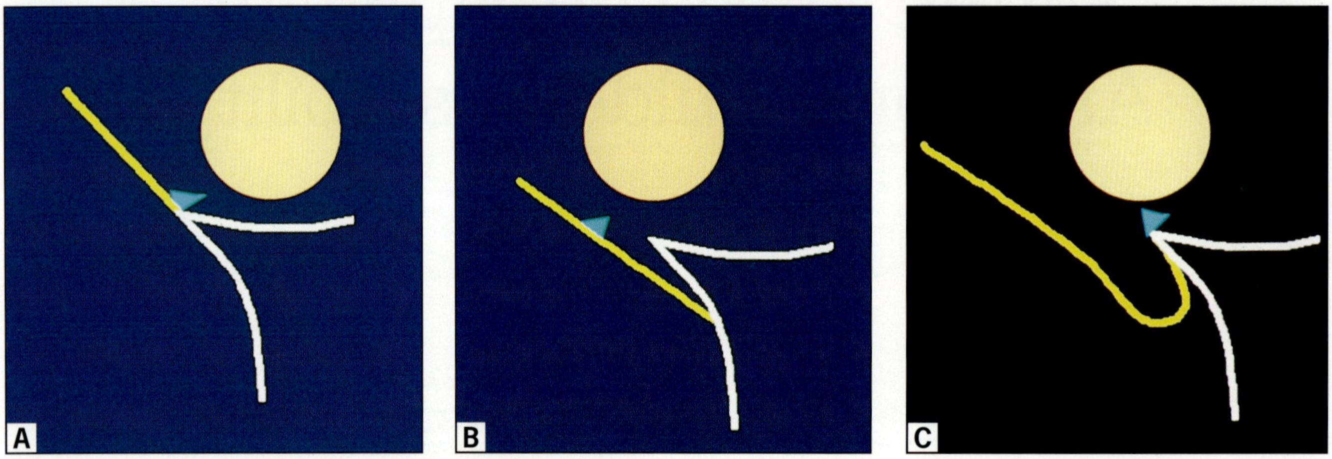

Figure 16-1. **A**, Normal anterior buttress effect of glenohumeral joint. **B**, **C**, Loss of normal buttress effect due to Bankart lesion or capsular redundancy.

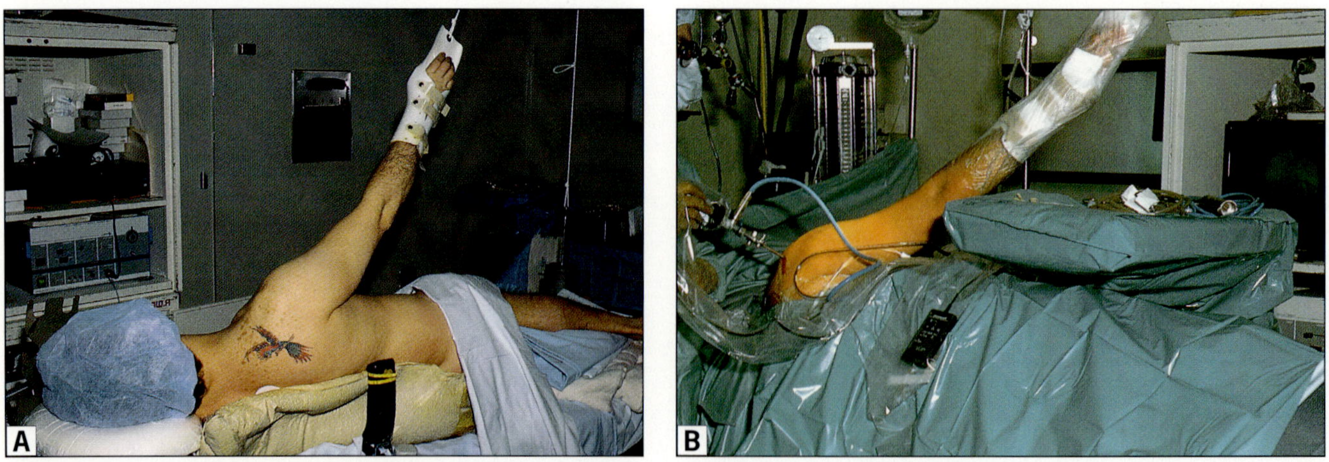

Figure 16-2. **A**, Patient in lateral decubitus position. **B**, Operative set-up with arthroscope inserted via posterior portal. (*From* Rose [27]; with permission.)

Arthroscopic Evaluation

The arthroscope is inserted through a standard posterior arthroscopic portal with inflow established through the arthroscopic cannula. The use of an arthroscopic pump facilitates visualization. Using a Wissinger rod placed through the arthroscopic cannula, a 7-mm inner diameter disposable cannula is inserted with the aid of a cannulated obturator through the triangular space bordered by the anterior glenoid rim, the superior edge of the subscapularis tendon, and the biceps tendon (Fig. 16-3). The cannula may be sutured to the skin anteriorly during the procedure to prevent inadvertent withdrawal. Outflow is controlled through the cannula's accessory portal, and all subsequent instrumentation is passed through the cannula. An arthroscopic examination of the shoulder is then performed. The presence or absence of a detached anterior glenohumeral ligament labral complex is determined (Fig. 16-4). The quality of tissues, the degree of separation, and amount of anterior or inferior capsular laxity is thoroughly assessed. Associated intra-articular pathology,*eg*, chondral damage, labral tears, loose bodies, and hypertrophic synovitis is evaluated and treated.

Preparation of Anterior Glenoid Neck

A motorized shaver or rasp is placed through the anterior cannula and soft tissue is removed from the anterior surface of the glenoid neck in the region of the Bankart lesion (Fig. 16-5). An abrader is then used to decorticate the anterior glenoid neck (Fig. 16-6). A second anterior arthroscopic portal placed superiorly [15] may be used to enhance anterior visualization.

Capsular Shift

A superior shift of the inferior glenohumeral ligament is then performed as required. A shoulder suture passer is used to pass multiple 0 or #1 monofilament, nonabsorbable (or absorbable) sutures through the superior band of the inferior glenohumeral ligament (Fig. 16-7). The suture end exiting from the tip of the suture passer is retrieved using a suture snare (Fig. 16-8) or a small

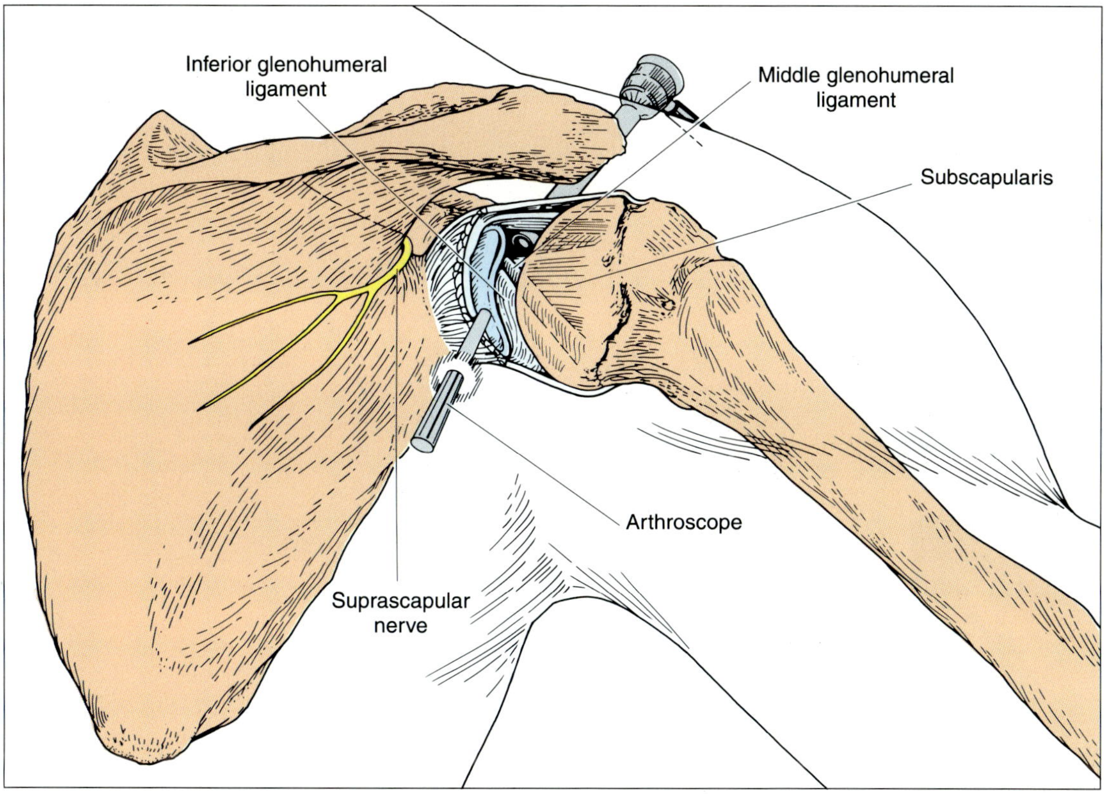

Figure 16-3. Arthroscopic anatomy of right shoulder, posterior view. (*From* Rose [27]; with permission.)

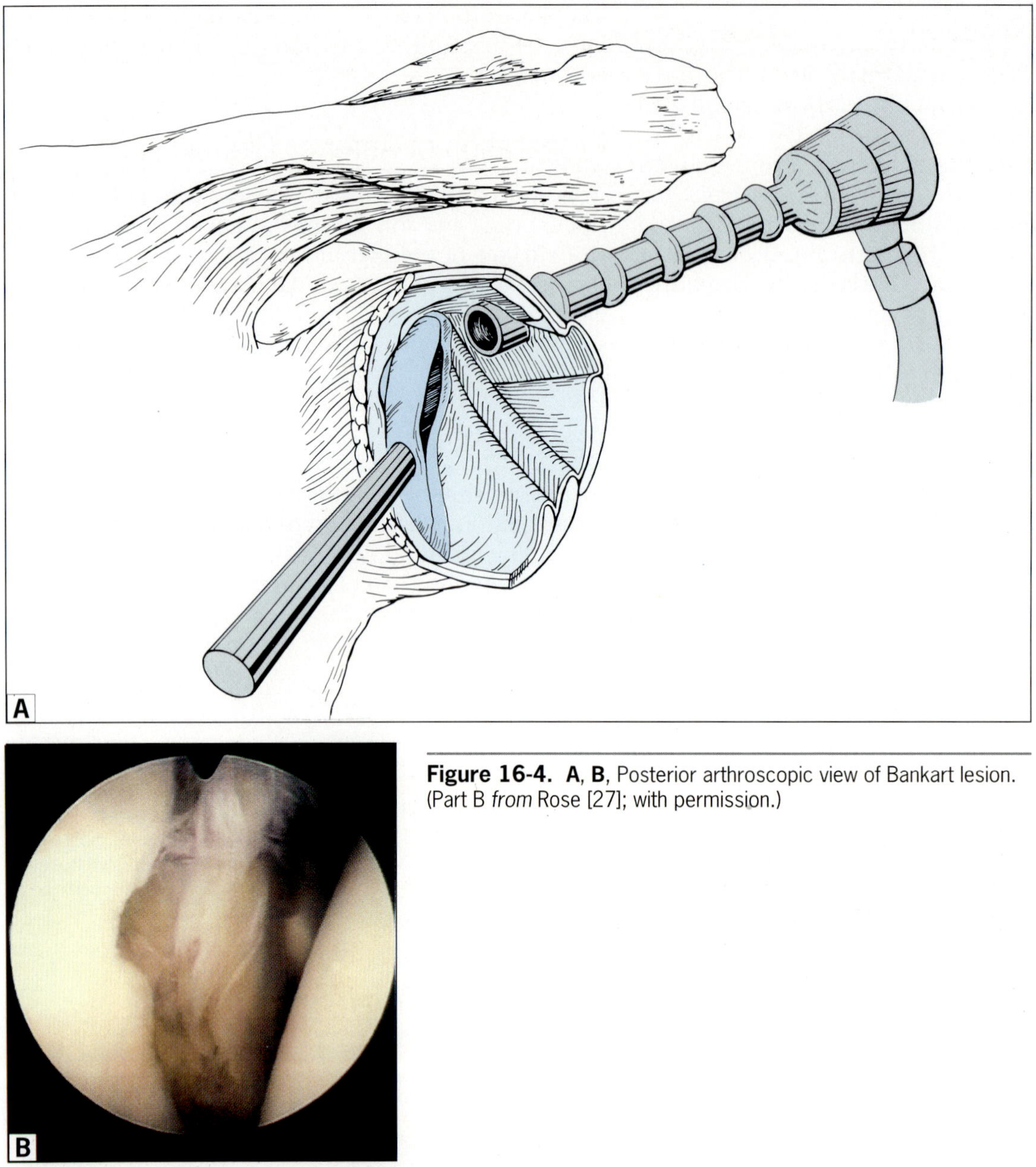

Figure 16-4. **A**, **B**, Posterior arthroscopic view of Bankart lesion. (Part B *from* Rose [27]; with permission.)

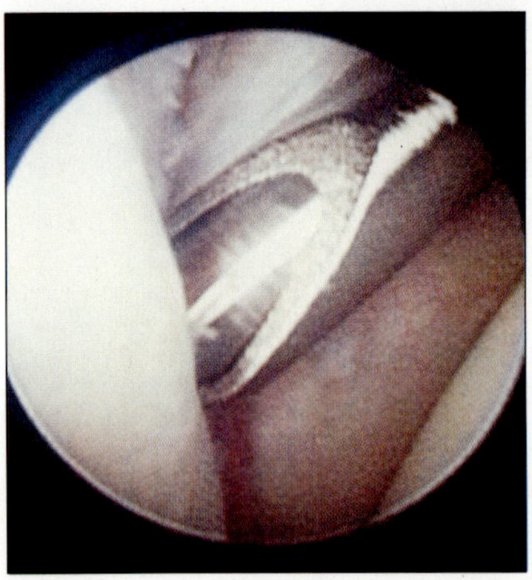

Figure 16-5. Soft-tissue debridement of anterior glenoid neck using a motorized shaver. (*From* Rose [27]; with permission.)

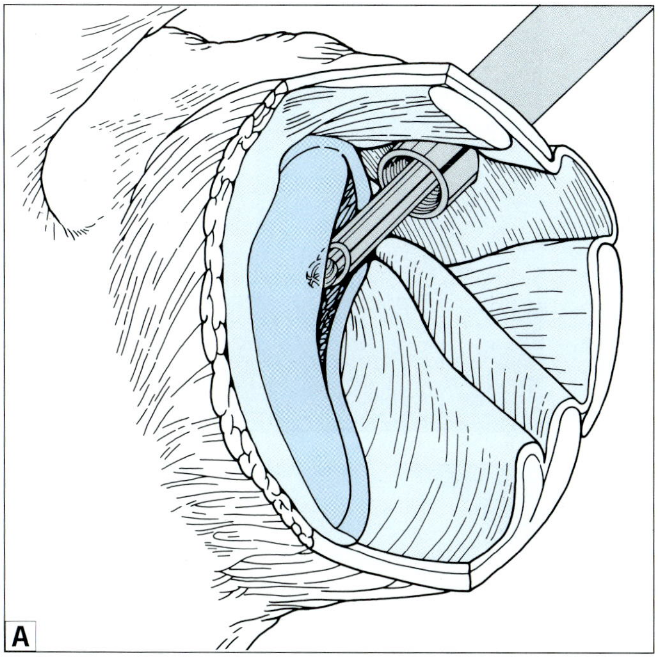

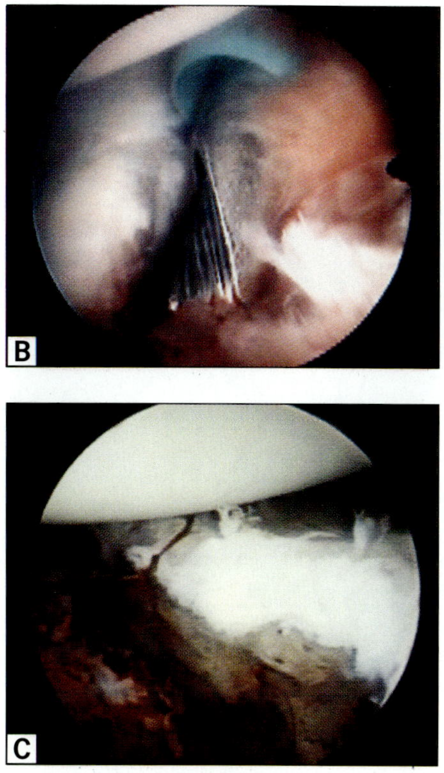

Figure 16-6. **A**, **B**, Decortication anterior glenoid neck using a motorized abrader. **C**, Anterior view of glenoid neck following abrasion. (Parts A and C *from* Rose [27]; with permission.)

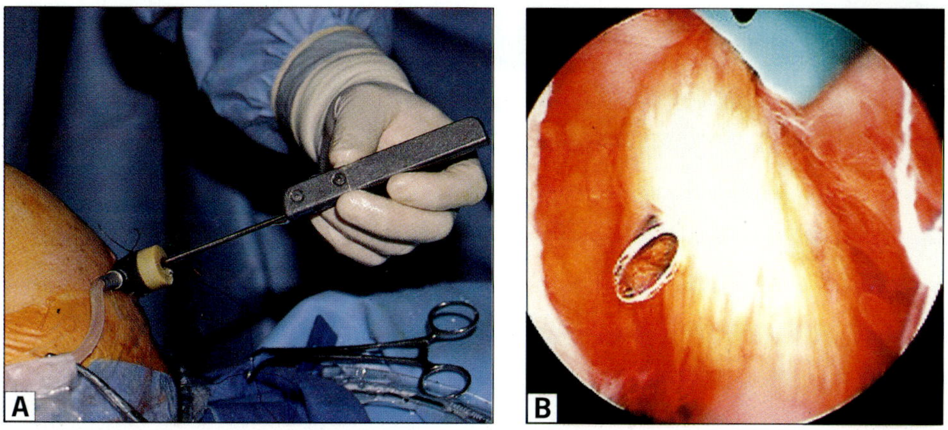

Figure 16-7. **A**, **B**, Spearing superior band of inferior glenohumeral ligament using a suture passer.

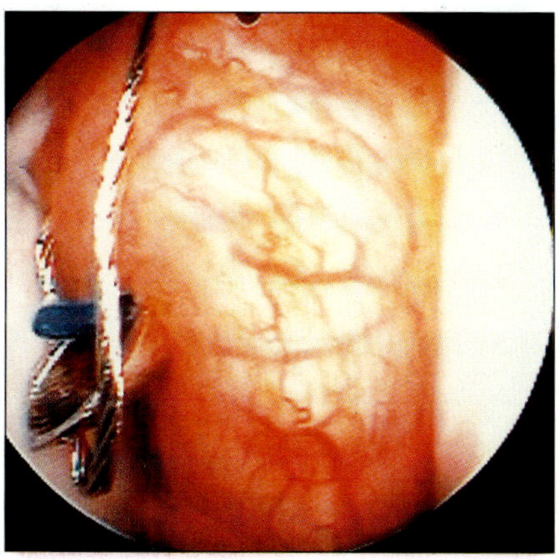

Figure 16-8. Retrieval of suture end from suture passer using a suture snare.

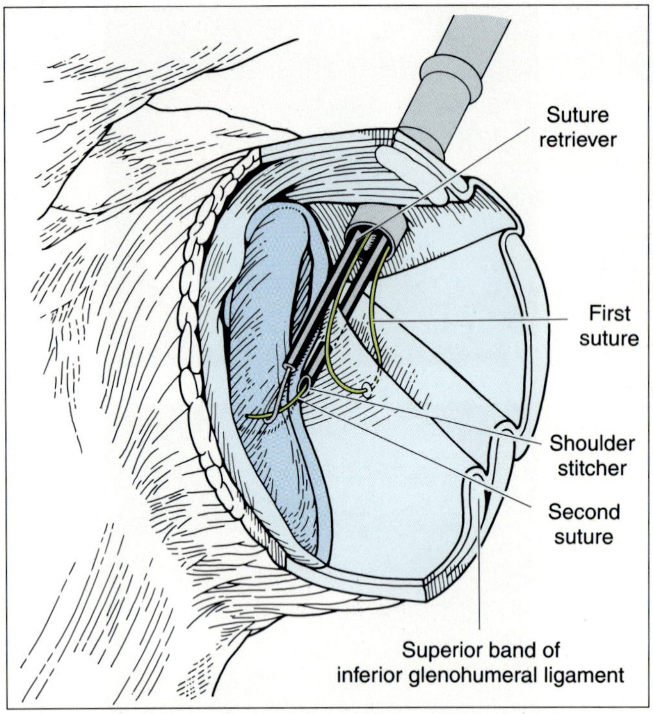

Figure 16-9. Suture passer and snare used to pass multiple sutures through superior band of inferior glenohumeral ligament via anterior cannula. (*From* Rose [27]; with permission.)

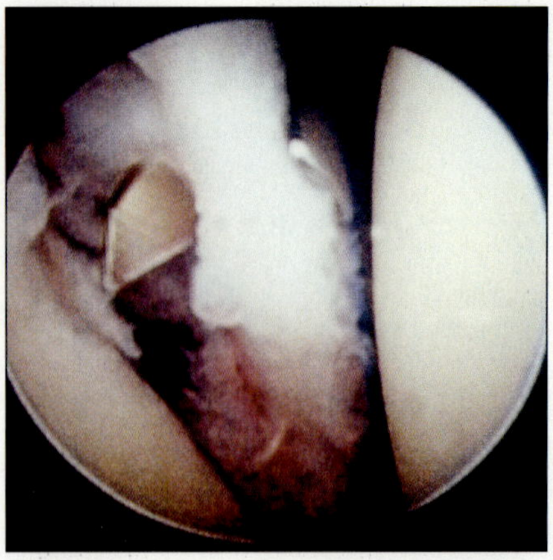

Figure 16-10. Spearing of detached glenohumeral ligament-labral complex with a suture pin.

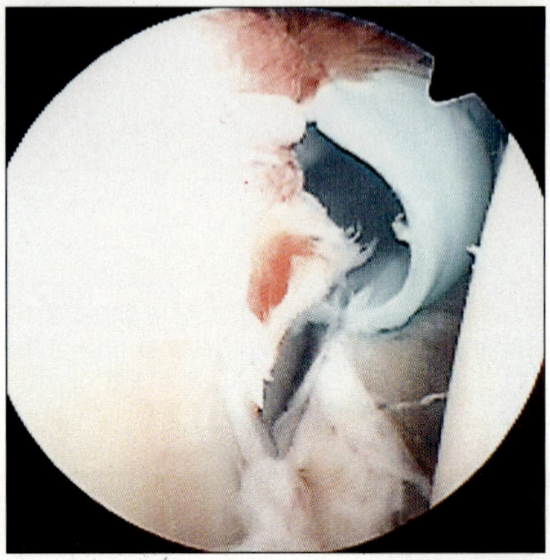

Figure 16-11. Glenohumeral ligament-labral complex advanced to anterior rim of glenoid using flanged pin cannula for placement.

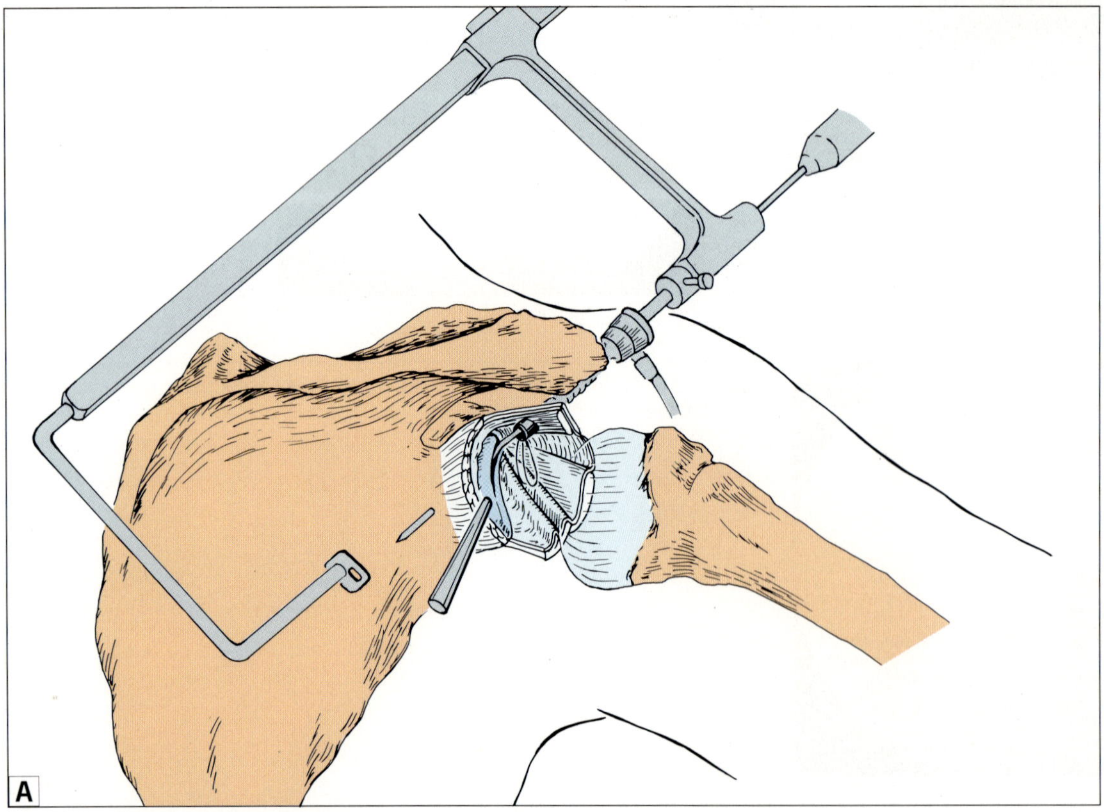

Figure 16-12. **A**, **B**, and **C**, Use of shoulder guide to direct posterior pin exit correlating arthroscopic view, surface anatomy, and horizontal cross-section of pin passage. (Part B *from* Rose [27]; with permission) (*continued*)

grasper and is brought out through the anterior cannula (Fig. 16-9). Both ends of each suture are clamped until later in the procedure.

Bankart Lesion Repair

Repair of the Bankart lesion using horizontal mattress sutures is then performed. The sharp end of a suture pin is passed via the anterior cannula through the detached glenohumeral ligament labral complex (Fig. 16-10). The suture pin cannula portion of the shoulder guide system is placed over the suture pin with its flange on the anterior edge of the glenoid articular surface (Fig. 16-11) to permit accurate placement and to prevent inadvertent medial migration of the suture pin. The tip of the suture pin may be gently tapped into the abraded bone surface of the anterior glenoid neck to enhance purchase.

The assembled shoulder guide is used to direct pin exit posteriorly toward a point approximately 4 to 5 cm inferior to the scapular spine and less than 15° medial to the articular surface of the glenoid (Fig. 16-12). The pin is drilled posteriorly through the glenoid neck and out through a small skin incision (Fig. 16-13). The shoulder guide, including the suture pin cannula, is removed. One end of a #1 nonabsorbable suture is placed through the hole in the trailing end of the suture pin, which is then advanced. A second braided suture may be used for additional insurance should a suture break during tying later in the procedure. Using the guide system, a second suture pin is placed in a similar fashion, with its posterior exit directed toward the first pin exit point (Fig. 16-14). Use of the guide system minimizes the risk of damage to the suprascapular nerve by accurately directing the suture pin and minimizes capture of soft tissue between the two pins. Maintaining the first pin within the glenoid neck while the second pin is drilled prevents inadvertent cutting of the sutures by the second pin. Soft tissue is retracted from between the two suture pins posteriorly (prior to the exit of the second pin through the soft tissue) by using a slotted cannula and obturator (Fig. 16-15). This method allows for later tying of the sutures down to the bone with minimal capture of soft tissue structures posteriorly. The other end of the braided suture is passed through the eye of the second suture pin anteriorly and both pins, together with the ends of

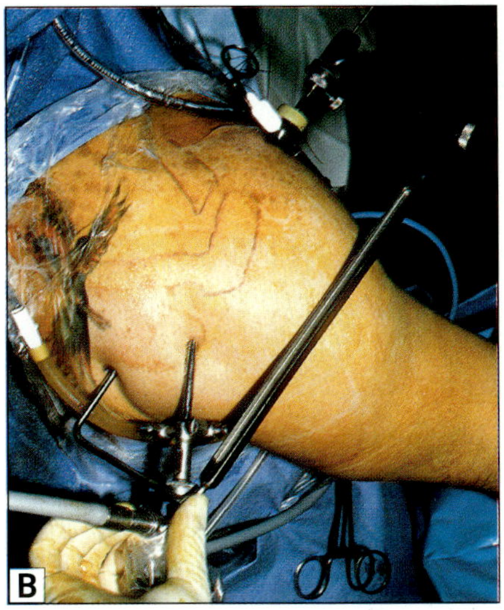

Figure 16-12.
B, C, *(continued)*

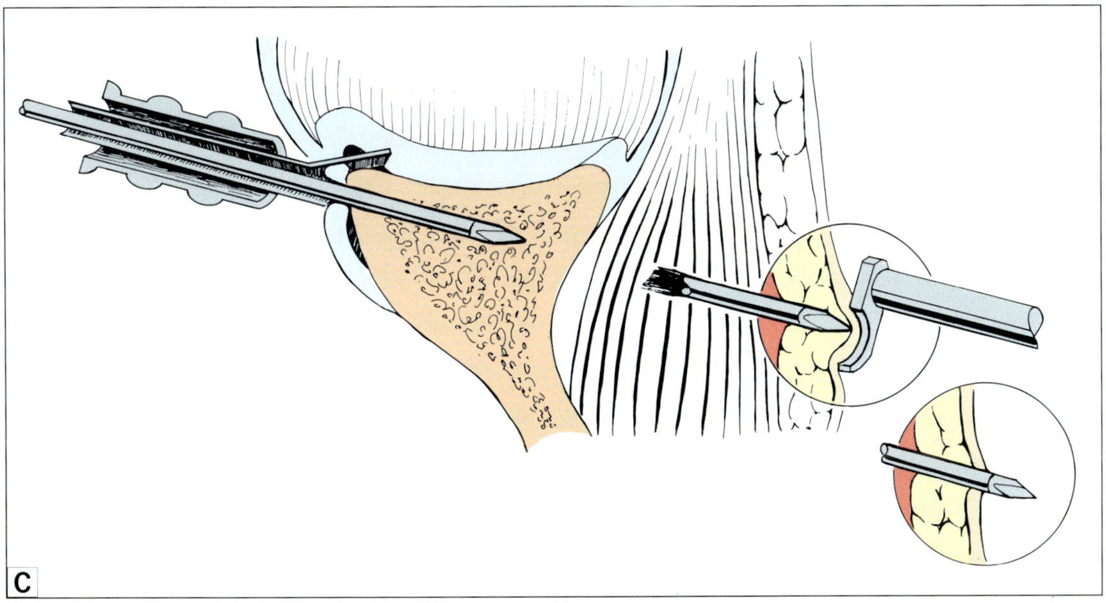

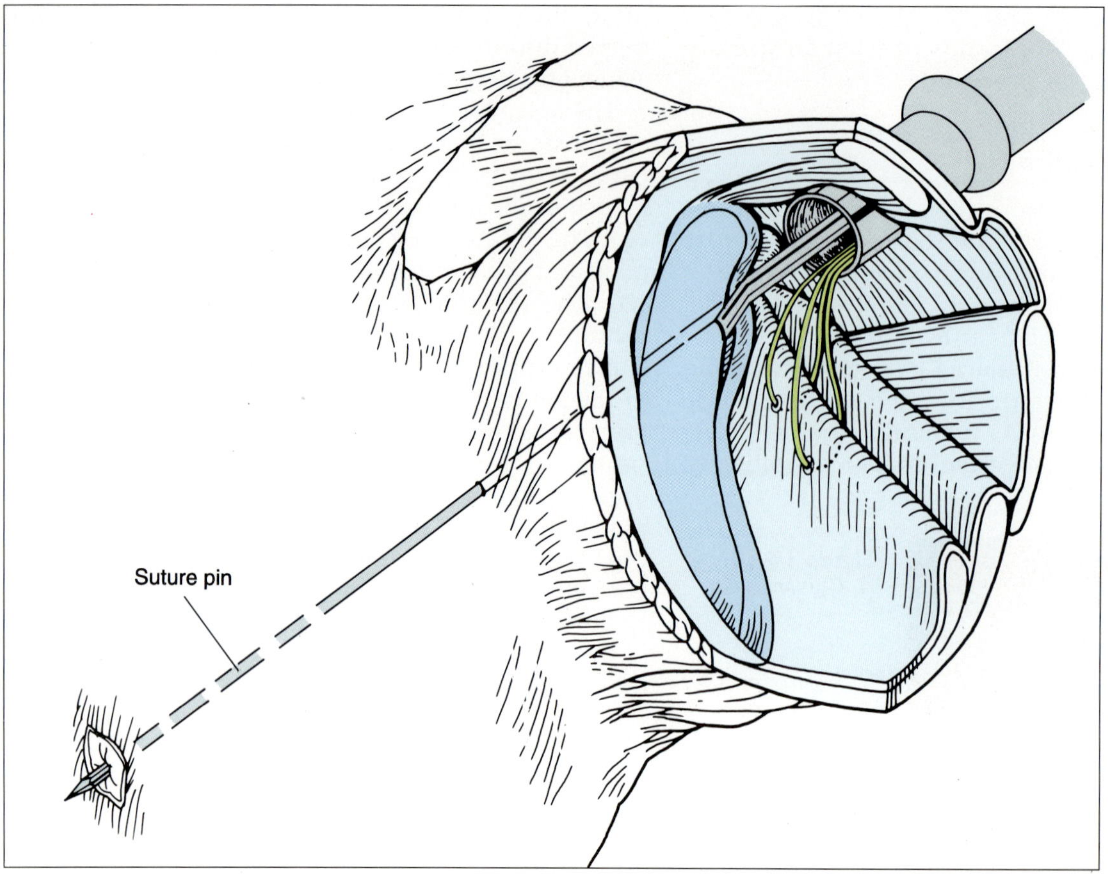

Figure 16-13. Transglenoid pin passage and posterior skin exit. (*From* Rose [27]; with permission.)

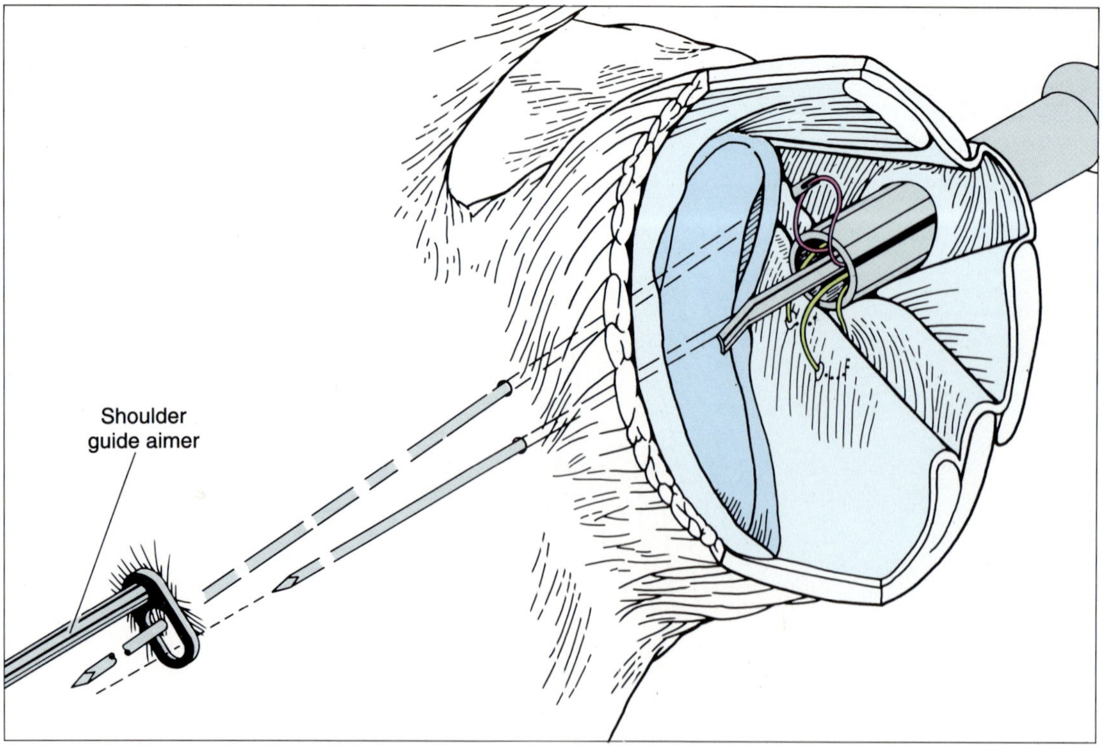

Figure 16-14. Second suture pin drilled transglenoid using shoulder guide to converge pins posteriorly. (*From* Rose [27]; with permission.)

the suture, are brought out posteriorly (Fig. 16-16). The multiple monofilament sutures placed earlier in the inferior glenohumeral ligament are also passed posteriorly via one or both of the suture pins.

After traction is removed and the upper extremity internally rotated, tension is placed on the suture ends posteriorly. The sutures are tied to themselves over the posterior cortex of the scapular neck, thus repairing the Bankart lesion and superiorly shifting the inferior glenohumeral ligament (Fig. 16-17). After the reconstruction is evaluated arthroscopically, all instruments are removed from the shoulder, and all incisions are closed.

POSTOPERATIVE MANAGEMENT

Postoperatively, the patient is maintained in a shoulder immobilizer for 3 to 4 weeks, allowing rotation to neutral, after which progressive range-of-motion and strengthening exercises are begun. Throwing and overhead sports are restricted for approximately 4 months. Contact sports are allowed at 6 months.

COMPLICATIONS AND PITFALLS

Arthroscopic suture stabilization procedures are technically demanding and not without their potential complications and pitfalls. Being aware of these complications helps to shorten the learning curve.

The use of suture pins can lead to inadvertent pin migration [16]. The newer, less flexible pins are helpful in avoiding this problem, as is the suture pin cannula. The cannula decreases the working length of the pin, while the flange on the cannula prevents medial migration of the pin prior to entry into the bone anteriorly.

The suprascapular nerve is at risk as the suture pins exit the scapular neck posteriorly. Injury to the nerve has recently been reported (Mologne and coworkers, Paper presented at Specialty Day Meeting, American Orthopaedic Society for Sports Medicine, New Orleans, 1994). By using a guide to direct pin exit posteriorly toward the "safe zone" [17], the likelihood of damage to the nerve can be significantly decreased, although not eliminated.

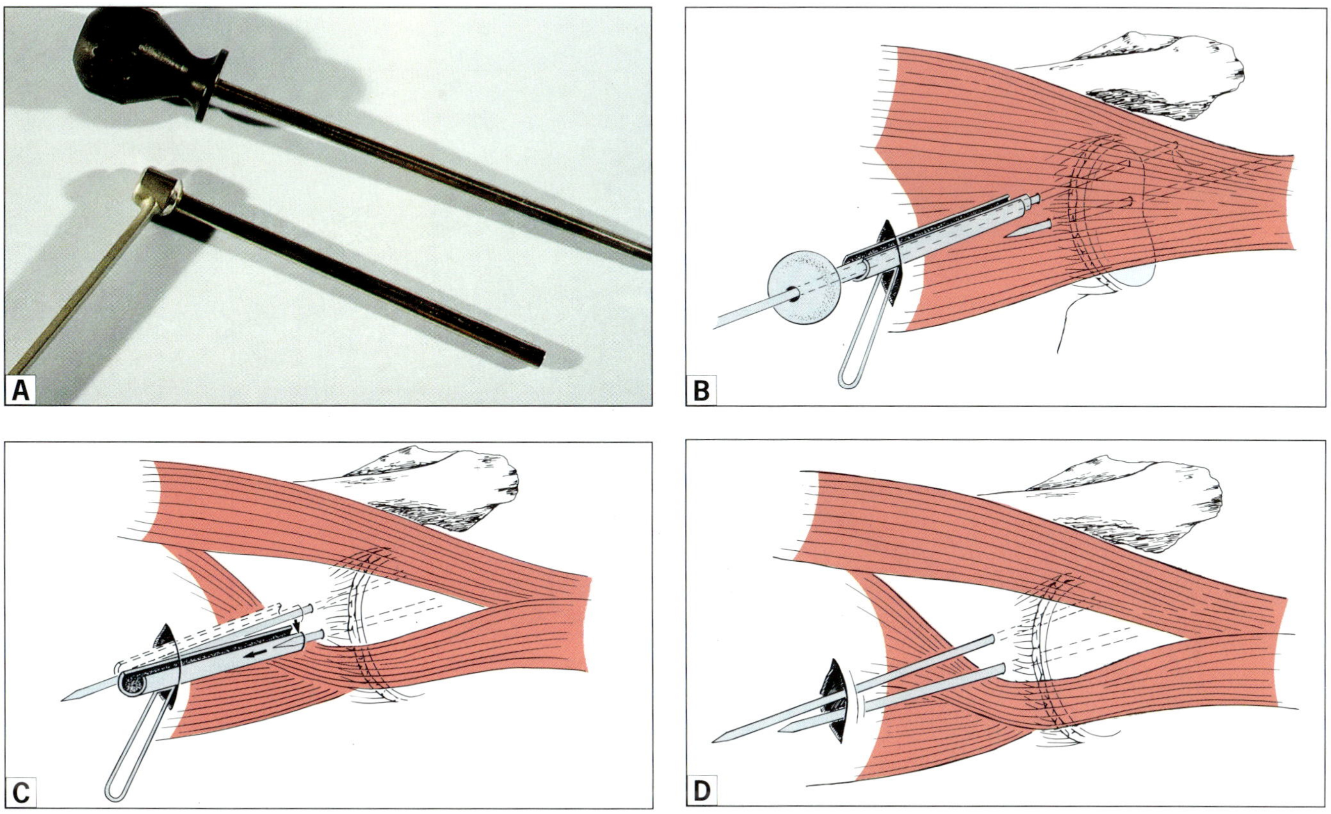

Figure 16-15. Slotted cannula and obturator, **A**, used to prevent capture of posterior soft tissue between pins, **B**, **C**, and **D**.

Careful dissection through the infraspinatus muscle and tying the sutures down to the bone avoids entrapment of the large muscle belly, especially if nonabsorbable sutures are preferred. Retraction of muscle from between the two pins prior to the second pin's passage through the infraspinatus helps to prevent entrapment of the infraspinatus. Absorbable sutures tied over the infraspinatus fascia have not been noted to have adverse consequences, however, by surgeons routinely using the technique [18,19].

Inappropriately medializing the repaired tissue anteriorly can result in a lack of restoration of the buttress. The use of a flanged pin cannula avoids this medialization by placing the suture pin entrance, and thus the soft-tissue repair, at the rim of the glenoid.

Adequate restoration of the inferior glenohumeral ligament tension by superior shift is important to the success of the procedure. Inappropriate tension may result in either recurrent instability [20] or restriction of full shoulder motion. Arthroscopic evaluation of this tension requires experience. More of a shift is usually required in the presence of an inferior component to shoulder luxation, or when the patient has generalized ligamentous laxity.

VARIATIONS OF PATHOLOGY

As one develops more experience with diagnostic arthroscopy of the shoulder, variations of pathology found in patients with anterior and anteroinferior luxation become more evident. After appropriate diagnosis, each shoulder's pathology should be specifically addressed.

When a Bankart lesion but no capsular redundancy is present (Fig. 16-18), mattress suturing of the Bankart lesion alone is performed. When capsular redundancy but no Bankart lesion is encountered (Fig. 16-19), the glenoid neck is debrided medial to the intact labrum, and a capsular shift is performed (Fig. 16-20). If a free labrum is encountered (Fig. 16-21), the hoop effect of the labrum is preserved by spearing the labrum and imbricating it in the repair.

If the glenohumeral ligaments are deficient or absent, the subscapularis tendon may be incorporated into the repair. However, many consider deficient ligaments to be a contraindication to arthroscopic repair.

Large Hill-Sachs lesions are not necessarily a contraindication to suture capsulorrhaphy as long as

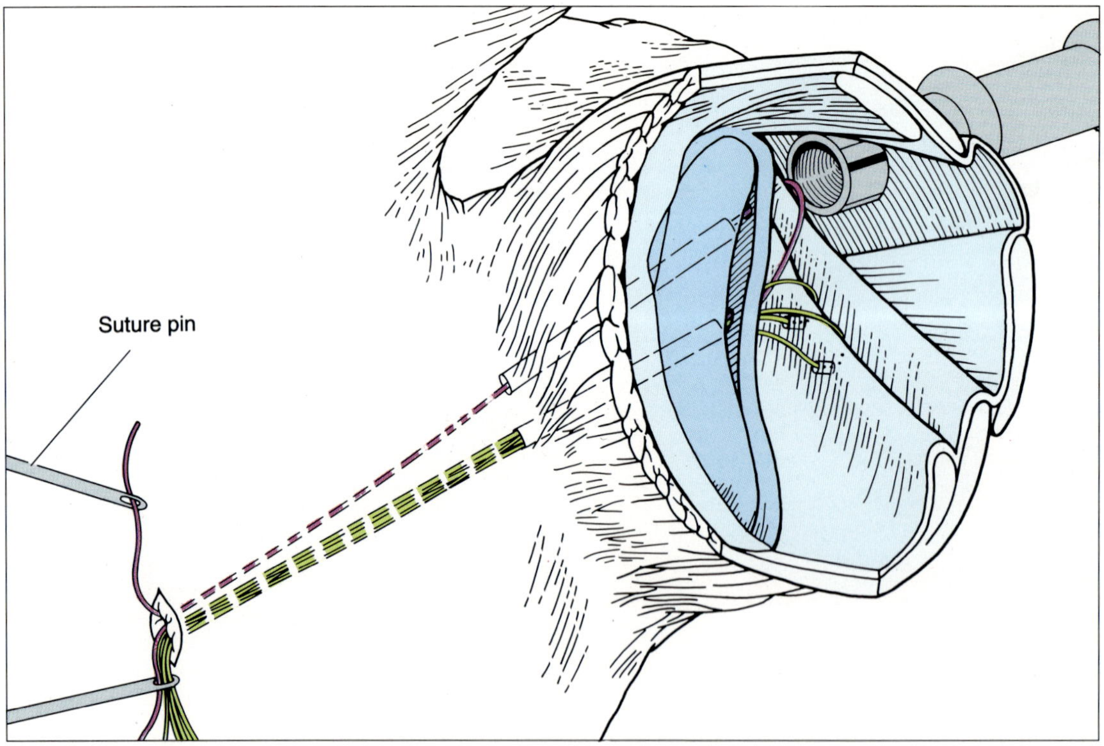

Figure 16-16. Suture pins brought out posteriorly together with ends of sutures. (*From* Rose [27]; with permission.)

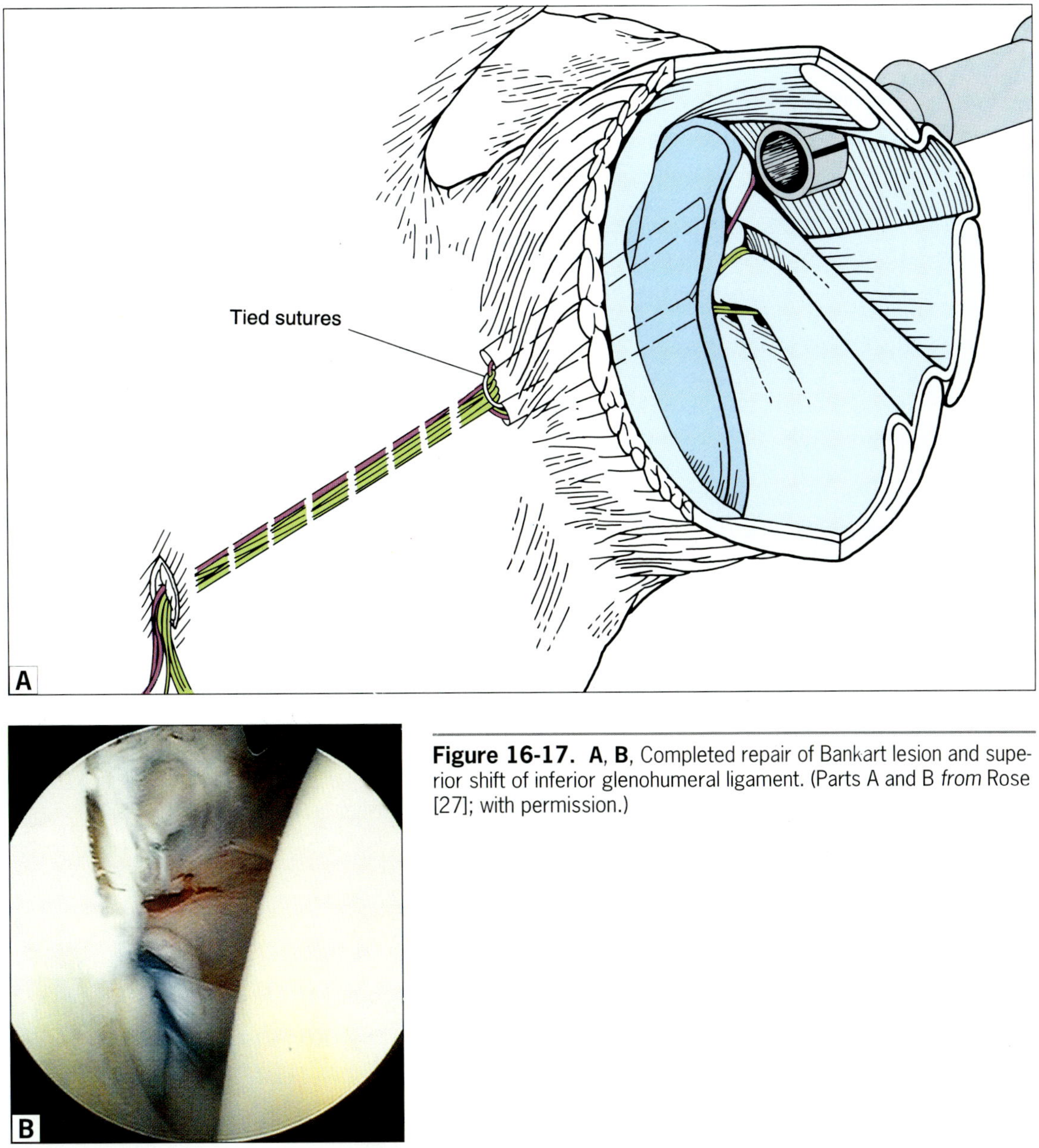

Figure 16-17. **A**, **B**, Completed repair of Bankart lesion and superior shift of inferior glenohumeral ligament. (Parts A and B *from* Rose [27]; with permission.)

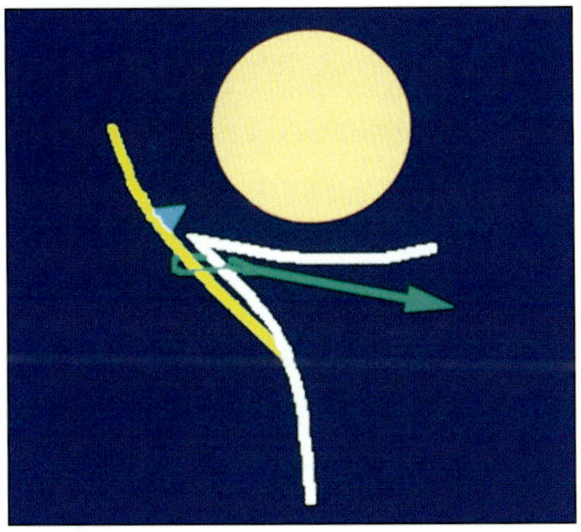

Figure 16-18. Repair of Bankart lesion to rim of glenoid.

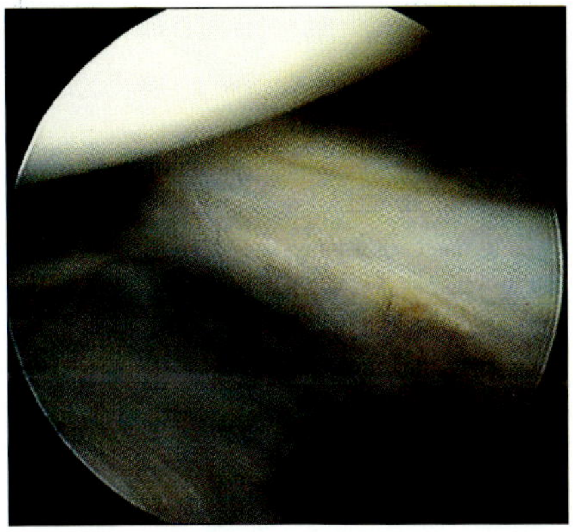

Figure 16-19. Capsular redundancy without Bankart lesion (anterior view).

the buttress effect can be re-established anteriorly by a combination of Bankart repair, capsular shift, or imbrication of the subscapularis tendon.

Small glenoid rim bony avulsions (Fig. 16-22) can be incorporated into the repair. Moderate or large rim defects are a contraindication to arthroscopic suture repair.

The anterior labral ligamentous periosteal sleeve avulsion (ALPSA) lesion described by Neviaser [21] is a medial reattachment of the detached glenohumeral ligament labral complex to the glenoid neck (Fig. 16-23), thus losing the buttress effect. This lesion is often not recognized. When encountered, the ligament-labral complex is sharply liberated from its medial attachment (Fig. 16-24) and advanced laterally to the glenoid rim where it is repaired.

With previously failed open or arthroscopic stabilization procedures, the advantage of an arthroscopic approach is that the pathology responsible for the failure can be evaluated and appropriately addressed, bypassing the often scarred and distorted anterior soft-tissue anatomy (Fig. 16-25).

RESULTS

As more experience is gained with arthroscopic transglenoid suture capsulorrhaphy procedures, there has been an increasing number of studies reporting on the results with varying degrees of success (Savoie, paper presented at the 12th Annual Meeting of the Arthroscopy Association of North America, Palm Desert, 1993) [18–20,24–26]. It is important to recognize that all transglenoid procedures are not the same. The techniques vary, depending on whether a capsular shift is performed, type of suture material used, posterior soft-tissue imbrication, and method of anterior suturing. Indications and patient selection have also been highly variable in the reported series.

The results of a study of 50 patients with a history of recurrent anterior or anteroinferior luxations who were available for a 2- to 6-year follow-up has recently been reported (Rose and coworkers, paper presented at the 12th Annual Meeting of the Arthroscopy Association of North America, Palm Desert, 1993). All patients indicated for surgery underwent arthroscopic transglenoid

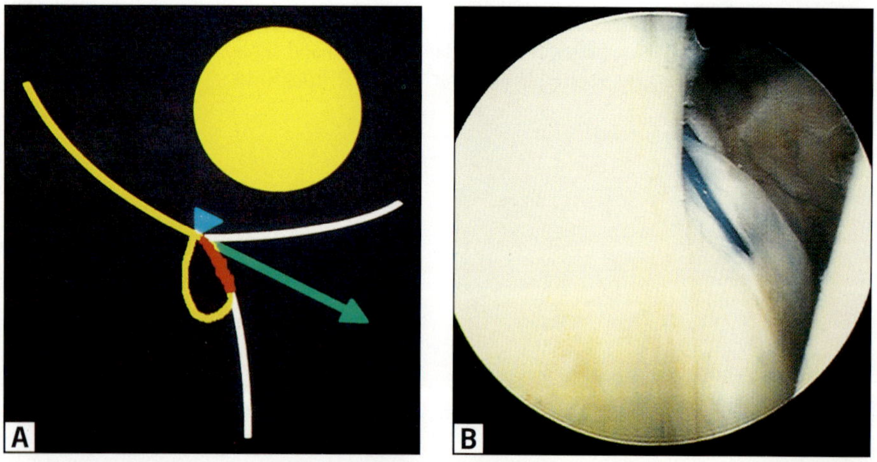

Figure 16-20. Superior shift of inferior glenohumeral ligament without Bankart repair when capsular redundancy is present without Bankart lesion. **A**, Horizontal cross-section. **B**, Arthroscopic view.

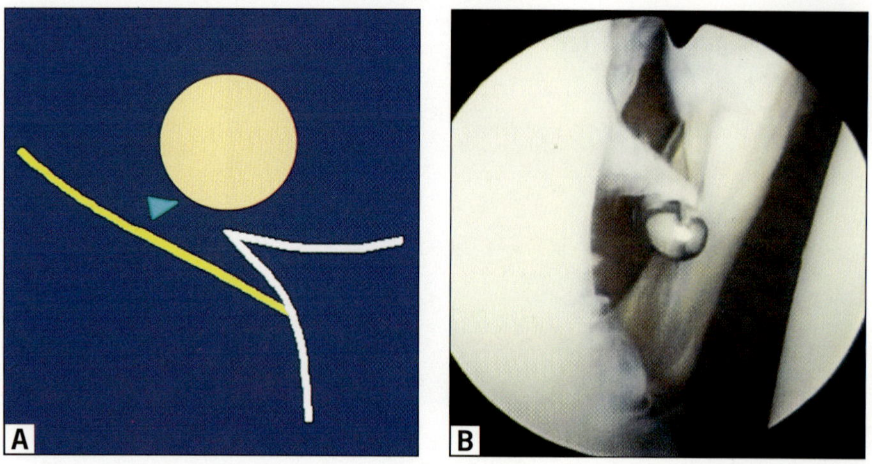

Figure 16-21. Free labrum unattached to either anterior glenoid rim or glenohumeral ligaments. **A**, Horizontal cross-section. **B**, Arthroscopic view.

suture capsulorrhaphy as described. Ten percent of the procedures were considered failures due to recurrent postoperative subluxation or dislocation.

Discussion

One of the most important factors for achieving success in shoulder reconstruction procedures, whether the procedure is performed open or arthroscopically, is to both recognize and correct the responsible pathology. The detached glenohumeral ligament labral complex, as well as any capsular redundancy, both need to be addressed. In reported series, when a capsular shift was performed, the failure rate was less than 16%. Failure to address this pathology has resulted in a higher failure rate [20,24].

A higher recurrence rate has also been reported in those patients involved with collision sports (Rose and coworkers, Paper presented at the 12th Annual Meeting of the Arthroscopy Association of North America, Palm Desert, 1993) [19,24], and in patients younger than 18 years old (Savoie, Paper presented at the 12th Annual Meeting of the Arthroscopy Association of North America, Palm Desert 1993). Among other factors, technical errors and suture materials that are different from those used in open procedures may also play a role.

The advantages of the arthroscopic procedure previously described are that a capsular shift and anatomic repair of the Bankart lesion are performed as required, strong, nonabsorbable sutures are used, and the sutures are tied down to bone, not over posterior soft tissue. An important advantage is that the procedure, as opposed to other arthroscopic or open techniques, does not rely on the bone integrity or quality of the anterior glenoid neck for fixation. The disadvantages include the learning curve and the potential complications from transglenoid pin passage.

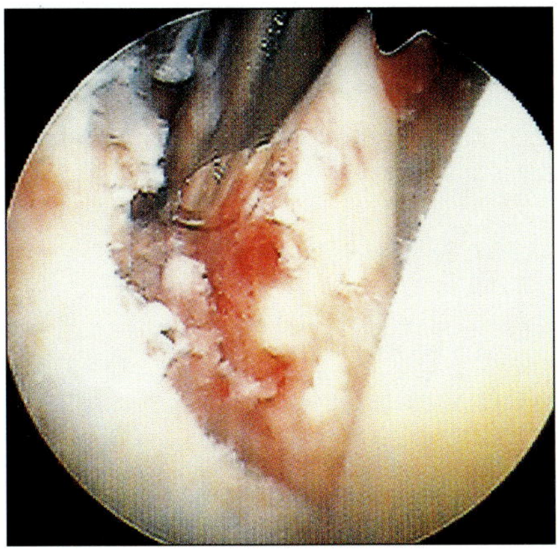

Figure 16-22. Bony Bankart lesion (capsular avulsion of anterior glenoid rim).

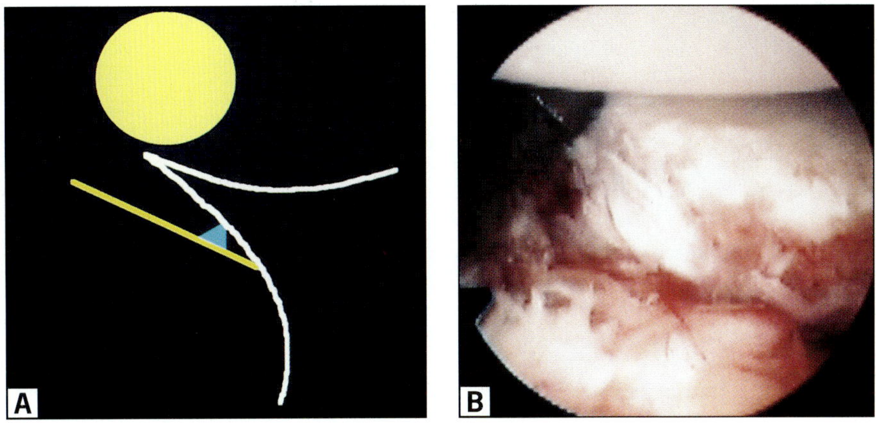

Figure 16-23. **A**, **B**, Anterior labral ligamentous periosteal sleeve avulsion lesion (anterior view).

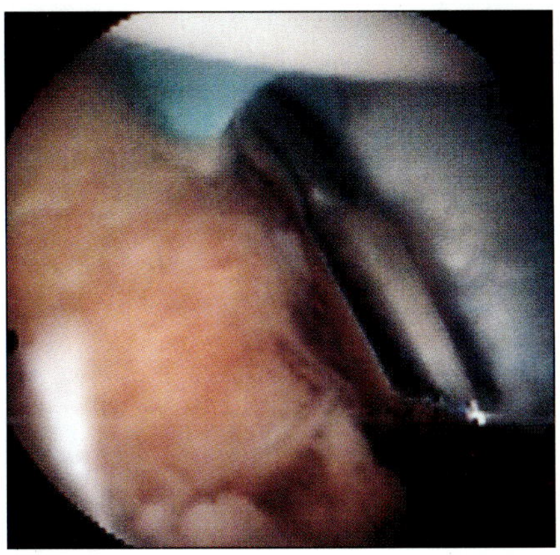

Figure 16-24. Liberation of anterior labral ligamentous periosteal sleeve avulsion lesion with sharp elevator (anterior view).

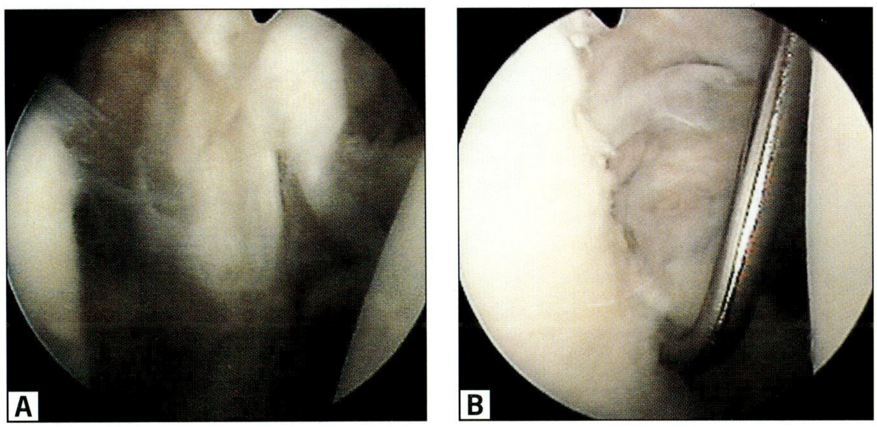

Figure 16-25. **A**, Bankart lesion in patient with a failed Bristow procedure. **B**, Following arthroscopic transglenoid suture repair of Bankart lesion.

Based on current arthroscopic experience, transglenoid suture capsulorrhaphy cannot be recommended for patients less than 18 years of age, those involved in upper extremity collision sports, those with a large glenoid rim defect or habitual luxators, or for those surgeons having a limited experience with operative arthroscopy of the shoulder. The procedure currently has an unresolved role in acute dislocations, multidirectional instability, those with previously failed open or arthroscopic repairs, and those with generalized joint hyperlaxity.

CONCLUSIONS

The role of arthroscopic procedures in the management of glenohumeral instability continues to evolve. Arthroscopic transglenoid suture capsulorrhaphy as described is an attractive and effective alternative for correcting the pathology of anterior and anteroinferior recurrent shoulder instability. The procedure is technically demanding. To achieve predictable results, recognition and addressment of the responsible pathology is essential, as is appropriate patient selection.

REFERENCES

1. Turkel SJ, Pannio MW, Marshall JL, *et al.*: Stabilizing mechanisms preventing anterior dislocation of the glenohumeral joint. *J Bone Joint Surg* 1981, 63A:1208–1217.
2. Rowe CR, Patel D, Southmayd WW: The Bankart procedure: a long-term end-result study. *J Bone Joint Surg* 1978, 60A:1–16.
3. Rowe CR, Zarins B, Ciullo JV: Recurrent anterior dislocation of the shoulder after surgical repair. *J Bone Joint Surg* 1984, 66A:159–168.
4. Jobe FW, Giangarra CE, Kvitne RS, *et al.*: Anterior capsulolabral reconstruction of the athlete in overhead sports. *Am J Sports Med* 1991, 19:429–434.
5. Rao JP, Francis AM, Hurley J, *et al.*: Treatment of recurrent anterior dislocation of the shoulder by Dutoit staple capsulorrhaphy: Results of long-term follow-up study. *Clin Orthop* 1986, 204:169–176.
6. Thomas SC, Matsen FA III: An approach to the repair of avulsion of the glenohumeral ligaments in the management of traumatic anterior glenohumeral instability. *J Bone Joint Surg* 1989, 71A:506–513.
7. Green MR, Christensen KP: Arthroscopic versus open Bankart procedures: a comparison of early morbidity and complications. *Arthroscopy* 1993, 9:371–374.
8. Johnson LL: The shoulder joint: an arthroscopist's perspective of anatomy and pathology. *Clin Orthop* 1987, 223:113–125.
9. Mathews LS, Vetter WL, Oneida SJ, *et al.*: Arthroscopic staple capsulorrhaphy for recurrent anterior shoulder instability. *Arthroscopy* 1988, 4:106–111.
10. Small MC: Complications in arthroscopic surgery performed by experienced arthroscopists. *Arthroscopy* 1988, 4:215– 221.
11. Snyder SJ, Strafford BB: Arthroscopic management of instability of the shoulder. *Orthopedics* 1993, 16:993–1002.
12. Luckey CA: Recurrent dislocation of the shoulder: Modification of Bankart capsulorrhaphy. *Am J Surg* 1949, 77:220–222.
13. Reider B, Inglis AE: The Bankart procedure modified by the use of proline pull-out sutures. *J Bone Joint Surg* 1982, 64A:628–629.
14. Gross RM, Fitzgibbons TC: Shoulder arthroscopy: a modified approach. *Arthroscopy* 1985, 1:156–159.
15. Laurencin LT, Deutsch A, O'Brien SJ, *et al.*:The superolateral portal for arthroscopy of the shoulder. *Arthroscopy* 1994, 10:255–258.
16. Shea KP, Jeffrey LL: Scapulothoracic penetration of a beath pin: an unusual complication of arthroscopic Bankart suture repair. *Arthroscopy* 1991, 7:115–117.
17. Bigliani LU, Dalsey RM, McCann PD, *et al.*: an anatomical study of the suprascapular nerve. *Arthroscopy* 1990, 4:301–305.
18. Caspari RB, Savoie FH: Arthroscopic reconstruction of the shoulder: the Bankart repair. In *Operative Arthroscopy*. Edited by McGinty JB. New York: Raven Press; 1991:507–515.
19. Morgan C, Bodenstab A: Arthroscopic transglenoid Bankart suture repair. *Oper Tech Orthop* 1991, 1:171–179.
20. Wolin PM: Arthroscopic glenoid labrum suture repair [Abstract]. *Orthop Trans* 1990, 14:597.
21. Neviaser TJ: The anterior labral ligamentous periosteal sleeve avulsion lesion: a cause of anterior instability of the shoulder. *Arthroscopy* 1993, 9:17.
22. Benedetto KP, Glotzer WW: Arthroscopic Bankart procedure by suture technique: Indications, techniques and results. *Arthroscopy* 1992, 8:111–115.
23. Goldberg BJ, Nirschl RP, McConnell JP, *et al.*: Arthroscopic transglenoid suture capsulolabral repairs: Preliminary results. *Am J Sports Med* 1993, 21:656–665.
24. Grana WA, Buckley PD, Yates CK: Arthroscopic Bankart suture repair. *Am J Sports Med*1993, 21:348–353.
25. Landsiedl F: Arthroscopic therapy of recurrent anterior luxation of the shoulder by capsular repair. *Arthroscopy* 1992, 8:296–304.
26. Maki NJ: Arthroscopic stabilization: suture technique. *Oper Tech Orthop* 1991, 1:180–183.
27. Rose DJ: Arthroscopic suture capsulorrhaphy for anterior shoulder instability. In *Techniques in Therapeutic Arthroscopy*. Edited by Parisien JS. New York: Raven Press; 1993:12.2–12.9.

17

CHAPTER

Arthroscopic Surgery for Soft-Tissue Lesions of the Ankle

J. SERGE PARISIEN

Ankle arthroscopy has rapidly become an important diagnostic and therapeutic procedure. Indications now include osteochondral and soft-tissue lesions. The latter includes mostly the synovium and to a lesser degree the capsule and ligamentous structures [1–5].

TYPES OF SYNOVIAL LESIONS

Nonspecific Chronic Synovitis

Ankle sprains and traumatic injuries to the ankle are the most common causes of nonspecific chronic synovitis [1–3,6,7, 8,9•,10–12]. Patients with the localized form of the lesion who have sustained an inversion injury of the ankle usually complain of continuous pain, intermittent swelling, and "giving way" for many months after the initial trauma. Tenderness over the anterolateral corner of the talus and lateral gutter is always present. There is usually no evidence of ligamentous disruption. Thorough clinical examination coupled with radiographs and—when indicated—computed tomography (CT) scans, magnetic resonance (MR) imaging, arthrograms, peroneal tenographies, inversion and eversion stresses, and sagittal stress tests will fail to demonstrate evidence of internal derangement such as ligamentous disruption impingement exostosis, transchondral fractures of the talus, sinus tarsi syndrome, peroneal tendinitis, or dislocation. This localized synovitis has been called anterior synovial or soft-tissue impingement of the ankle [6–8,9•,10–12]. It can also be present on the medial aspect of the ankle following a sprain (Fig. 17-1). This localized synovitis has also been reported less frequently at the posterior aspect of the joint, the so-called posterior soft-tissue impingement [13•]. Guhl and Stone [8,14] have implicated some other very rare lesions such as a hypertrophied transverse tibiofibular ligament (Fig. 17-2), the meniscus of the ankle, and a pathologic labrum of the posterior aspect of the ankle.

The so-called meniscoid lesion of the anterolateral aspect of the ankle was described by Wolin and coworkers [12] in 1950 as a mass of hyalinized connective tissue from the talofibular joint area that could cause pain and swelling from repeated catching of the tissue in this limited space. Open surgical excision was the treatment of choice. Guhl and Stone [8,14] are of the impression that this meniscoid lesion may represent an advanced form of synovial impingement. More recently, Bassett and coworkers [15] reported the thickening and hypertrophy of the inferior slip of the anterior tibiofibular ligament as another cause of impingement at the anterolateral aspect of the ankle.

Arthroscopy can provide dramatic responses for patients with localized soft-tissue impingement whose symptoms are not relieved by conservative measures of at least 3 months: physical therapy, the use of anti-inflammatory medications, steroid injections, or even the use of orthotics when valgus heels and pronation are present. Pathologic findings such as hypertrophic localized synovitis are sometimes associated with chondromalacic areas of the tibial or talar dome.

Patients with diffuse nonspecific chronic synovitis usually have a long history of chronic ankle sprain or repetitive trauma. Chondromalacic areas, loose chondral fragments, and generalized synovial hypertrophy are present.

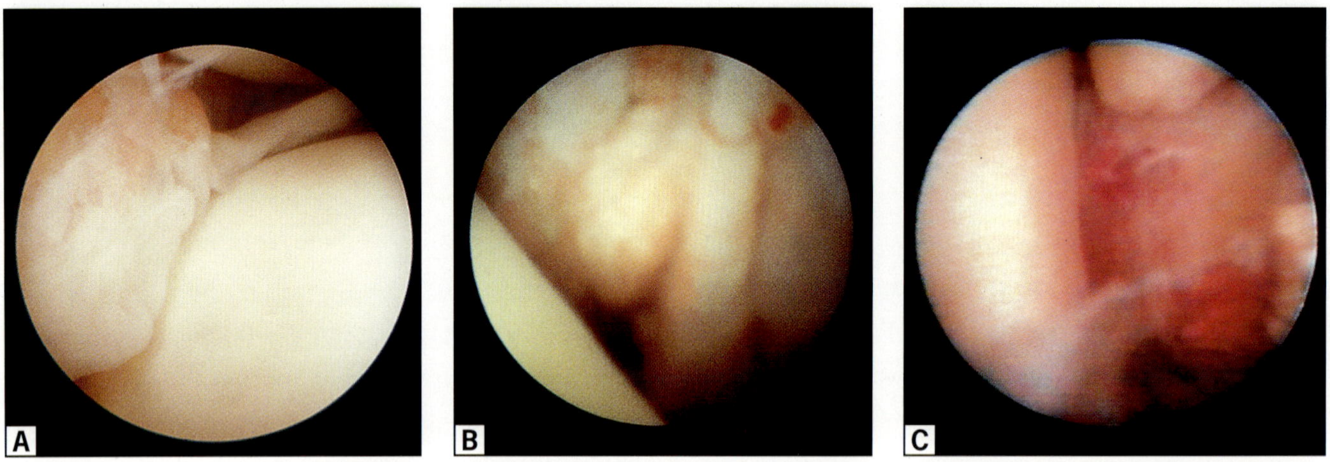

Figure 17-1. **A**, Synovial impingement of the anterolateral aspect of the right ankle. **B**, Synovial impingement of the anterolateral aspect of the left ankle. **C**, Synovial hypertrophy of the medial talomalleolar space causing pain and swelling in the right ankle.

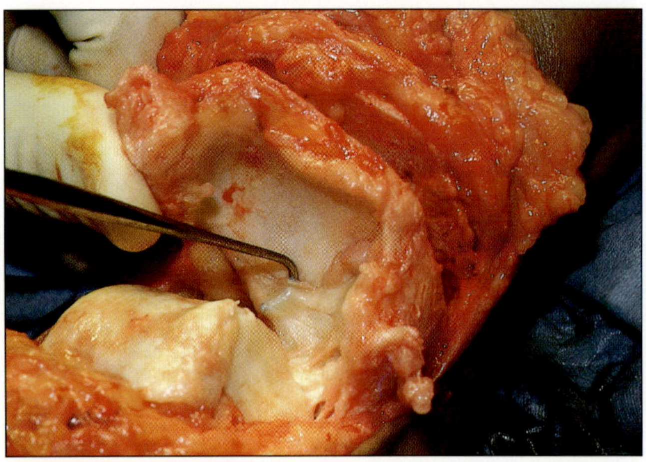

Figure 17-2. Anatomic dissection of a left ankle showing the transverse ligament. This ligament should not be confused with an abnormal posterior fibrous band.

Arthrofibrosis

Following a sprain or direct trauma to the ankle joint, localized adhesions can develop on the lateral or medial aspect of the ankle. Patients usually experience localized tenderness, pain after walking on uneven ground, and discomfort from forced dorsiflexion or plantar flexion. Adhesions of the distal tibiofibular syndesmosis have also been reported by Pritsch and coworkers [16•] in patients suffering from chronic ankle pain after undisplaced ankle fractures. Diffuse arthrofibrosis can occasionally follow ankle sprains, previous surgical procedures, or long periods of immobilization for ankle and leg fractures. The patients are usually disabled owing to pain and limitation of range of motion. Multiple sheets of adhesions can be seen in the anterior compartment as well as in the medial and lateral talomalleolar spaces (Fig. 17-3). Various degrees of articular cartilage damage can be seen arthroscopically with a reactive synovitis.

Pigmented Villonodular Synovitis

Pigmented villonodular synovitis is believed to be a benign synovial disorder. The localized form of the lesion is usually found in the knee, but it can also affect the ankle and can present itself as a solitary, well-circumscribed lesion associated with an otherwise normal synovium [17,18••]. According to Jaffe and coworkers [19], it is probably a hyperplastic process of reactive and inflammatory origin. X-chromosome inactivation analysis in patients who have pigmented villonodular synovitis have shown that the lesion was polyclonal in origin and was therefore more likely to be a reactive process rather than a true neoplasm [20]. Clinical presentation includes internal derangement with intermittent swelling and locking. Arthroscopically, brown or yellow components may be visible on the surface of the lesion (Fig. 17-4).

The diffuse form of pigmented villonodular synovitis is not as commonly seen in the ankles

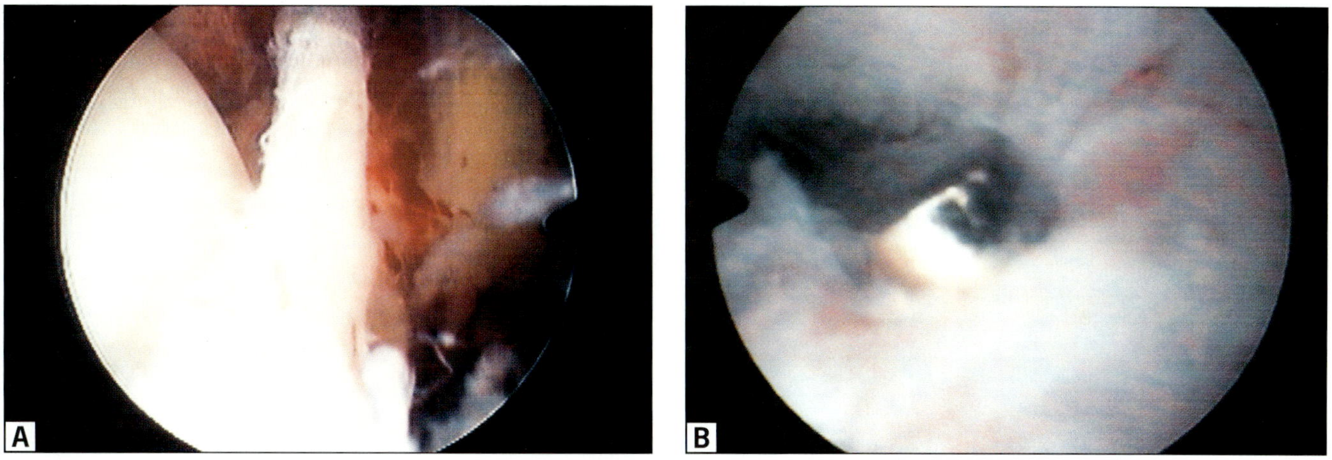

Figure 17-3. **A**, Adhesive band shown in the anterior aspect of the left ankle with some reactive synovitis. **B**, Note the large sheet of adhesions seen on the anterior aspect of the right ankle.

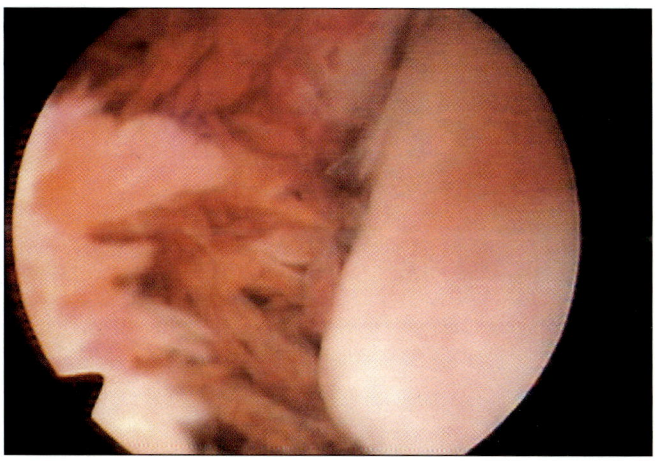

Figure 17-4. Arthroscopic view of a diffused pigmented villonodular synovitis of the right ankle.

compared with its presence in the knee joint. There is a mahogany brown effusion associated with ankle pain. Arthrograms may show nodular masses. MR imaging is very helpful in the diagnosis of both forms (Fig. 17-5) [18••]. The findings on MR imaging are owing to the hemosiderin deposition that causes a decrease in signal intensity on both T_1- and T_2-weighted images. Arthroscopic surgery is usually curative in the localized form. In the diffuse form, complete synovectomy with some form of distraction using the posterolateral portal and the two anterior portals will lessen the chances of recurrence.

Synovial Chondromatosis

Synovial chondromatosis, an uncommon disorder of the ankle, is a monoarticular condition with formation of multiple cartilage bodies secondary to metaplastic transformation of the subintimal connective tissue of the synovium. Milgram [21] has described the three phases of this disorder.

1. An active intrasynovial phase with the absence of loose bodies
2. A transitional phase characterized by active synovial disease and formation of loose bodies
3. A burn-out phase without intrasynovial activity with the ankle joint filled with several or multiple osteochondral bodies

Because there is no osteoid involvement in the early stages, radiographs and scans, except for arthrograms, CT scans, and MR images, are not helpful. In the later stages, loose bodies and degenerative changes can be detected on a radiograph. (Fig. 17-6).

Arthroscopic surgery in the burn-out phases will consist only of removal of all loose osteochondral fragments. Distraction and the use of the posterolateral portal may be necessary. When there is still activity, a synovectomy should complete the procedure.

Inflammatory or Rheumatoid Synovitis

Rheumatoid synovitis is a chronic systemic inflammatory disease that is usually polyarticular when it affects the ankle. It causes pain, limitation of motion, and swelling. It is characterized by hypertrophy and hyperplasia of the synovial cells with villous papillary formation. During the active phase of the disease, it may have an inflamed boggy appearance. The hypertrophied synovium can cause damage to the articular surface of the talus and tibial plafond (Fig. 17-7). Because of the zones of surface necrosis, many synovial villi may have a creamy yellowish appearance referred to as *rice bodies*. A preoperative work-up using CT scans and MR imaging can help locate the synovitis. When in the presence of a single-joint flare, the possibility of a local sepsis, fractures, hemarthrosis, or even malignancy has to be ruled out. Borg and

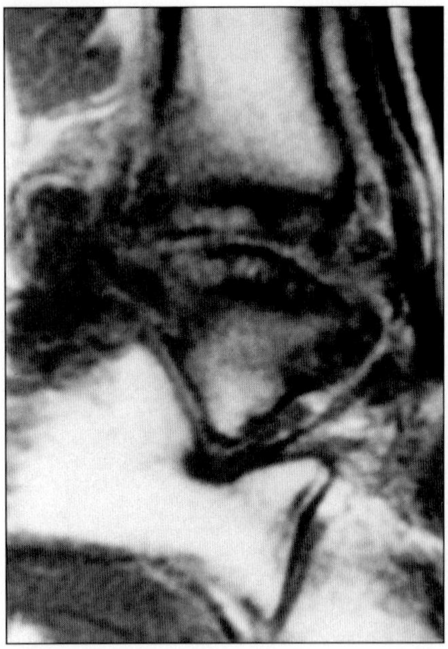

Figure 17-5. Magnetic resonance image of an ankle with pigmented villonodular synovitis. (Photo courtesy of Dr. Javier Beltran).

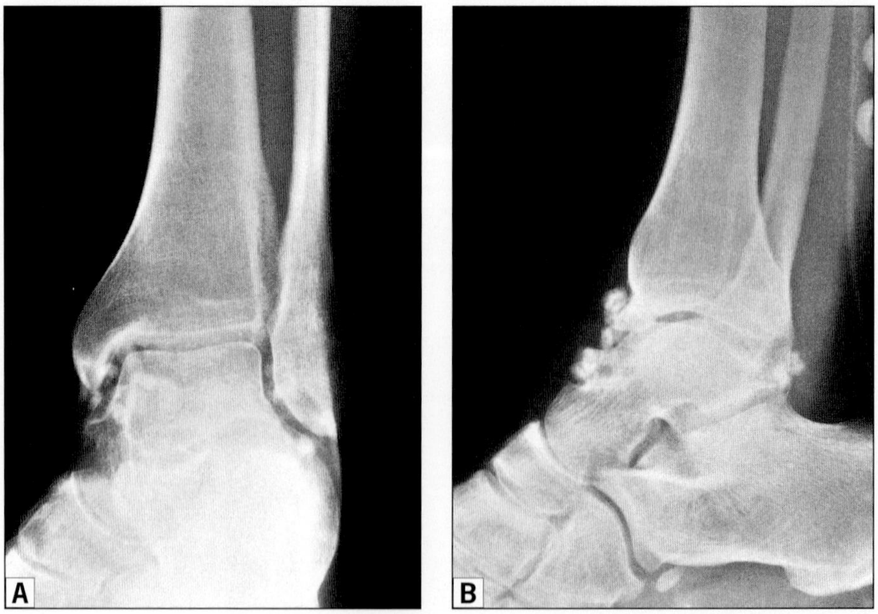

Figure 17-6. **A**, Anteroposterior radiograph view of synovial osteochondromatosis of the left ankle. **B**, Lateral radiograph view of synovial osteochondromatosis.

coworkers [22•] have reported a case of synovial sarcoma in a patient with rheumatoid arthritis. A similar patient who was treated for rheumatoid arthritis was referred to us for arthroscopy. The diagnosis of synovial sarcoma was done at that time.

Better results can be obtained by performing early synovectomy on patients with rheumatoid arthritis of the ankles before the development of bone and articular lesions, rather than late synovectomy.

Infectious Synovitis

As in the knee, arthroscopy can be useful in the diagnosis and management of pyarthrosis of the ankle (Fig. 17-8). Debridement of necrotic synovium can be performed and drainage tubes can be applied. The administration of appropriate antibiotics after culture and sensitivity of the purulent material and a proper rehabilitation regimen with non–weight-bearing ambulation for 6 weeks will insure satisfactory results [8,23].

Chronic Ligamentous Instability

Arthroscopic examination of the ankle has been useful when done before ligamentous reconstruction procedures. The presence of articular cartilage lesions, which may cause persistent pain following reconstruction, can be ascertained [23,24•].

In selected situations, Hawkins [25] has described, with promising results, an arthroscopic technique for stabilization of chronic lateral instability using staples or the Mitek anchor (Mitek Surgical Products, Westwood, MA).

Hemophilic Synovitis

Recurrent bleeding episodes in hemophilic patients are thought to be secondary, in part, to mechanical entrapment of the diffuse synovial proliferation. Arthroscopic synovectomy has been reported as very effective in controlling the rate of bleeding episodes while preserving the range of motion of the involved

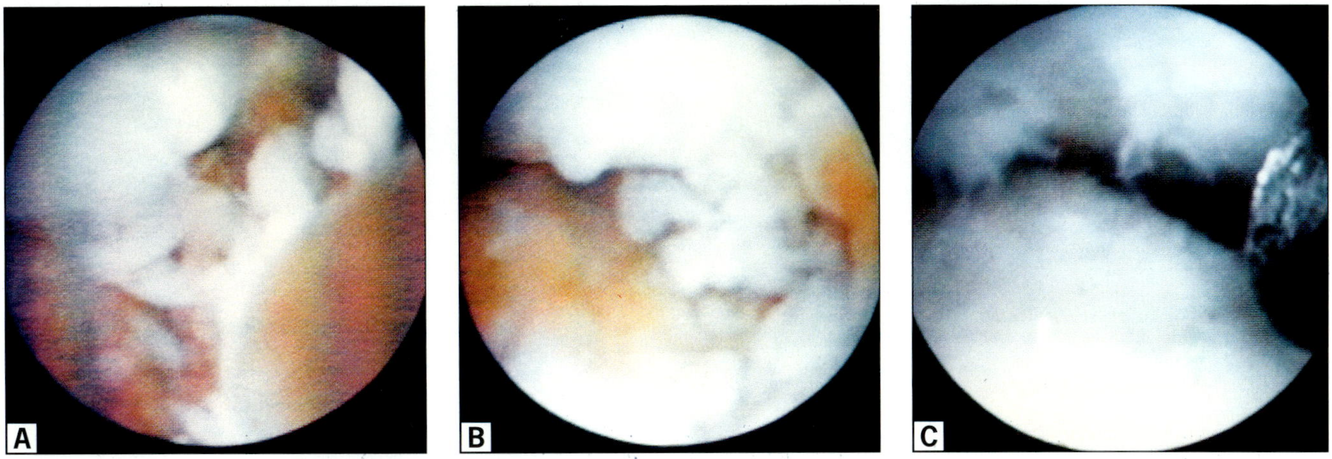

Figure 17-7. **A**, **B** Two arthroscopic views of synovectomy for rheumatoid arthritis of the right ankle. **C**, Arthroscopic view following synovectomy for rheumatoid arthritis of the right ankle.

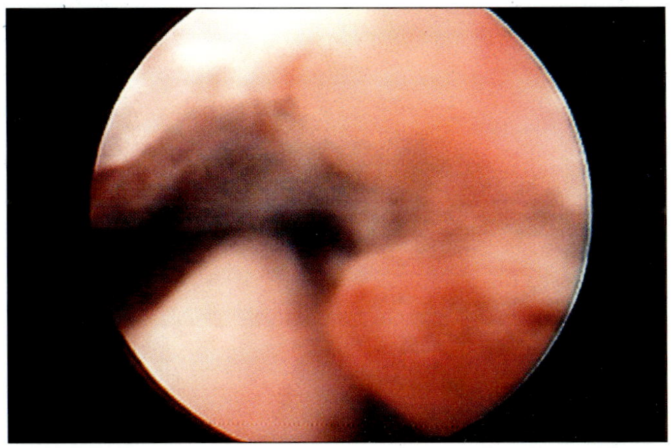

Figure 17-8. Arthroscopic view of pyarthrosis of the ankle joint.

joint. This procedure is best done very early, before failure of medical management, because synovectomy cannot reverse the established degenerative changes of the joint. Few reported series are available on the use of this procedure in adults [26,27]. Recently, it has been found to be a viable option in children provided there is absence of autoantibody, patient compliance during the postoperative period, and absence of HIV [28]. In his series of 28 joints (17 ankles, eight knees, and three elbows with a mean follow-up time of 28 months) Busch and coworkers [28] reported a tenfold decrease in bleeding without complications such as infection.

ARTHROSCOPIC TECHNIQUE

Arthroscopic surgery of the ankle is performed under general, spinal, or epidural anesthesia. The patient is placed supine with a leg holder immobilizing the involved ankle (Fig. 17-9). A tourniquet is placed over the thigh for possible use during the procedure. A bolster is placed under the buttock to allow easy access to the medial lateral and posterolateral aspects of the ankle. Another bolster placed underneath the heel area will facilitate manual distraction. A 4-mm, 30° arthroscope or a short 2.7-mm, 30° arthroscope with a wide-angle lens can be used. Full-radius blades or Whisker blades (2.9 mm or 3.5 mm) are very useful (Fig. 17-10 and 17-11). The two anterior portals are used for the arthroscope and instruments. The posterolateral portal can be used if necessary for the inflow cannula.

For localized, anterior soft-tissue lesions, the two anterior portals are all that are needed. No mechanical traction is necessary. Small basket scissors may be necessary to incise tough scar tissues before their excision with motorized instruments (Fig. 17-12–17-14). The large 3.5-mm blade can be used in the anterior

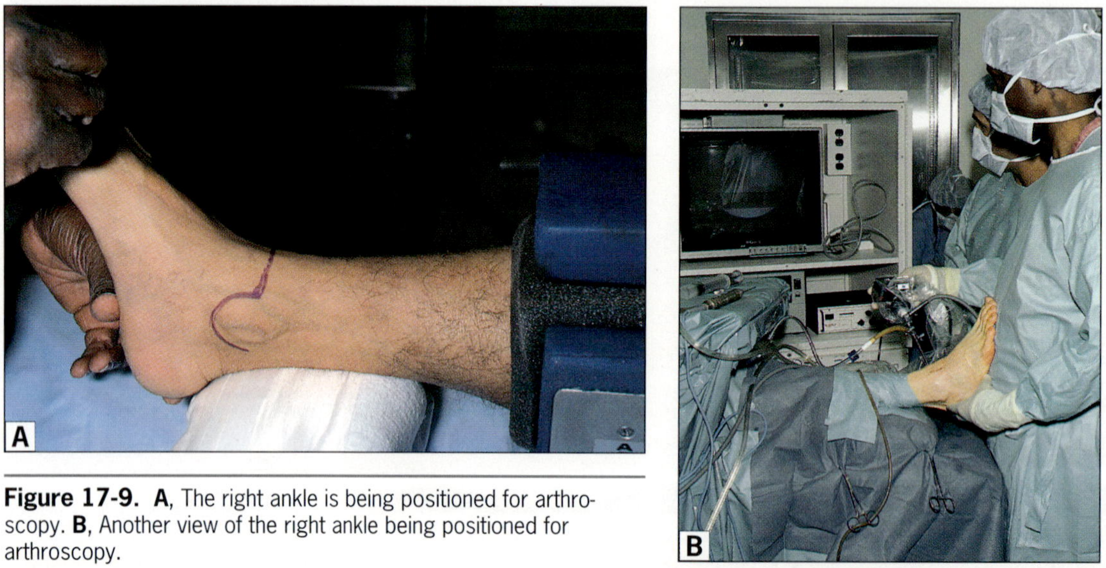

Figure 17-9. **A**, The right ankle is being positioned for arthroscopy. **B**, Another view of the right ankle being positioned for arthroscopy.

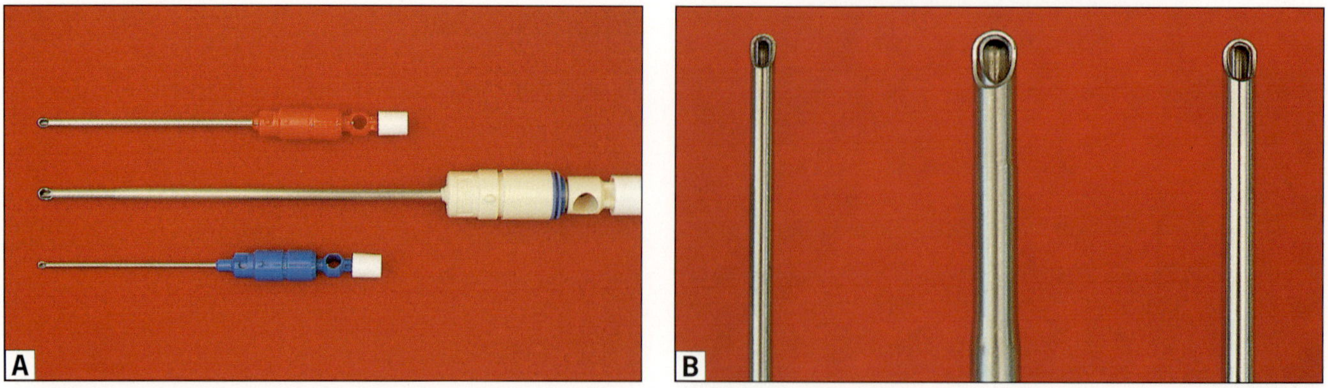

Figure 17-10. **A**, Full-radius blades, 3.5 mm, 2.9 mm, and 2 mm. **B**, Close-up of the full-radius blades. *(continued)*

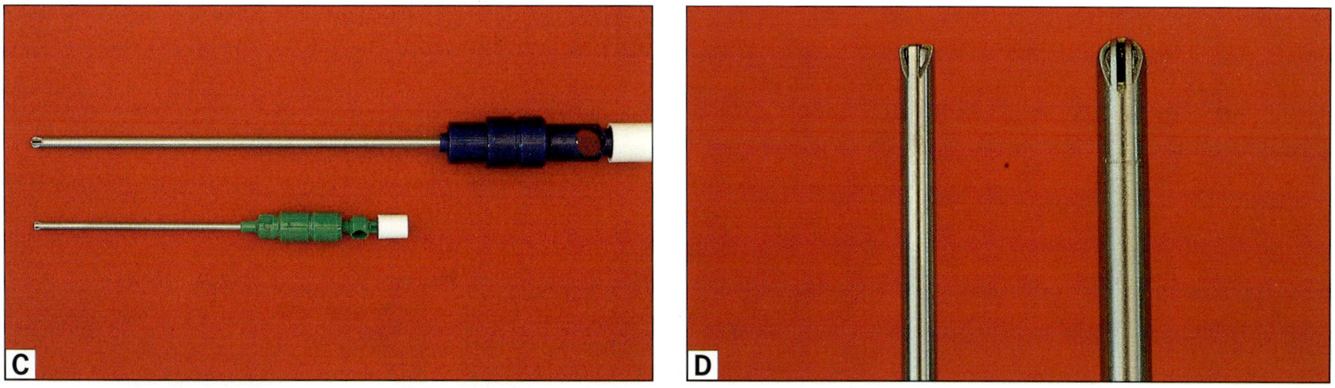

Figure 17-10 (*continued*) **C**, Whisker blades, 4.5 mm and 2.9 mm. **D**, Close-up of Whisker blades.

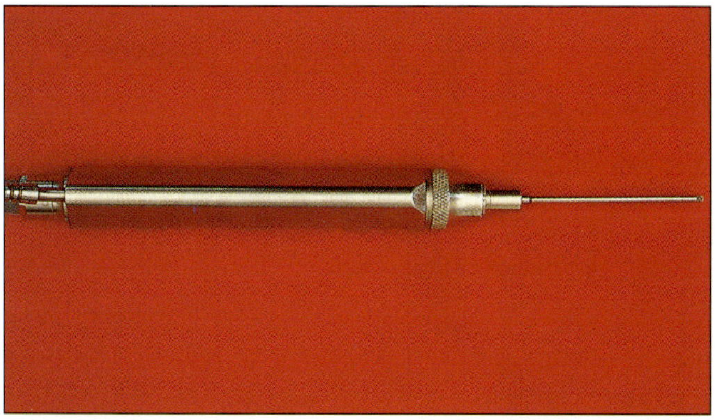

Figure 17-11. Small motorized shaver.

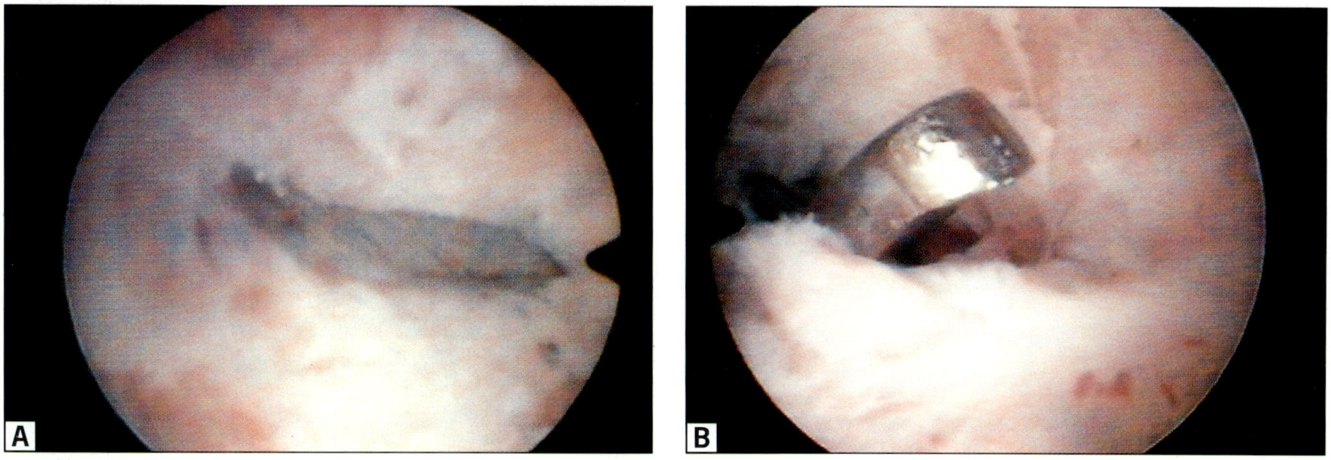

Figure 17-12. **A**, An arthroscopic knife is excising a large sheet of adhesions around the anterior aspect of the right ankle. **B**, Basket forceps complete the excision of adhesions.

pouch, with the 2.9-mm blade reserved for the talomalleolar spaces and posterior pouch. When the synovium is very friable as in rheumatoid arthritis, it is preferable to use the Whisker blade to avoid aggressive debridement of the soft-tissue layer that is very close to the anterior and posteromedial neurovascular structures.

Diffuse soft-tissue lesions of the ankle may require the use of a distractor, preferably the noninvasive type, with or without an infusion pump (Figs. 17-15). Instrumentation through the posterolateral portal will allow complete joint debridement (Fig. 17-16).

Prophylactic antibiotics are used because of the extensive nature of the procedure. Postoperatively, a

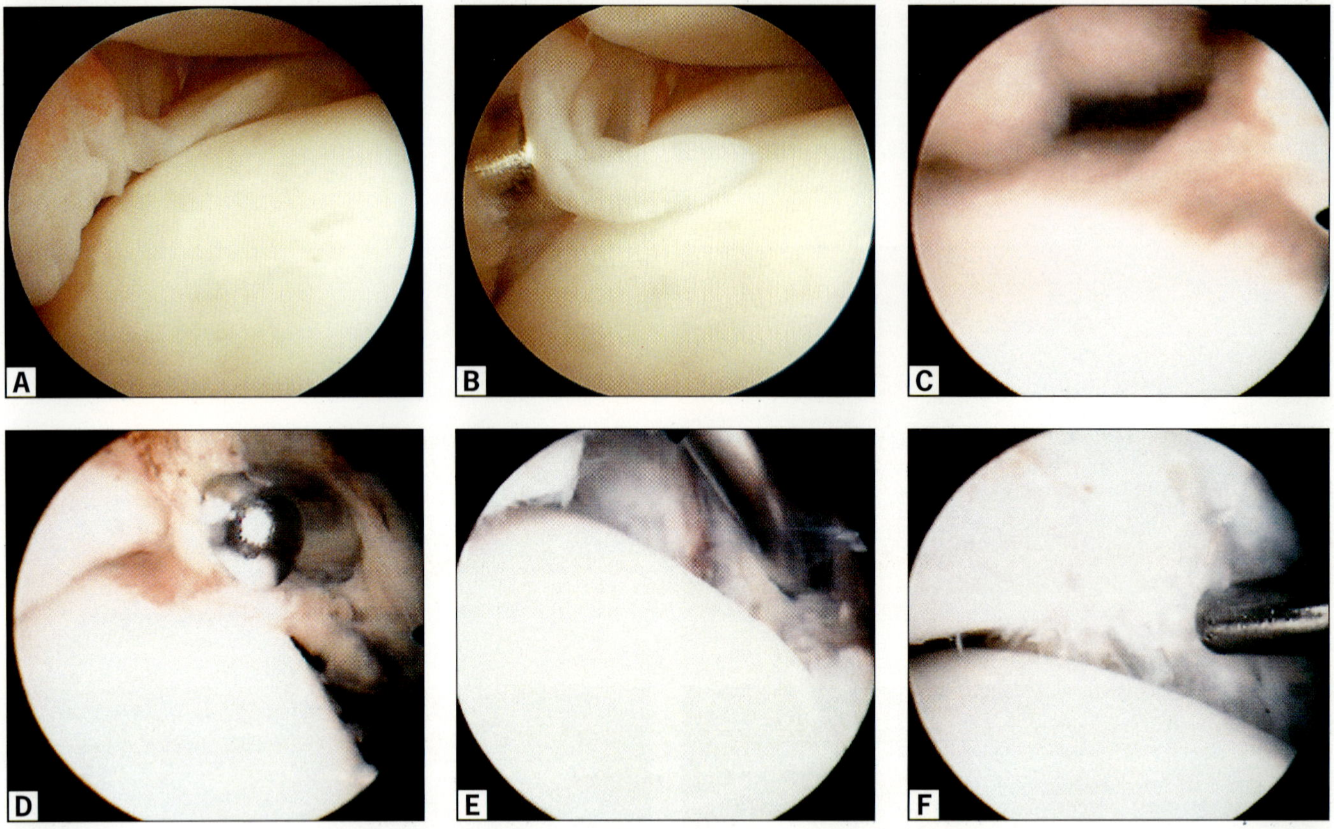

Figure 17-13. **A**, Synovial impingement of the right ankle. **B**, The motorized shaver is excising hypertrophic synovial tissue in a patient with soft-tissue impingement of the anterolateral aspect of the right ankle. **C–F**, Steps of arthroscopic debridement in synovial impingement of the anterolateral aspect of the left ankle.

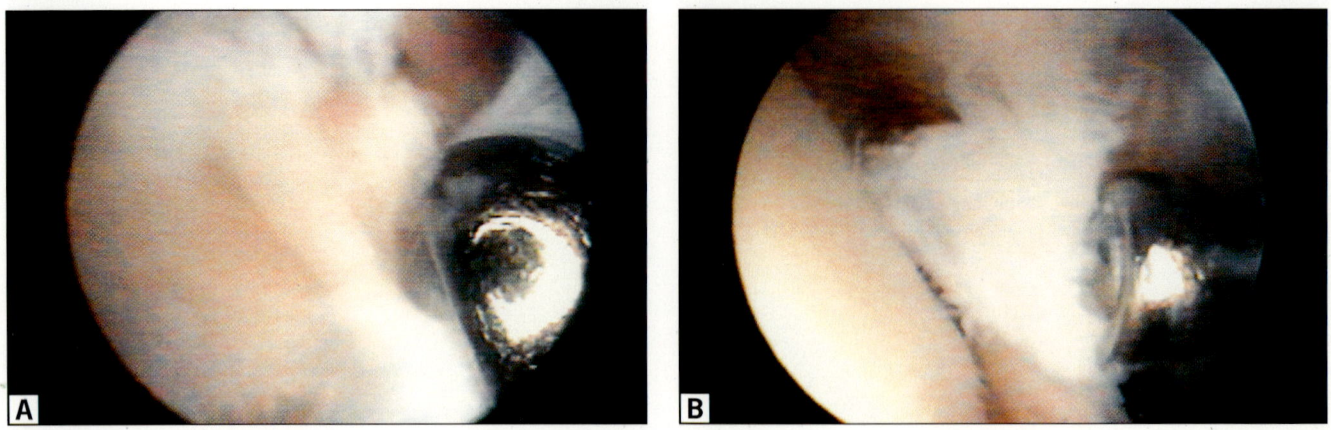

Figure 17-14. **A**, Motorized shaver excising adhesions of the medial aspect of the right ankle. **B**, Motorized shaver completing the excision of adhesions.

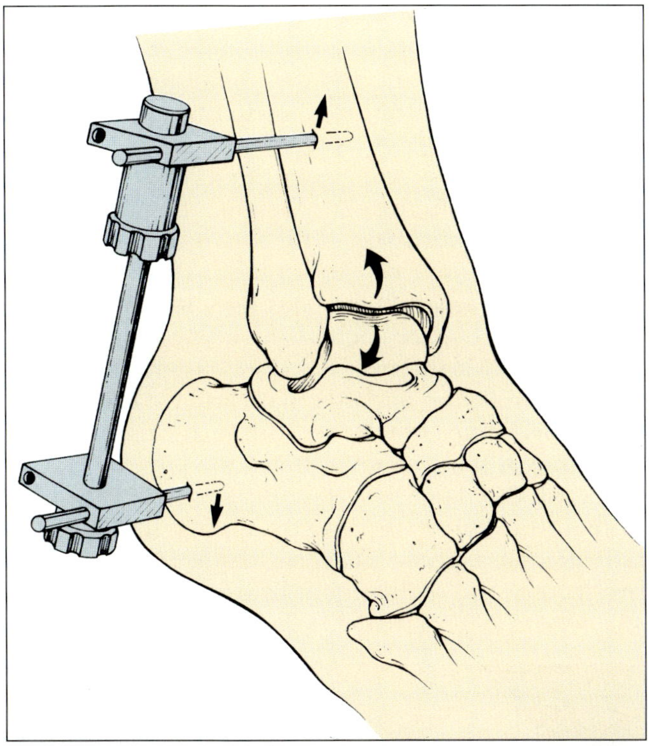

Figure 17-15. Invasive distraction with pins placed laterally.

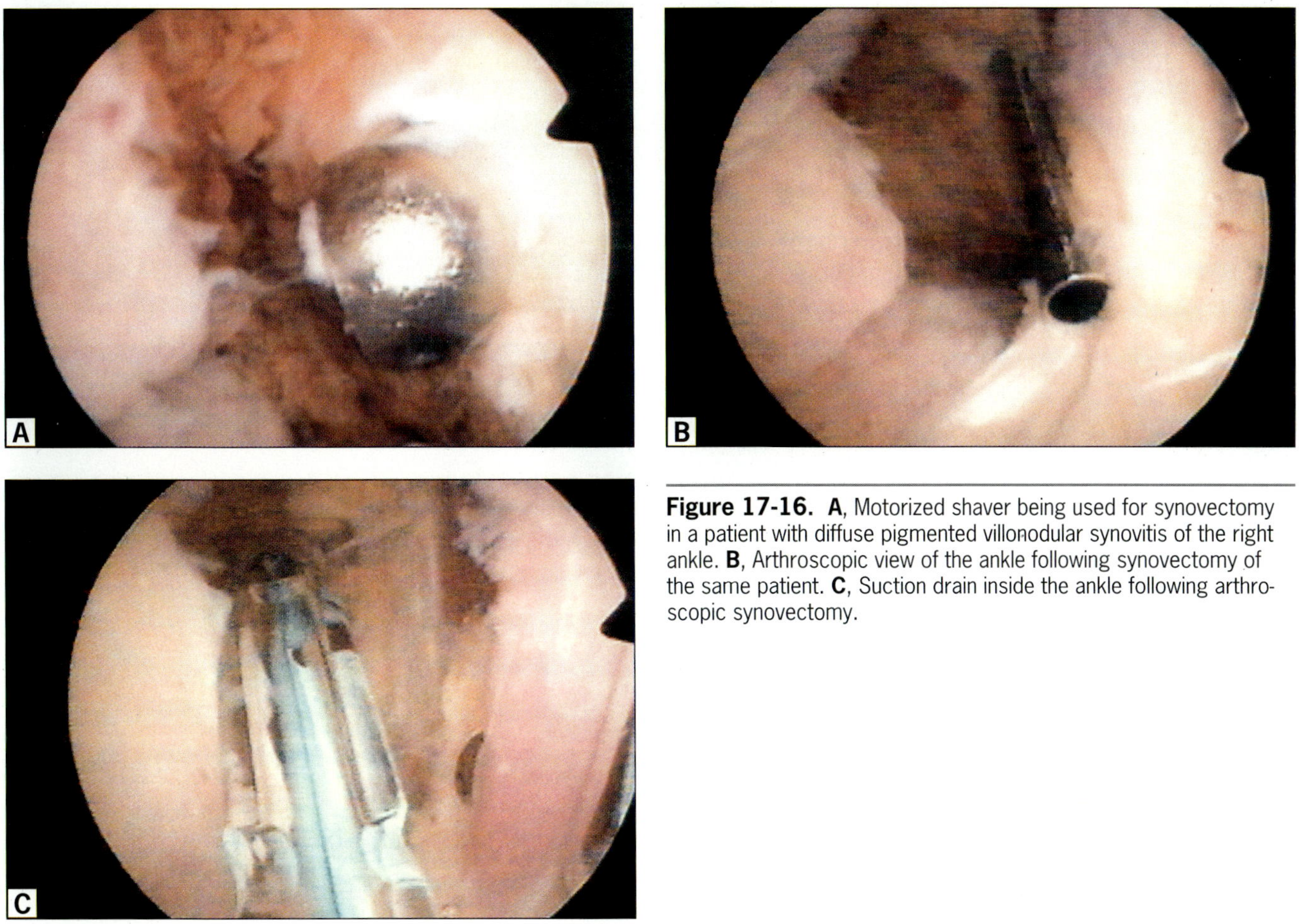

Figure 17-16. **A**, Motorized shaver being used for synovectomy in a patient with diffuse pigmented villonodular synovitis of the right ankle. **B**, Arthroscopic view of the ankle following synovectomy of the same patient. **C**, Suction drain inside the ankle following arthroscopic synovectomy.

drain is applied followed by a compression dressing. Partial weight bearing with crutches for a few days with a gradual return to daily activity is advisable.

Techniques for Instability

Two anterior portals are needed. After a diagnostic evaluation of the ankle joint is performed to rule out the presence of loose bodies and damage to the articular cartilage (usually at the medial corner of the tibia) joint debridement is done with small motorized instrumentation. An area approximately 6 mm or 8 mm in diameter is abraded 1 cm anterior to the tip of the fibula with a small burr. The use of a 70° arthroscope medially will obviate the need for an accessory lateral portal to perform the abrasion. A skin incision is made over the anterior talofibular ligament. Care needs to be taken not to involve any sensory nerves in the area. The staple is placed at a right angle into the talus, creating a plication of the stretched capsuloligament structure into the abraded area of the talus (Fig. 17-17). The foot is held in a neutral position in a posterior splint. After removal of the stitches within 1 week, a short leg cast is applied for 6 more weeks.

Laser Technique

Syndesmodic disruptions usually secondary to external rotation injury of the ankles is not as common as the lateral ligamentous injury. The diagnosis of this entity can be confirmed by a positive external rotation stress test and increased activity in a bone scan. Disruption of the posterior inferior tibiofibular and interosseous ligaments associated with chondral fracture of the posterolateral aspect of the tibial plafond are present. Despite conservative treatment consisting of the use of a brace, an intensive rehabilitation program, and the administration of anti-inflammatory medication, persistent symptoms may require surgery.

Ogilvie-Harris and coworkers have recently reported successful results following the arthroscopic resection of the torn area of the interosseous ligament, with debridement of the articular damage of the posterolateral aspect of the talus [29•,30•]. Access to a confined joint space such as the ankle can be easily facilitated with the use of a small laser hand piece. Synovial resection and articular cartilage contouring can be performed with ease. Although earlier reports have shown some complications, the potential benefits of the CO_2 laser have recently been demonstrated in regard to knee surgery. Its application to ankle arthroscopic surgery has been hampered because of two factors: the requirement of a gas or air medium,

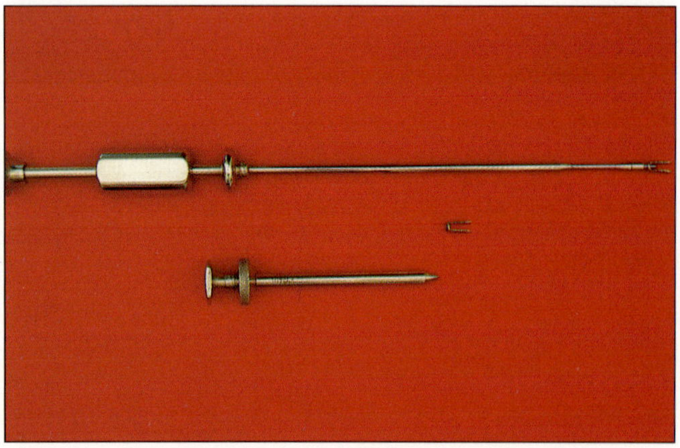

Figure 17-17. Staple used for fixation of a torn anterior talofibular ligament.

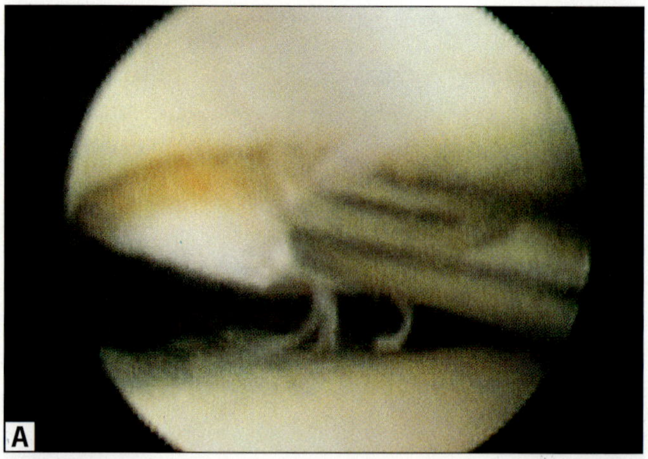

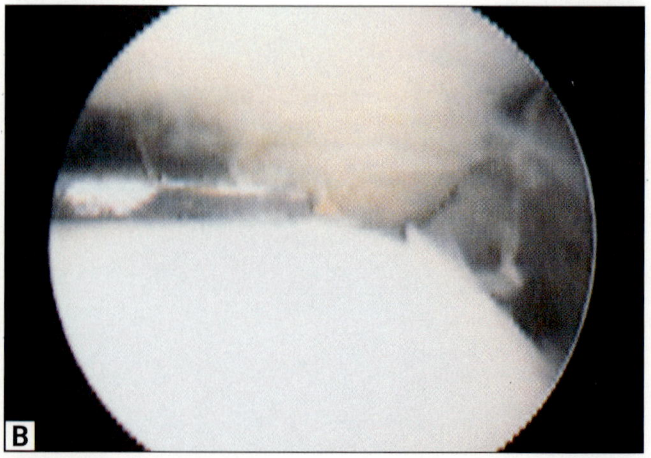

Figure 17-18. **A**, Laser probe being used for synovectomy for a patient with synovial impingement lesion of the ankle. **B**, laser probe debriding a chondromalacic lesion of the ankle. (Photos courtesy of Dr. S. Abelow)

and its inability to be fiberoptically transmitted. Because the holmium:yttrium-aluminum-garnet (Ho:YAG) laser can be used in normal saline and transmitted through a fiber with a beam in almost close contact with the tissue, it has the potential of being an effective tool in arthroscopic surgery (Fig. 17-18) [33]. The use of lasers in the clinical setting seems to have the most promise for synovectomy, chondroplasty, excision of osteochondritis dissecans, and fibrous tissue [34].

Because of the expense, the use of medical lasers is presently prohibitive. However, in the future, more useful roles for lasers in the arthroscopic management of ankle pathology will be found.

REFERENCES AND RECOMMENDED READING

Recently published papers of particular interest have been highlighted as:

- • Of interest
- •• Of outstanding interest

1. Cerrulli G, Caraffa A, Buompadre V, *et al.*: Operative arthroscopy of the ankle. *Arthroscopy* 1992, 8:537–540.

2. Feder KS, Schonholtz GJ: Ankle arthroscopy: Review and long term results. *Foot Ankle Int* 1992, 13:382–385.

3. Phillips BB: Arthroscopy of the ankle. *Oper Tech Sports Med* 1994, 2:71–80.

4. Parisien JS: Techniques for soft tissue and osteochondral lesions of the ankle. In *Techniques in Therapeutic Arthroscopy. Edited by Parisien JS. New York: Raven Press; 1993:17-1–17-17.*

5. Parisien JS: Arthroscopic surgery of the ankle. In *Arthroscopic Surgery* Edited by Parisien JS. New York: McGraw Hill; 1988, 259–281.

6. Thein R, Eichenblat M: Arthroscopic treatment of sports-related synovitis of the ankle. *Am J Sports Med* 1992, 20:496–498.

7. Ferkel RD, Karzel RP, Del Pizzo W, *et al.*: Arthroscopic treatment of anterolateral impingement of the ankle. *Am J Sports Med* 1991, 19:440–446.

8. Guhl JF, Stone JW: Soft tissue pathology. In *Foot and Ankle Arthroscopy*, edn 2. Edited by Guhl JF: Thorofare, NJ: Slack Inc., 1993, 83–105.

9.• Meislin RJ, Rose DJ, Parisien JS, *et al.*: Arthroscopic treatment of synovial impingement of the ankle. *Am J Sports Med* 1993, 21:186–189.

Results of 29 cases of operative arthroscopy for synovial impingement at 25-month follow-up revealed 26 patients with excellent or good results.

10. Biedert R: Anterior ankle pain in sports medicine: Etiology and indications for arthroscopy. *Arch Orthop Trauma Surg* 1991, 110:293–297.

11. McCarroll JR, Schrader JW, Shelbourne KD, *et al.*: Meniscoid lesions of the ankle in soccer players. *Am J Sports Med* 1987, 15:255–257.

12. Wolin I, Glassman F, Sidman S: Internal derangement of the talofibular component of the ankle. *Surg Gynecol Obstet* 1950, 91:193–200.

13.• Liu SH, Mirzayan R: Posteromedial ankle impingement. *Arthroscopy* 1993, 9:709–711.

Arthroscopic debridement of the hypertrophic tissue was proven successful in a patient who presented soft-tissue impingement in the posteromedial aspect of the ankle.

14. Stone JW, Guhl JF: Meniscoid lesions of the ankle. *Clin Sports Med* 1991, 10:661–676.

15. Bassett FH, Gates HS, Billys JB, *et al.*: Talar impingement by the anteroinferior tibiofibular ligament. A cause of chronic pain in the ankle after inversion sprain. *J Bone Joint Surg* 1990, 72A:55–59.

16.• Pritsch M, Lokiec F, Sali M, *et al.*: Adhesions of distal tibiofibular syndesmosis. A cause of chronic ankle pain after fracture. *Clin Orthop* 1993, 289:220–222.

Adhesion of the distal tibiofibular syndesmosis was found to be the cause of chronic ankle pain in 11 of 19 patients suffering from chronic ankle pain after an uncomplicated fracture of the ankle. Arthroscopic resection resolved the symptoms in all 11 patients.

17. Green A, Sutherland W, Trafton PG: Localized nodular synovitis of the ankle: a case report. *Foot ankle* 1991, 12:47–51.

18.•• Konrath GA, Shifrin LZ, Nahigian K: Magnetic resonance imaging in the diagnosis of localized pigmented villonodular synovitis of the ankle: a case report. *Foot Ankle* 1994, 15:84–87.

Preoperative MR imaging was found to be useful in the diagnosis of localized pigmented villonodular synovitis and in the planning for surgery.

19. Jaffe HL, Lichenstein L, Sutro CJ: Pigmented villonodular synovitis bursitis and tenosynovitis: a discussion of the synovial and bursal equivalents of the tenosynovial lesion commonly denoted as xanthoma, xantrogranuloma, giant cell tumor, or myeloplaxoma of the tendon sheath with some consideration of this tendon sheath lesion itself. *Arch Pathol* 1941, 31:731–765.

20. Sakkers RJB, DeJong JD, Van Der Beul RO: X-chromosome inactivation in patients who have pigmented villonodular synovitis. *J Bone Joint Surg* 1991, 73A:1532–1536.

21. Milgram JW: Synovial osteochondromatosis: a histological study of 31 cases. *J Bone Joint Surg* 1977, 59A:792–801.

22.• Borg AA, Wynn-Jones C, Dawes PT: Synovial sarcoma manifesting as a single joint flare in rheumatoid arthritis. *Clin Rheumatol* 1993, 12:89–92.

A case of a 69-year-old woman with rheumatoid arthritis revealed that the swelling in the left ankle was due to a synovial sarcoma.

23. Parisien JS, Shaffer B: Arthroscopic management of pyarthrosis. *Clin Orthop* 1992, 275:243–247.

24.• Taga I, Shino K, Inoue M, *et al.*: Articular cartilage lesions in ankles with lateral ligament injury: an arthroscopic study. *Am J Sports Med* 1993, 21:120–127.

Thirty-one ankles in 31 patients with lateral ligament injury were examined arthroscopically. Nine patients were freshly injured; the other 22 had chronic injuries. It was noted that the longer the time elapsed from the initial injury, the more severe the associated chondral lesions became.

25. Hawkins RB: Arthroscopic repair for chronic lateral ankle instability. In *Foot and Ankle Arthroscopy*, edn 2. Edited by Guhl J. Thorofare, NJ: Slack Inc.; 1993:155–160.

26. Klein KS, Aland CM, Kim HC, *et al.*: Long term follow-up of arthroscopic synovectomy from chronic hemophilic synovitis. *Arthroscopy* 1987, 3:230–236.

27. Wiedel JD: Arthroscopic synovectomy for chronic hemophilic synovitis of the knee. *Arthroscopy* 1985, 1:205–209.

28. Busch M, Swayze OS, Kurczynski EM: Role of arthroscopic synovectomy in the treatment of children with hemophilia. *Orthop Trans* 1994, 17:1030.

29.• Ogilvie-Harris DJ, Reed SC, Hedman TP: Disruption of ankle syndesmosis: biomechanical study of the ligamentous restraints. *Arthroscopy* 1994, 10:558–560.

The relative importance of the four component ligaments of the distal tibiofibular syndesmosis was studied in eight fresh-frozen cadavar specimens. The percentage resistance of 2 mm of displacement of the syndesmosis was tested for each ligament on a hydraulic test system.

30.• Ogilvie-Harris DJ, Reed SC: Disruption of the ankle syndesmosis: diagnosis and treatment by arthroscopic surgery. *Arthroscopy* 1994, 10:561–568.

The authors report the follow-up results of 17 patients treated arthroscopically by resection of the torn portion of the interosseous ligament and the chondral fracture. Most patients benefited from the procedure with significant improvement in symptoms and activity levels.

31. Smith JB, Nance TA: Laser energy in arthroscopic surgery. In *Arthroscopic Surgery* Edited by Parisien JS. New York: McGraw Hill; 1988:325–330.

32. Garrick JG, Kandel N: The CO_2 laser in arthroscopy. *Arthroscopy* 1991, 7:129–137.

33. Smith C, Dillingham M, Fanton G: The use of lasers in ankle arthroscopy. In *Foot and Ankle Arthroscopy*, edn 2. Edited by Guhl J. Thorofare, NJ: Slack Inc.; 1993:189–196.

34. Vangsness CT, Ghaderi B, Saadatmanesh V: Lasers in arthroscopic surgery. In *Current Techniques in Arthroscopy.* Edited by Parisien JS. Philadelphia: Current Medicine; 1993, 1–8.

18

CHAPTER

Arthroscopically Assisted Ankle Arthrodesis

CHAMP L. BAKER, JR.
ANDREW A. BROOKS

Surgical arthrodesis of the ankle is a proven and highly effective procedure for relief of disabling tibiotalar arthritis [1–4]. Surgical indications include disabling pain and loss of motion in the ankle, which are often secondary to degenerative osteoarthritis, rheumatoid arthritis, or most commonly, posttraumatic arthritis.

Arthroscopically assisted fusion is indicated for patients with poor skin conditions who therefore may have an increased risk of complications with an open procedure. At particular risk are patients who have posttraumatic arthritis from open fractures and patients with peripheral vascular disease or diabetes. The arthroscopic procedure is only indicated for patients who have minimal or no varus-valgus ankle deformity because it is essentially an *in situ* fusion. However, equinus positioning can be corrected using this technique.

Among the many advantages of an arthroscopically assisted tibiotalar arthrodesis is a shortened hospital stay. The procedure can be performed on either an outpatient basis or as an overnight-stay procedure because postoperative pain is markedly reduced compared with that of an open procedure. As mentioned previously, surgical complications secondary to skin problems are diminished and surgical morbidity is reduced. In addition, studies have shown that the rate of bony union is more rapid than that of an open procedure.

The disadvantages of the arthroscopic technique are primarily associated with surgery in patients who have a marked varus or valgus deformity. The hindfoot cannot be easily translated posteriorly to fit properly under the tibia for improved gait after ankle fusion [5]. The procedure is very equipment intensive, and there is a significant learning curve for the average arthroscopist. Initially, operating time may be lengthened. This procedure should be attempted only by surgeons who are experienced in ankle arthroscopy and who are familiar with arthrodesis as an open procedure.

TECHNIQUE

The technique of arthroscopically assisted tibiotalar fusion is similar to that of the open procedure advocated by Morgan and coworkers [2]. All articular surfaces and a portion of the underlying subchondral bone are removed. The ankle is placed in a neutral or slight valgus position [6]. The fusion site is then fixed internally with two 6.5-mm cancellous screws that are introduced percutaneously.

The arthroscopic procedure is usually done under spinal or general anesthesia, and depending on the surgeon's preference, it may be done with or without a tourniquet. The patient is placed in the supine position with a sandbag under the buttock of the involved extremity to prevent external rotation of the ankle. The thigh is placed in a leg holder and the end of the table is flexed so that the lower leg is placed in a gravity-dependent position (Fig. 18-1). During surgery, the lower leg can be extended to allow the use of fluoroscopy to monitor the procedure (Fig. 18-2). After the leg is prepared and draped, the outlines of the tibiotalar joint and the medial and lateral malleoli are marked with a pen and the anteromedial and anterolateral portals are identified.

Traction is extremely important during a tibiotalar arthrodesis. With the most commonly used invasive traction, 5-mm distractor pins are placed in the distal tibia and the calcaneus from a lateral direction [7] (Fig. 18-3). Medially, the distractor pins may be placed in the tibia and in the talus as described by Morgan [8]. The distal pin should be inserted with a 30° distal inclination so that when distraction is applied, the pins will be parallel. Lateral fixation is preferred because technically it is easier to apply. Commercial distractors are available and most have calibrations to monitor the amount of displacement (Fig. 18-4). Twenty-five lbs is generally believed to be a safe distraction force.

An alternative to invasive distraction is noninvasive distraction as advocated by Guhl [9]. We have found this to be effective in some ankles, but for those with very limited motion, invasive distraction has been proven best for visualizing the joint and allowing access for joint debridement. A pump is also helpful for distending the joint and often can eliminate the need for a third (posterolateral) portal.

The operative arthroscope can be either a 30° angled arthroscope or the smaller 2.7-mm arthroscope. Standard motorized instruments, such as synovial resectors and burrs, can be used to remove the articular cartilage. A ring curette or bevelled curette is useful for scraping the articular cartilage from the joint and cleaning out the medial and lateral gutters. A video camera documents the diseased joint. A C-arm image intensifier is

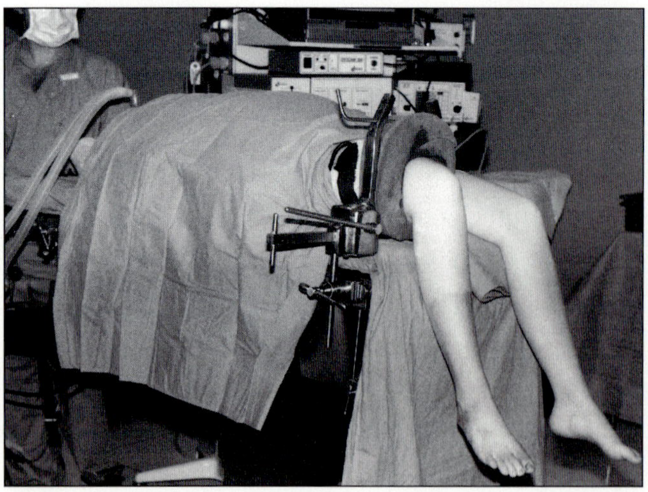

Figure 18-1. Patient positioning for arthroscopically assisted ankle fusion.

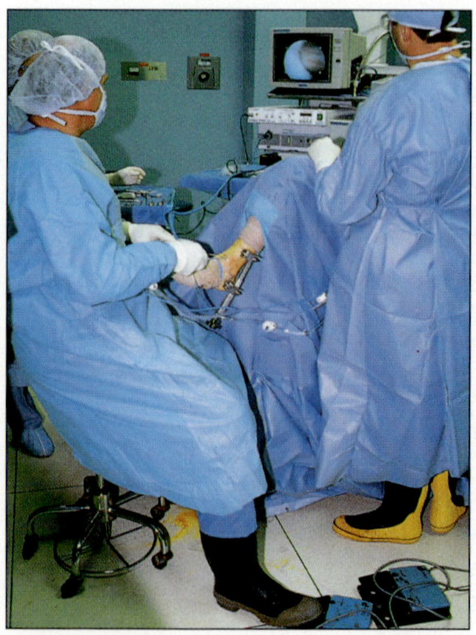

Figure 18-2. Operating room set-up. This arrangement allows comfortable positioning for the surgeon and easy access for imaging.

used to aid in the placement of the fixating cancellous screws. The 6.5-mm cannulated cancellous screws with short threads are preferred for fixation (Table 18-1).

After the leg has been prepared and draped and the portals have been marked, the tourniquet is inflated. Using an 18-gauge needle, the surgeon attempts to distend the joint with 10 cm^3 of saline introduced through the anterolateral portal. If the arthritic condition of the ankle limits joint distension, mechanical distraction must be used to create space between the tibia and talus and the joint is distended through the anteromedial portal if necessary (Fig. 18-5). The stan-

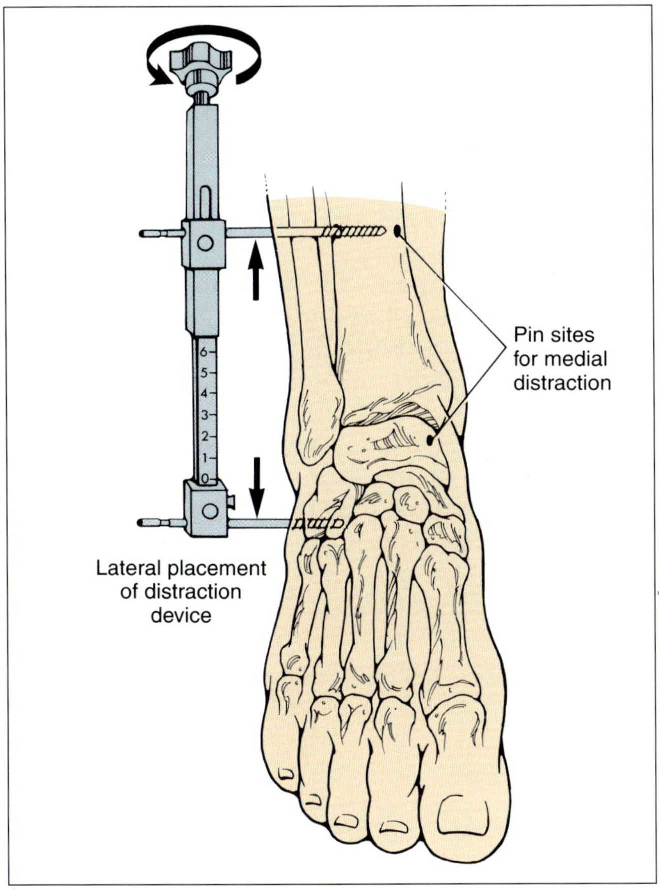

Figure 18-3. With lateral distraction, the pins are placed in the distal tibia and the calcaneus. With medial distraction, pins are placed in the tibia and in the talus. (*Adapted from* Baker and Graham [14]; with permission).

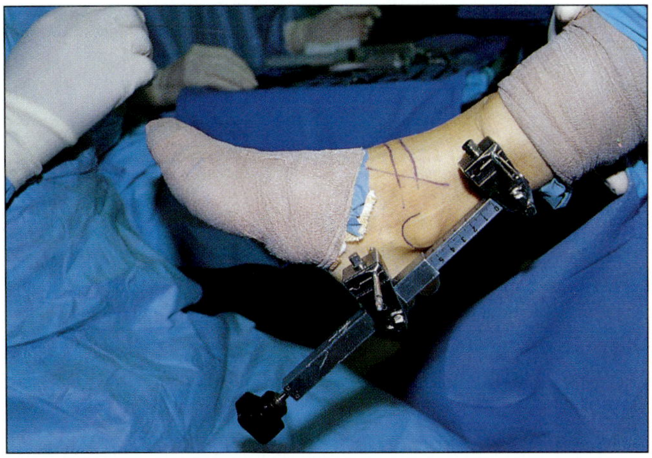

Figure 18-4. Invasive distraction. The distractor is applied laterally.

Table 18-1 Equipment required for arthroscopically assisted ankle arthrodesis

Standard 4-mm diameter video arthroscope with 30° lens
High flow pump system for irrigation
High speed arthroscopic shaver and burr
Sharp cup and ring curettes
Skeletal distraction device
Cannulated 6.5-mm cancellous screw system
Image intensifier

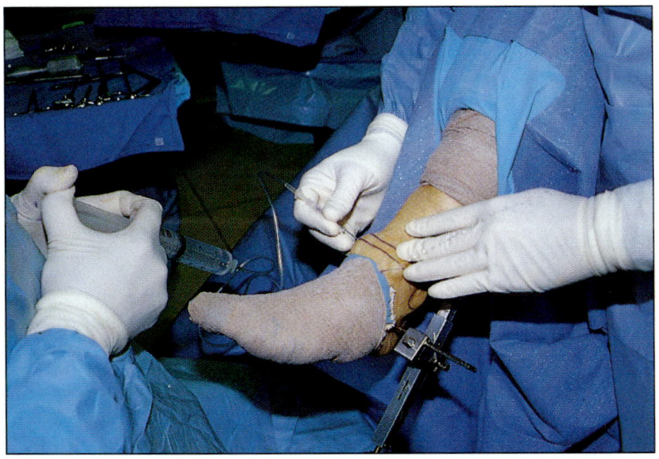

Figure 18-5. The surgeon distends the joint through the anterolateral or, in some ankles, the anteromedial portal.

dard anterolateral portal is made at the level of the tibiotalar joint lateral to the common extensor tendons. A #11 blade knife is used to make a transverse incision in the skin. A hemostat is used to spread the soft tissues, thereby avoiding damage to the cutaneous sensory nerves. The arthroscopic cannula with a blunt trocar is used to enter the joint.

An anteromedial portal is then established under direct visualization. This portal is located at the level of the tibiotalar joint, medial to the anterior tibial tendon and lateral to the saphenous vein (Fig. 18-6). A second stab incision is made and a cannula is inserted through this portal, which is then used as an operating portal.

A third portal is often needed for inflow, especially if a pump is not being used. Once the joint is distended, the posterolateral portal is more easily established. An 18-gauge needle is brought into the joint at the level of the tibiotalar joint, which is proximal to the distal fibula. The entry site is medial or lateral to the Achilles tendon and medial to the sural nerve. An image intensifier can be helpful in localizing this portal.

Initially, an arthroscopic evaluation is performed to ascertain the status of the tibiotalar surface. When visualization of the joint is difficult because of thickened synovium, a motorized resector can be introduced through either the medial or lateral portal to debride the soft tissue. Once the joint is able to be seen adequately, the pathologic condition of the ankle is readily identifiable (Fig. 18-7). Loss of articular cartilage is accompanied by bone spurs and bridge osteophytes that must be debrided or removed to allow for a congruous tibiotalar approximation. Systematic debridement of all remaining articular cartilage of the talus, tibial plafond, and medial and lateral talomalleolar surfaces is performed. Care is taken to debride the area back to the posterior capsule. If the patient's foot is in an equinus position because bridge and anterior tibial or talar osteophytes are present, the arthroscope can be inserted through the posterolateral portal for viewing, and the shaver or burr can be placed in one of the anterior portals. Removal of the osteophytes allows the foot to be brought to a more neutral position.

It is extremely important to clean out the medial and lateral gutters to allow approximation of the talus to the tibia and fibula. A ring curette or wide spoon curette is very helpful to perform this scraping of the articular cartilage. This portion of the procedure can

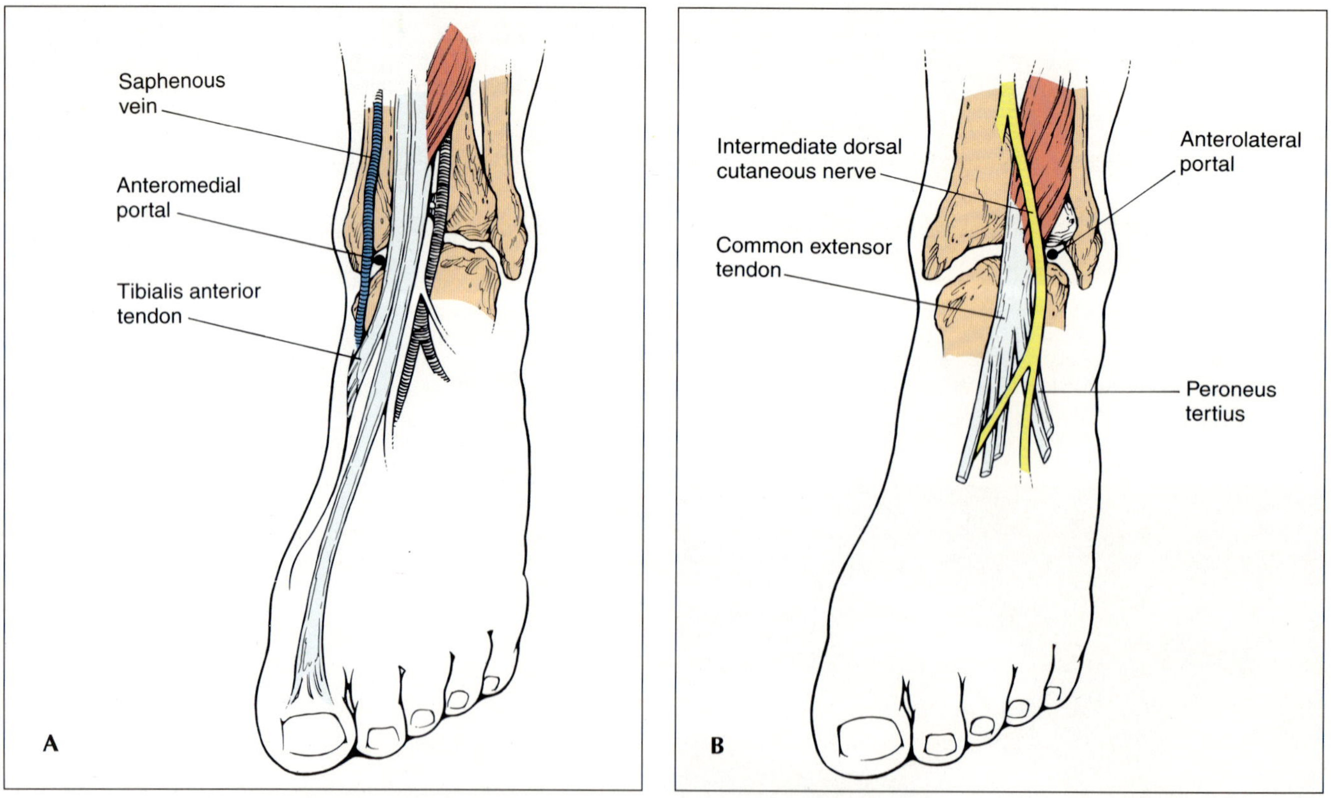

Figure 18-6. **A**, **B** Anatomy of the standard anterolateral and anteromedial arthroscopic portals. (*Adapted from* Baker and Graham [14]; with permission).

even be done by hand with the arthroscope out of the joint, because articular surface scraping is done to remove cartilage down to subchondral bone.

Care must be taken to avoid removing too much bone in one area, which would prevent congruence between the bony surfaces. A motorized shaver is then used to abrade the remaining bone to obtain raw bleeding surfaces (Fig. 18-8).

This surgical technique allows the arthroscope to be changed from the medial to the lateral portal or to the posterior portal with the shaver or burr placed in the opposite portal for adequate viewing and denuding of the bone. The image intensifier can be used to confirm adequate removal of osteophytes and subchondral bone.

FIXATION

Cannulated 6.5-mm cancellous screws are used for fixation. Guidepins are placed percutaneously from the metaphyseal area of the tibia into the talus and from the metaphyseal area of the fibula into the body of the talus. The angle of the pins can be marked on the skin after confirming the position fluoroscopically and the pins can be inserted free hand. Ferkel (Personal communication) has developed a mini-vector guide system that allows accurate placement of the pins (Fig. 18-9). The tips of the pins can be seen penetrating the distal tibia and the lateral malleolus arthroscopically.

Once the position of the pins has been confirmed both arthroscopically and with the image intensifier, the distractor is released and all arthroscopic equipment is removed. The ankle is then reduced under fluoroscopic control, and the proper position of neutral and minimal hindfoot valgus is confirmed. The guidepins are then advanced into the talus while avoiding penetration into the subtalar joint. Pin depth is confirmed using the image intensifier. The proper length screw is selected by using the measuring device and then the holes are tapped over the guidewires

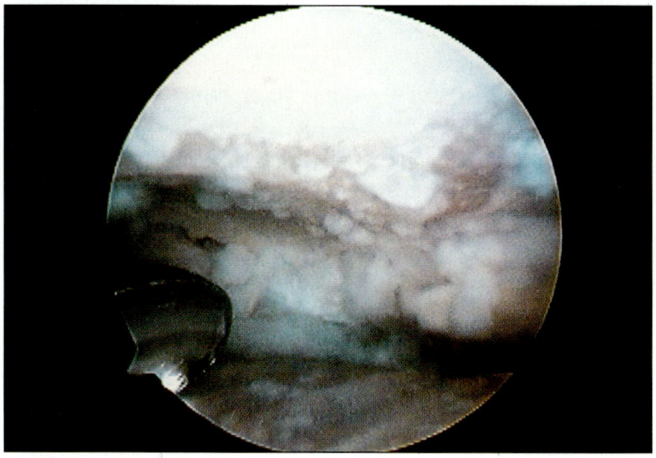

Figure 18-7. Arthroscopic view of a right ankle joint after synovectomy. This patient has rheumatoid arthritis.

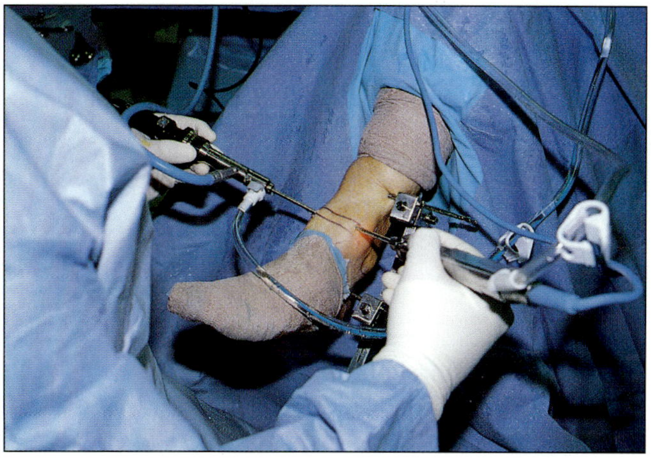

Figure 18-8. With the arthroscope in the anteromedial portal, a motorized resector is introduced through the anterolateral portal to abrade the joint surfaces.

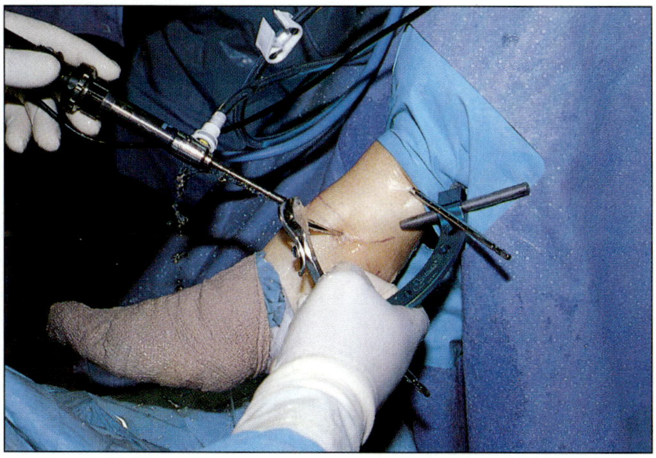

Figure 18-9. Application of mini-vector guide for pin placement.

and the screws are tightened into place. Proper position is confirmed radiographically (Fig. 18-10) or fluoroscopically (Fig. 18-11).

Incisions are closed with nylon sutures, a bulky dressing is applied, and the ankle is then placed in a U-shaped splint. The patient is hospitalized overnight with the ankle elevated and on ice and is usually discharged the following morning. The patient maintains toe-touch weight bearing for the first week. At 1 week after surgery, the splint is removed and a short walking cast is applied to the leg. The cast is changed at 4 to 6 weeks, and the patient's leg is placed in a removable walking boot and allowed full weight-bearing movement. Use of the walking boot is discontinued when the patient has painless gait, and the radiographs show bridging callous across the fusion site.

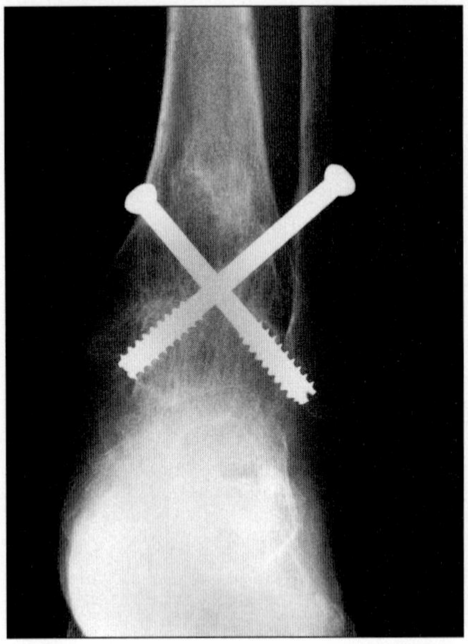

Figure 18-10. Anteroposterior view showing placement of screws.

RESULTS

Published results of this technique of ankle arthrodesis have been good. In 1990, Glick and coworkers [10] reported on 35 arthroscopic ankle fusions. Most were performed as same-day surgery. Radiographic union was evident at a mean of 8 weeks (range, 6–11 weeks) when crossed screws were used for fixation. Two patients developed nonunions. One of these patients developed a dorsalis pedis pseudoaneurysm secondary to use of an anterocentral approach.

Tasto [11] reported his results with 10 patients who were treated over an 18-month period. Nine united uneventfully, and one patient had a delayed union that was thought to be secondary to pre-existing avascular necrosis of the talus. Average time to union in his series was 8.5 weeks. The average hospital stay was 1 day.

Dent and coworkers [12•] performed arthroscopic ankle fusions in eight patients: two had rheumatoid arthritis and six had posttraumatic arthritis. Average follow-up in this series was 24 months. Clinical union was achieved in all patients, however, only four patients showed radiographic union.

Recently, Ogilvie-Harris and coworkers [13••] reviewed cases of 19 patients who underwent this procedure for osteoarthrosis of the ankle. At 2 years of follow-up, they rated their results in these patients as excellent in 12, good in four, fair in two, and poor in one. Two of their patients developed nonunions that ultimately required an open procedure. Median hospital stay in this series was 1 day. Ten patients had radiographic evidence of union by the second postoperative month, five by the third postoperative month, one by the fifth month, and one by the sixth month. Two patients had nonunions.

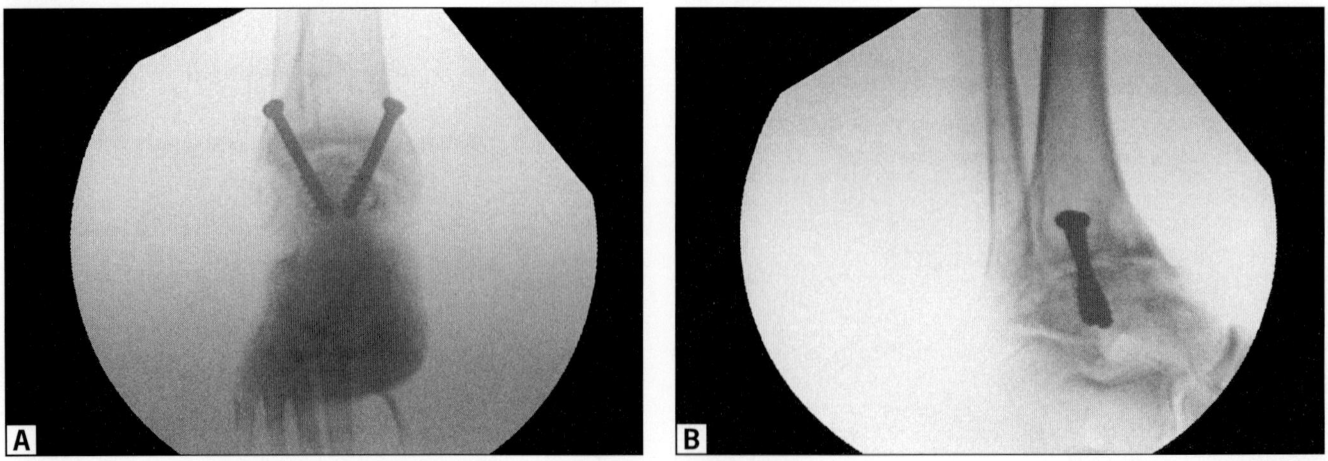

Figure 18-11. The position of the screws is confirmed fluoroscopically. **A**, Anteroposterior view. **B**, Lateral view.

Conclusion

Arthroscopically assisted ankle arthrodesis is a safe and effective technique for achieving rapid fusion of the ankle joint. It is indicated in patients who require *in situ* fusion and who may have a poor skin condition or compromised vascularity. It is minimally invasive and can be performed as outpatient or overnight-stay surgery. The procedure is technically demanding and should only be performed in properly selected patients by skilled arthroscopic surgeons. The procedure can be used in patients in lieu of an open tibiotalar fusion but is not indicated in all patients and should be used selectively.

References and Recommended Reading

Papers of interest, published recently, have been highlighted as

- • Of special interest
- •• Of outstanding interest

1. Mazur JM, Schwartz E, Simon SR: Ankle arthrodesis. Long-term follow-up with gait analysis. *J Bone Joint Surg* 1979, 61-A:964–975.
2. Morgan CD, Henke JA, Bailey RW, *et al.*: Long-term results of tibiotalar arthrodesis. *J Bone Joint Surg* 1985, 67-A:546–550.
3. Lynch AF, Bourne RB, Rorabech CH: The long-term results of ankle arthrodesis. *J Bone Joint Surg* 1988, 70-B:113–116.
4. Scranton PE, Jr.: An overview of ankle arthrodesis. *Clin Orthop* 1991, 268:96–101.
5. Holt ES, Hansen ST, Mayo KA, *et al.*: Ankle arthrodesis using internal screw fixation. *Clin Orthop* 1991, 268:21–28.
6. Buck P. Morrey BF, Chao EYS: The optimum position of arthrodesis of the ankle: a gait study of the knee and ankle. *J Bone Joint Surg* 1987, 69-A:1052–1062.
7. Guhl JF: Portals and techniques. In *Ankle Arthroscopy: Pathology and Surgical Techniques.* Edited by Guhl JF. Thorofare, NJ: Slack; 1988:49.
8. Morgan CD: Arthroscopic tibiotalar arthrodesis. In *Ankle Arthroscopy: Pathology and Surgical Techniques.* Edited by Guhl JF. Thorofare, NJ: Slack, Inc.; 1988:119.
9. Guhl JF: New concepts (distraction) in ankle arthroscopy. *Arthroscopy* 1988, 4:160–167.
10. Glick JM, Sampson TG, Myerson MS, *et al.*: Arthroscopic skills ankle arthrodesis. [Abstract]. *Arthroscopy* 1990, 6:155.
11. Tasto JP: Arthroscopic ankle arthrodesis utilizing a soft tissue distraction technique. *Arthroscopy* 1991, 7:314.
12.• Dent CM, Patil M, Fairclough JA: Arthroscopic ankle arthrodesis. *J Bone Joint Surg* 1993, 75-B:830–832.

A high rate of fusion was achieved in this small group of carefully selected patients. The technique was used only on patients with slight deformities and no avascular necrosis of the talar dome.

13.•• Ogilvie-Harris DJ, Lieberman I, Fitsialos D: Arthroscopically assisted arthrodesis for osteoarthrotic ankles. *J Bone Joint Surg* 1993, 75-A:1167–1174.

This article describes the authors' arthroscopic technique of ankle fusion. A comprehensive discussion of the indications for the procedure and its advantages and disadvantages follows a detailed description of the technique. The authors emphasize that arthroscopic arthrodesis does not permit correction of deformity.

14. Baker CL, Graham JM, Jr.: Current concepts in ankle arthroscopy. *Orthopedics* 1993, 16:1028–1029.

19

CHAPTER

Avoiding Possible Complications Associated With Ankle Arthroscopy

J. SERGE PARISIEN

Over the past decade, improved instrumentation and better visualization have led to an increased use of arthroscopy in the successful management of many synovial, chondral, and osteochondral lesions of the ankle. The challenge of ankle arthroscopy comes from the small size of the joint and the close proximity of the neurovascular structures surrounding it.

In general, complications associated with arthroscopic surgery vary from 0.6% to 8.2% [1,2]. A prospective study collecting responses from experienced arthroscopists revealed an overall incidence rate of 1.68% [3].

Very few series are available describing the occurrence of complications associated with ankle arthroscopy. Guhl [4] reported a complication rate of 11.1%, with 2.86% being complications directly associated with the distraction technique. In their series of 58 ankles, Martin and coworkers [5] reported a rate of 15%. Barber and coworkers [6], reporting on their early experience, mentioned a postoperative complication rate of 17%. However, Small [3], in his report on complications related to arthroscopies performed by experienced arthroscopists, mentioned only one complication in 146 ankle procedures—an incidence of 0.58%.

Some complications, such as thrombophlebitis and pulmonary embolism, can occur occasionally and are not specific to the ankle. Guhl [4] claims that the infection rate following ankle arthroscopy is higher than in most other joints. Although it has not been my experience, I concur with Guhl that prophylactic antibiotic therapy is advisable for patients who will undergo potentially long, complicated procedures or for patients who have undergone previous surgery. When intra-articular infection occurs, the management is by arthroscopic means, along with appropriate parental antibiotics.

The most commonly reported complication associated with ankle arthroscopy is neurologic in nature [7••], with the least common being the hemarthrosis. According to Barber [6], articular cartilage abrasion is probably the most unreported complication associated with ankle arthroscopy. Ferkel and coworkers [8•], in a retrospective review of 600 patients, revealed an overall complication rate of 7.5%. Twenty-five complications (4.2%) were neurological.

In this chapter, two categories of complications associated with ankle arthroscopy will be analyzed: those associated with technique and those associated with specific procedures.

COMPLICATIONS ASSOCIATED WITH TECHNIQUE

Portal Placement

In creating portals for ankle arthroscopy, cutaneous nerves, veins, and tendons around the ankle are at risk. The *anteromedial portal* is located approximately 1 cm distal to the joint line and medial to the tibialis anticus tendon. Anatomical studies have found that this portal is in close proximity to the saphenous nerve and vein (Fig. 19-1). If an accessory medial portal is developed (Fig. 19-2), it should not be placed too close to the previously basic medial portal. This step should minimize skin maceration.

The *anterolateral portal* is placed lateral to the peroneus tertius and common extensor tendon, approximately 1 cm distal to the joint line. This portal is in close proximity to the intermediate branch of the superficial peroneal nerve. This nerve can be seen or

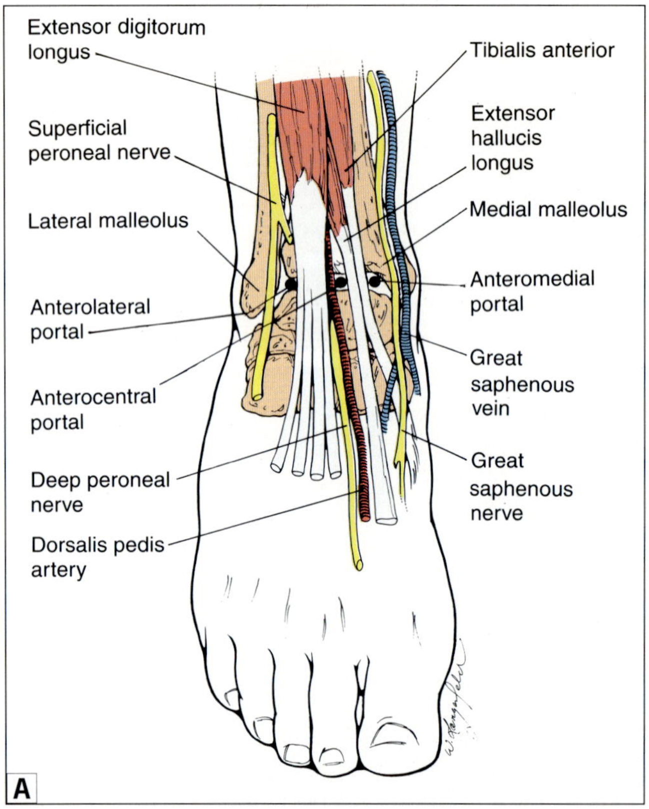

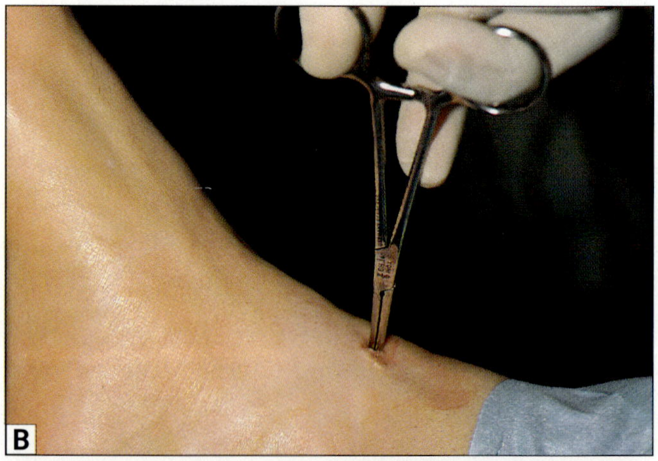

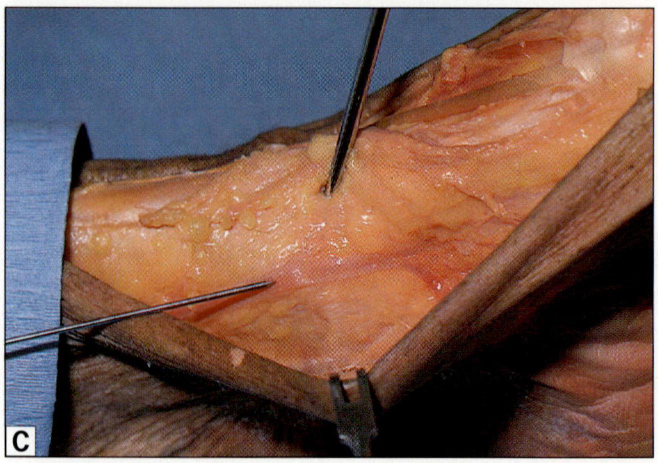

Figure 19-1. A, The anterior portals. **B**, A small hemostat is used to spread the vertical incision at the site of the anteromedial portal. **C**, An anatomic dissection of the left ankle shows the relationship of the anteromedial portal to the saphenous nerve and vein.

palpated by placing the ankle in forced inversion. Visualization can be obtained through transillumination as well (Fig. 19-3). This portal can also be developed by placing a needle from outside-in or by tenting the skin with a blunt obturator through the anteromedial portal (Fig. 19-4).

The *posterolateral portal,* which is close in proximity to the sural nerve, is located behind the peroneal tendons and close to the Achilles tendon (Fig. 19-5). Its entrance is placed approximately 1 cm above the tip of the lateral malleolus. It can be developed by using a spinal needle in this posterior location while being viewed with the arthroscope anteriorly. With the joint distracted, this posterolateral portal can be developed from inside-out with a K-wire or smooth rod passing from an anterior portal and tenting the

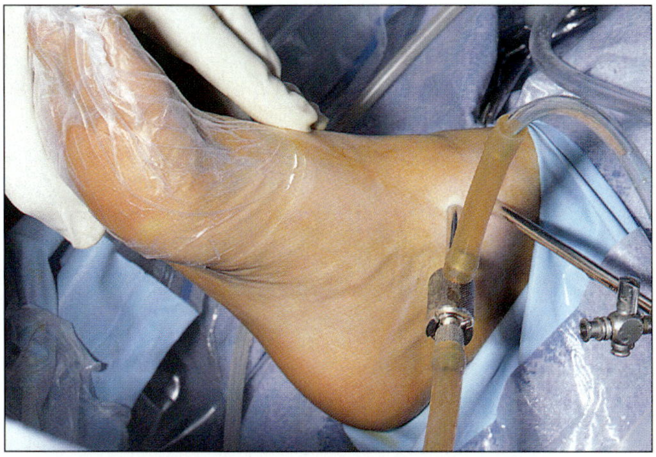

Figure 19-2. The accessory medial portal used for the insertion of the pump cannula.

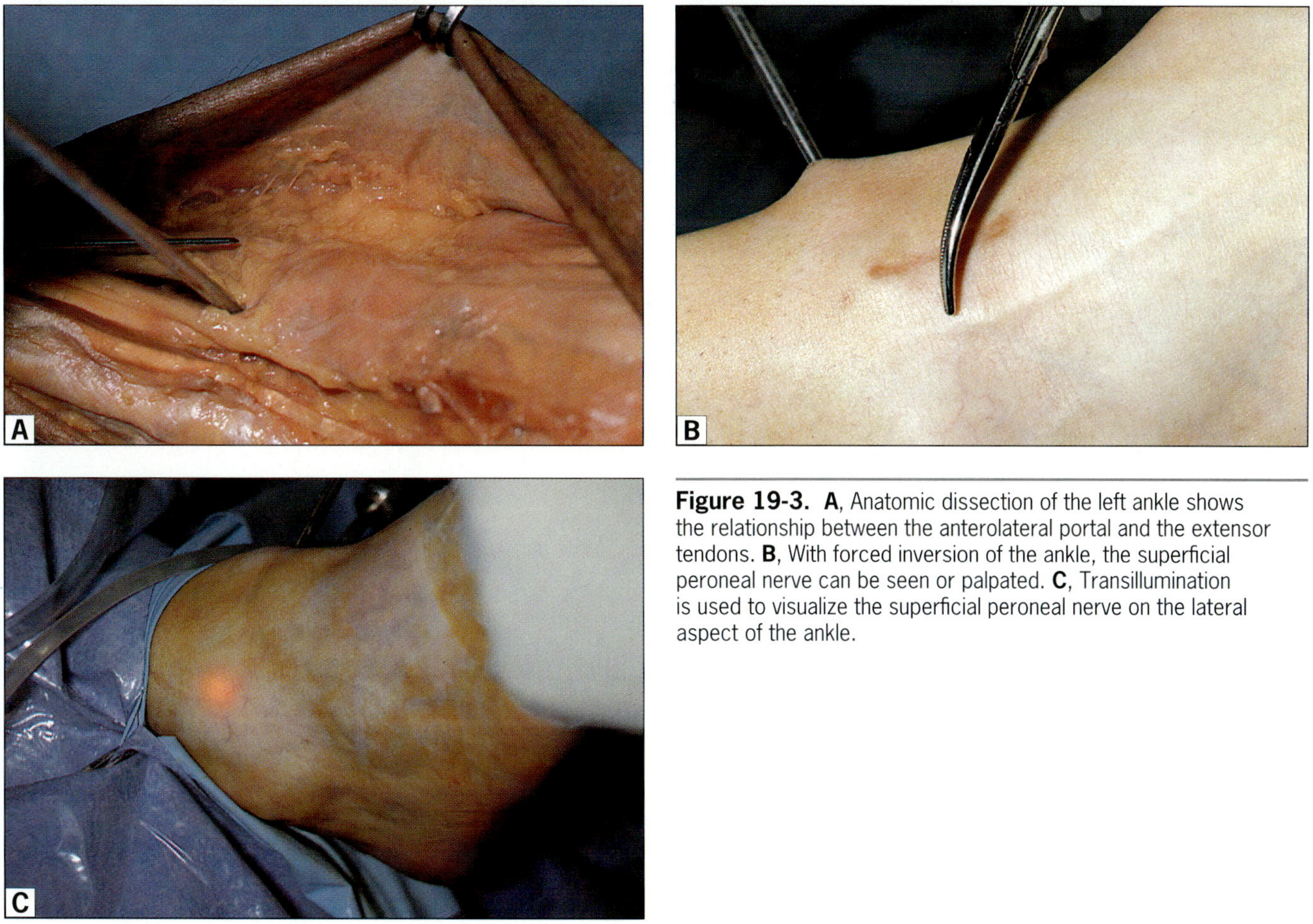

Figure 19-3. A, Anatomic dissection of the left ankle shows the relationship between the anterolateral portal and the extensor tendons. **B**, With forced inversion of the ankle, the superficial peroneal nerve can be seen or palpated. **C**, Transillumination is used to visualize the superficial peroneal nerve on the lateral aspect of the ankle.

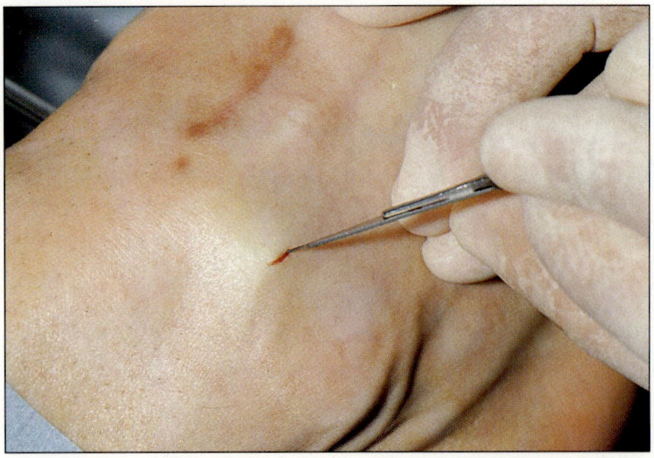

Figure 19-4. The anterolateral portal can be developed by tenting the skin with a smooth obturator, which is introduced through the anteromedial portal.

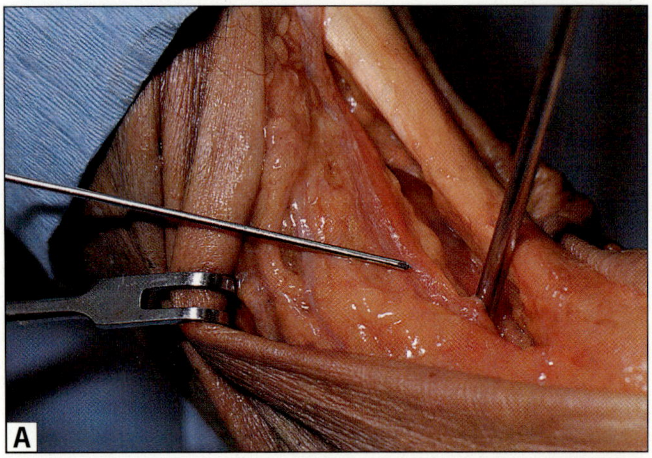

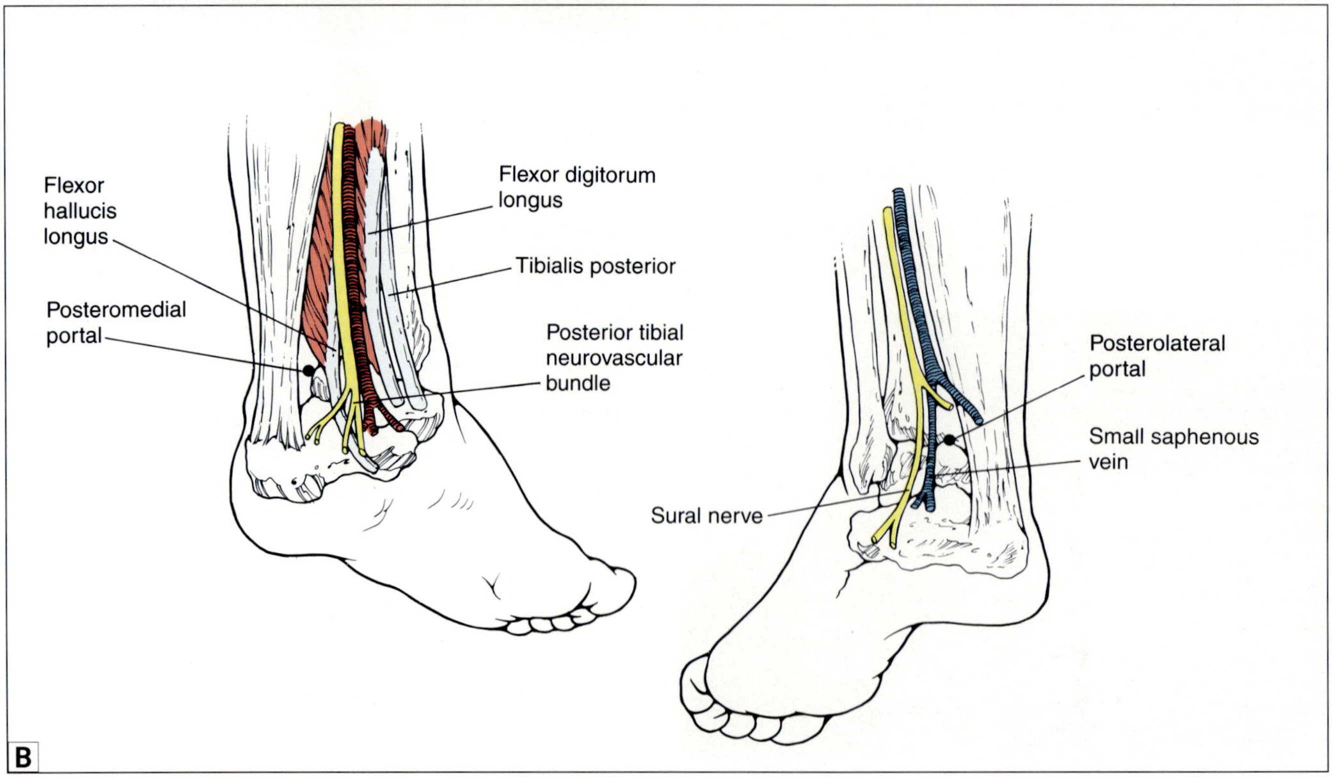

Figure 19-5. **A**, Posterior dissection of the left ankle showing the relationship of the posterolateral portal to the sural nerve. **B**, Posterolateral and posteromedial portals.

skin posteriorly. One should avoid a too distal location of this portal in order to avoid the posterior aspect of the subtalar joint (Figs. 19-6 and 19-7).

The two other portals that have been described—the *posteromedial* and the *central portals*—are not recommended for routine use in arthroscopic surgery of the ankle because of their close proximity to the neurovascular structures of the anterior and posteromedial aspects of the joint.

Transmalleolar portals, medial and lateral, were described by Guhl [4] in order to gain better access to a posteriorly located lesion of the talus. Kirshner wire, 0.062 inches in diameter, can be used through the medial malleolus for drilling intact lesions of the talus (Fig. 19-8). A larger canal has also been advocated by Guhl [4] for placement of instrumentation and bone grafting (Fig. 19-9).

In my experience, I have not found any practical use for the transmalleolar approach. The benefits of using this portal should be weighed against the possibility of stress fractures, pin tract infections, and arthrofibrosis.

The morbidity associated with the standard portals can be minimized or avoided by taking these few steps:

- Mark the skin with a sterile pencil to delineate the important anatomical structures at the start of the procedure before distortion of the land marks by swelling and extravasation of fluid occur.
- Make vertical skin incisions to avoid damage to cutaneous nerves and vessels. A small blunt hemostat can be used to spread the incision down to the capsule.
- Do not make unnecessary portals adjacent to existing ones to avoid skin maceration and necrosis.

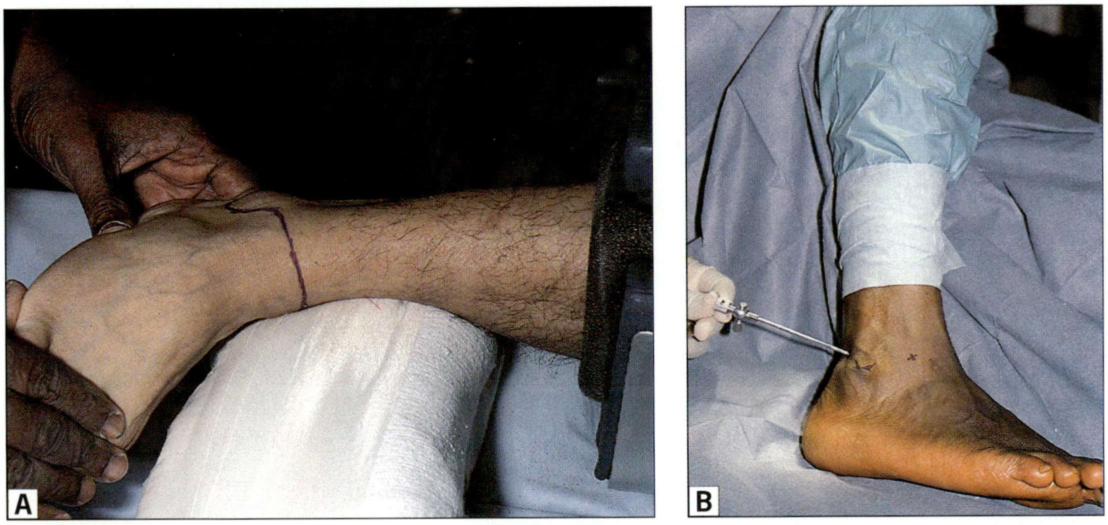

Figure 19-6. A, With the patient in a semi-supine position, the posterolateral aspect of the ankle is made accessible for placement of the posterolateral portal. **B**, The posterolateral portal is located in the space between the Achilles tendon and peroneal tendons. This portal is more distal than the corresponding anterolateral portal and is placed adjacent to the lateral border of the Achilles tendon.

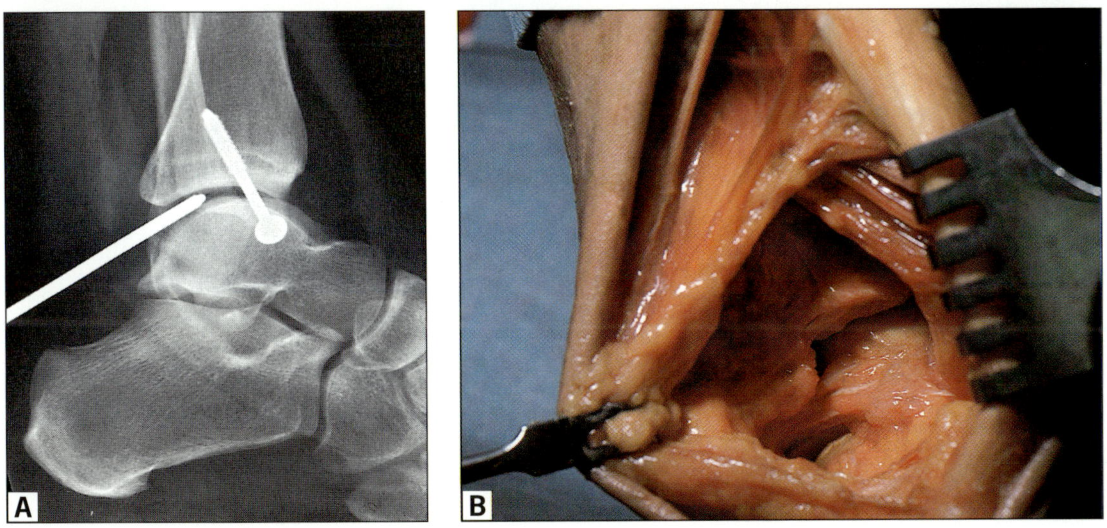

Figure 19-7. A, Radiograph of a cadaver specimen shows the position of the arthroscope through the posterolateral portal. **B**, Anatomic dissection of the left ankle shows the close proximity of the posterior portal to the posterior subtalar joint.

Invasive and Noninvasive Mechanical Distraction

The purpose of distraction in ankle arthroscopy is to increase the space in order to better view, triangulate, and manipulate the instruments. Different types of distraction can be used from a simple sling attached to the ankle to the more complicated invasive pin distraction introduced by Guhl [9]. Guhl advocates the use of 3/16-in threaded pins for distraction, which are placed through the tibia and os calcis laterally. Proximally, the pin should be inserted 1.5 in above the ankle and 1 to 1.5 cm posterior to the anterior crest of the tibia through one cortex. Distally, it is placed in the lateral aspect of the calcaneus, 0.5-in anterior and 0.5-in superior to the posterior cortex and inferior cortex of the bone, respectively. Injury to the sural nerve should be avoided when developing the distal placement of the pin. A downward position of the distal pin, approximately 20° to 25° into the lateral cortex of the os calcis is recommended so that the pins end up in a parallel position. This is because the distraction is applied to only one side of the joint. A locking nut used on the distal pin will prevent the distractor from slipping off the pin. If the distraction apparatus is placed medially, the distal pin is usually placed into the talus, inferior and slightly anterior to the tip of the medial malleolus. Placing the pin in any posterior position can cause injury to the neurovascular structures and posterior tendon (Fig. 19-10).

Potential complications of invasive mechanical distraction include broken pins, pin tract problems, neurovascular damage, and fractures. Guhl [4,9] noted that paraesthesias and neuromas appear to be the most serious types of complications.

Albert and coworkers [10] studied the efficacy of ankle distraction—the strain on four ankle ligaments and the tibiotalar joint opening resulting from distraction force—in various foot positions. Their study revealed that it was important to avoid distraction forces

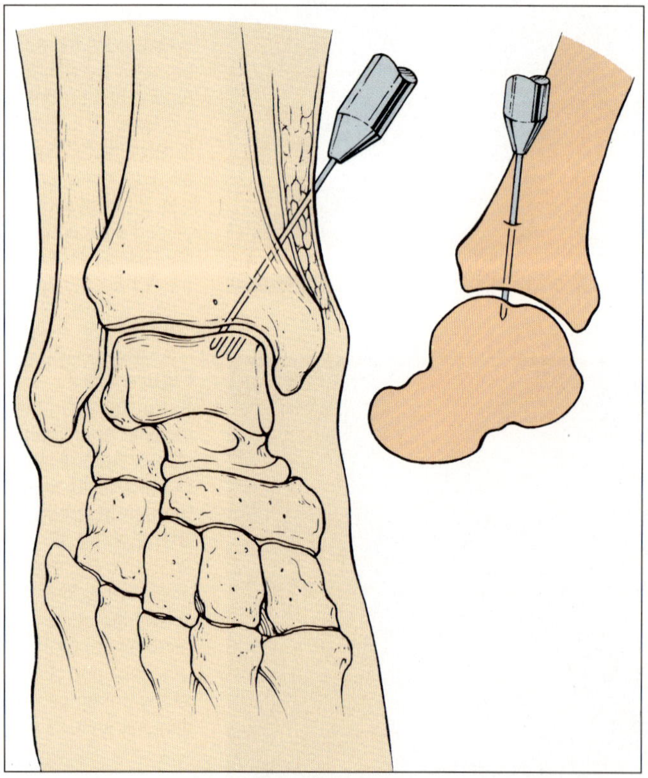

Figure 19-8. Transmalleolar drilling of the posteromedial lesion of the talus.

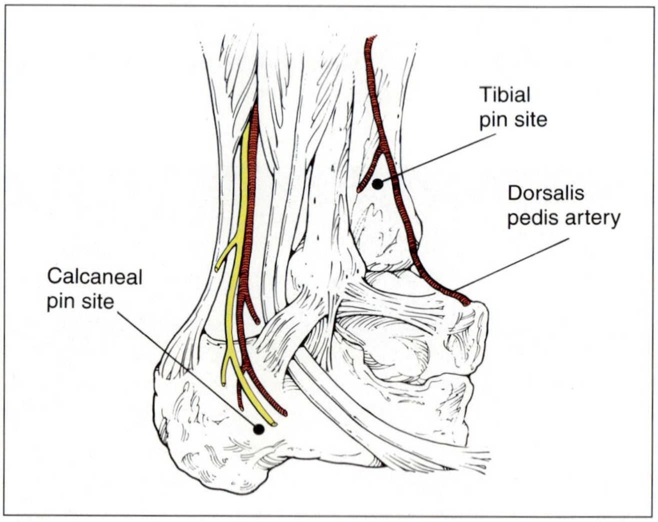

Figure 19-9. Lateral placement of the mechanical distractor.

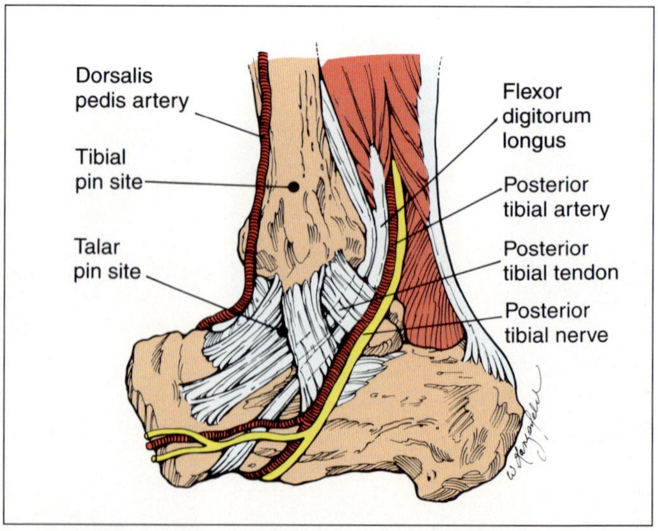

Figure 19-10. Medial placement of the mechanical distractor.

greater than 90 N while distracting the ankle in the 20° dorsiflexion position. Greater forces may lead to calcaneofibular ligament injury. They also found that forces greater than 135 N can cause pin bending and bony calcaneal damage. The safest method of distraction was to use forces less than 135 N with the ankle in the neutral position. Invasive distraction is not indicated in open epiphysis, localized infection, and osteopenia.

To avoid problems associated with the invasive method, distraction can be applied using sterile disposable straps over the ankle. A multimode distraction technique is also now available that allows for the use of the same mechanical distractor without the strain gauge in a noninvasive mode (Fig. 19-11).

Regarding noninvasive distraction (Fig. 19-12), a recent study by Dowdy and coworkers [11•] recommended 25 lbs of traction for 1 hour when using noninvasive ankle distraction apparatus. By increasing the distraction time and force, symptoms of paraesthesias may occur. The superficial and deep peroneal nerves, and to a lesser extent the sural nerve, seem to be affected by this increase.

Incision

Although not very common, sinus and fistula formation can occur. The most common site for fistula formation is around the anterior portals. The tell-tale signs of fistula occurrence are a slow healing portal, erythema, and a large amount of drainage of sterile synovial fluid. It is important to carefully treat these patients with local debridement of the fistula, followed by immobilization of the ankle, to avoid the occurrence of secondary pyarthrosis.

Triangulation and repeated interchanging of the instrumentation are potential causes for sinus formation. The use of plastic cannulas can reduce the likelihood of sinus formation (Fig. 19-13).

Retained foreign bodies, such as chondral debris, can lead to an area of chronic discomfort or even the formation of a granuloma. This can be avoided by a thorough lavage of the joint before closure and the use of a suction cannula to remove loose fragments.

Finally, when closing incisions around the ankle, one has to be careful to include only the skin to avoid catching subcutaneous superficial nerves in the sutures.

Instrument Failure

It is important to consistently check, properly maintain, and sharpen the surgical instruments—particularly the curettes, rasps, knives, and basket scissors—so that the risk of breaking during a procedure is reduced. In a situation where the instrument breaks off, the outflow of saline must be closed and inflow must be maintained when the gravity system is in use. This will keep the joint distended and reduce the risk of migration. Magnetic retrievers will facilitate extraction (Fig. 19-14).

Pumps with a small cannula and small infusion tubing are now available for the ankle joint (Fig. 19-15). When they are being used, frequent visualization of the pump cannula and palpation of the extremity will help reduce the risk of extravasation. If the tip of any instrument breaks off, it is recommended to switch to an overhead irrigation system to avoid quick migration of this foreign body.

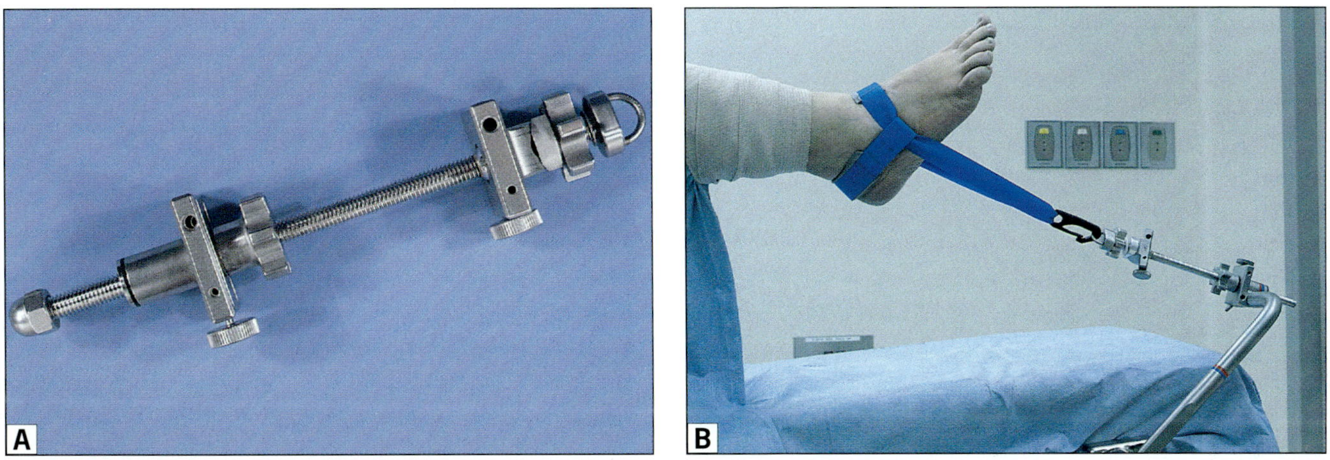

Figure 19-11. **A**, **B**, Multimode mechanical distractor. (Photos courtesy of Dr. J.F. Guhl.)

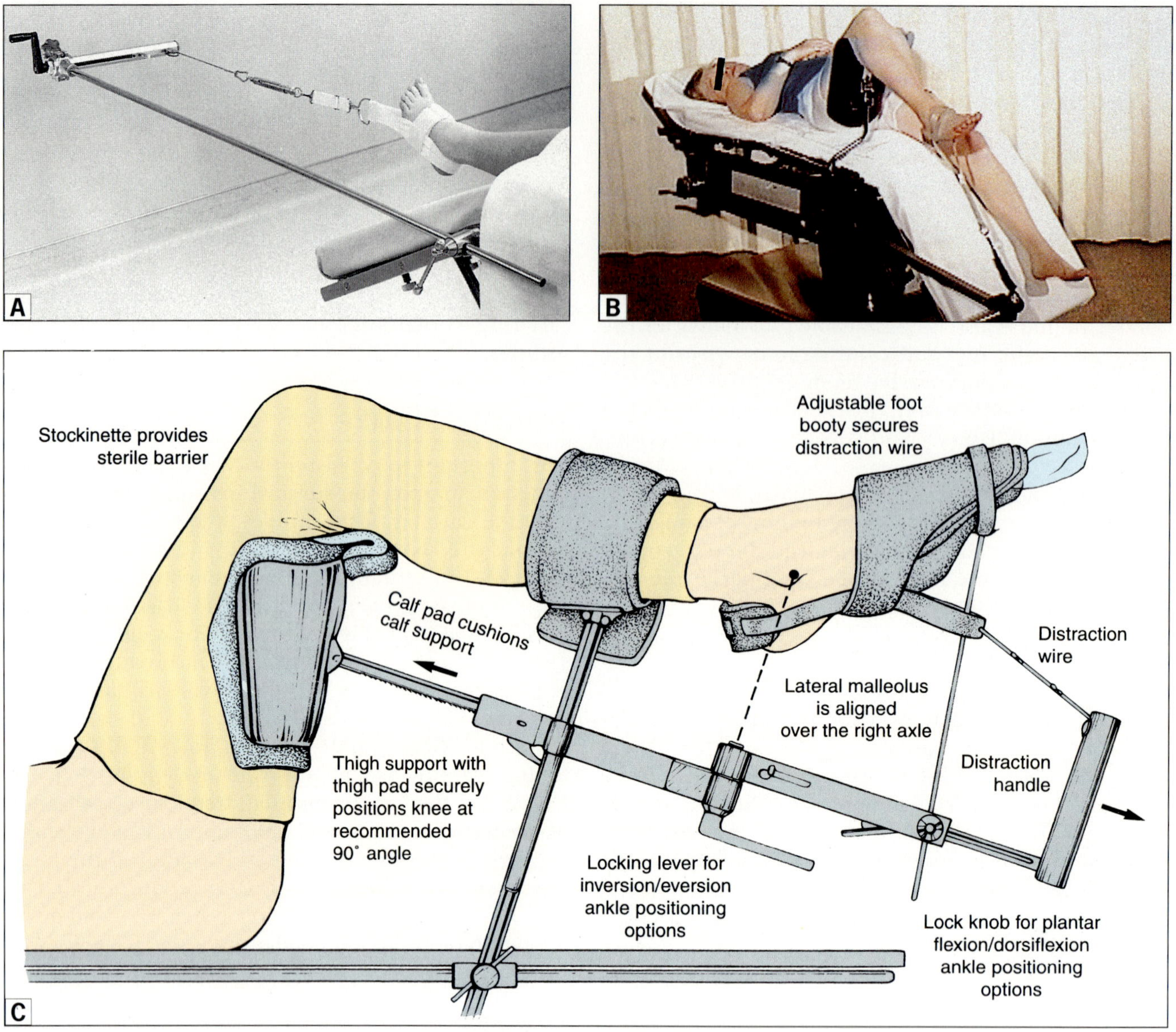

Figure 19-12. **A**, Noninvasive distraction. (Photo courtesy of Zimmer Inc., Warsaw, IN). **B**, Noninvasive distraction. (Photo courtesy of Dr. J. Laico.) **C**, Noninvasive distraction (Smith & Nephew Dyonics, Andover, MA.)

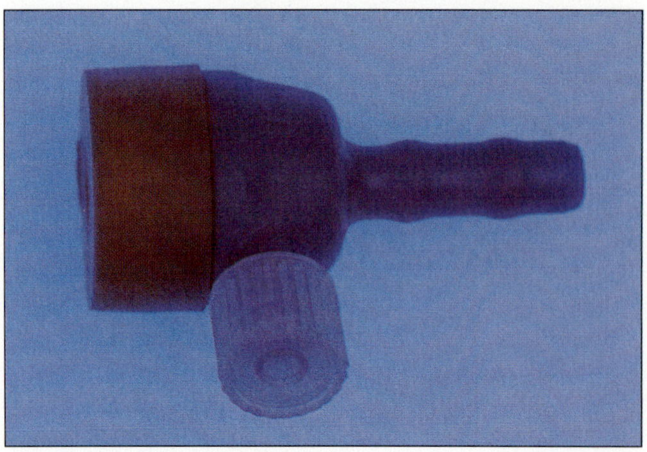

Figure 19-13. Plastic disposable cannula with side port that can be used in ankle arthroscopy.

Complications Associated With Specific Procedures

Synovial Lesions

Synovial lesions can be either localized or diffuse. Two anterior portals are used for the scope and instruments. To avoid potential complications, a 70° arthroscope is used for the opposite portal. This allows for better visualization.

A small motorized blade should be used in the recesses of the ankle for debridement. When the synovium is very friable, as in rheumatoid arthritis, it is preferable to use the Whisker blade to avoid aggressive debridement of the soft-tissue layer that is very close to the anterior and posteromedial neurovascular structures. Use of a hemovac is recommended (if debridement has been extensive) with a compression dressing. Crutch ambulation with partial ambulation may be necessary to prevent postoperative effusion.

Osteochondral Lesions

The osteochondral lesions that are amenable to arthroscopic debridement are: transchondral fractures of the talar dome, osteochondritis dissecans lesions, impingement exostosis, osteochondral lesions of the tibial plafond, loose bodies, and the sequelae of fractures with chronic symptoms. Some arthroscopists prefer to use some form of distraction for better visualization of the posteriorly located lesion. However, it must be kept in mind that most of these lesions, although posterior, are accessible with plantar flexion with some manual distraction. Small instruments and a 70° arthroscope will facilitate the procedure (Figs. 19-16 to 19-19).

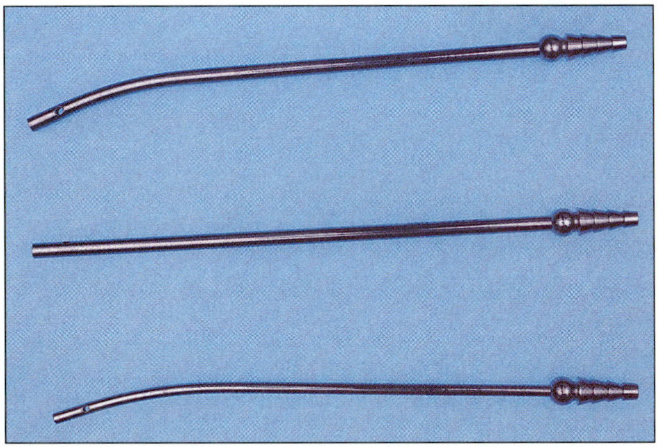

Figure 19-14. Magnetic retrievers for extraction of broken instruments.

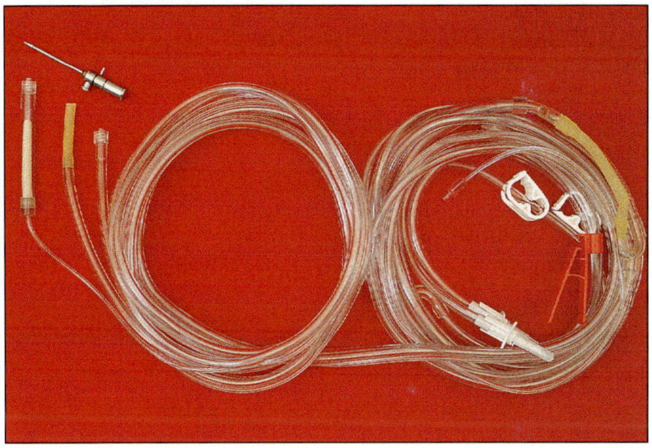

Figure 19-15. Small pump cannula and small infusion tubing used for ankle arthroscopy.

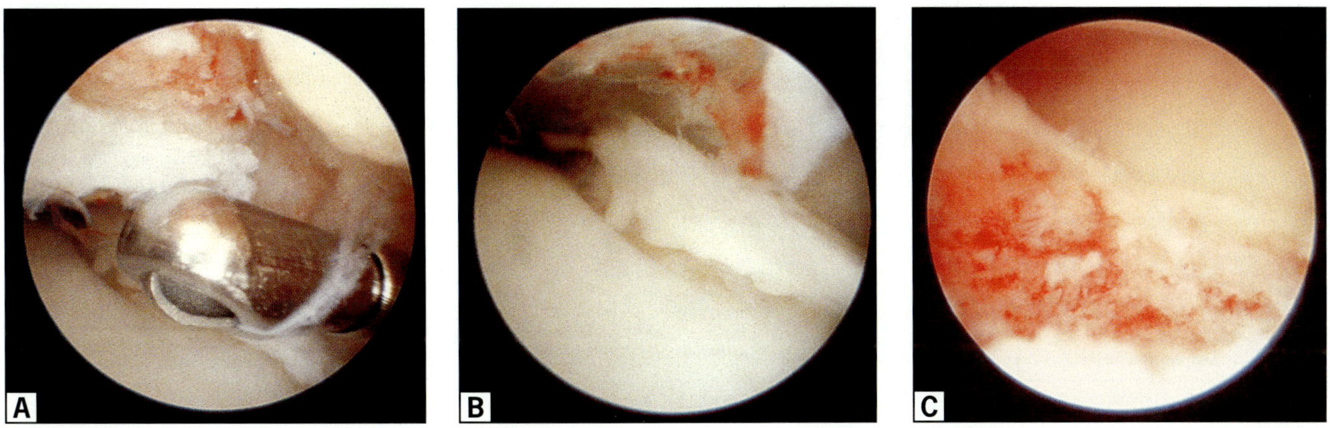

Figure 19-16. Arthroscopic debridement of an osteochondral lesion in a talus fracture. **A**, Transchondral fracture of the talus of the right ankle located posteromedially. A small motorized shaver is used to perform synovectomy to improve visualization of the lesion. **B**, With the assistant placing the ankle in forced plantar flexion, over a bolster placed underneath the patient's heel, the lesion becomes more accessible. **C**, Osteochondral bed following excision of lesion and curettage with small hand instruments.

Following the excision of an osteochondral lesion of the talus, careful probing is important to make sure the debridement is complete.

Also, the exostosis of the anterior aspect of the ankle needs to be evaluated from the two anterior portals to ascertain the adequacy of the excision.

Arthroscopic Ankle Arthrodesis

Arthroscopy has been shown to be useful for patients who need to undergo arthroscopic ankle arthrodesis. The advantages of the closed technique are less morbidity and a shorter hospitalization. However, the

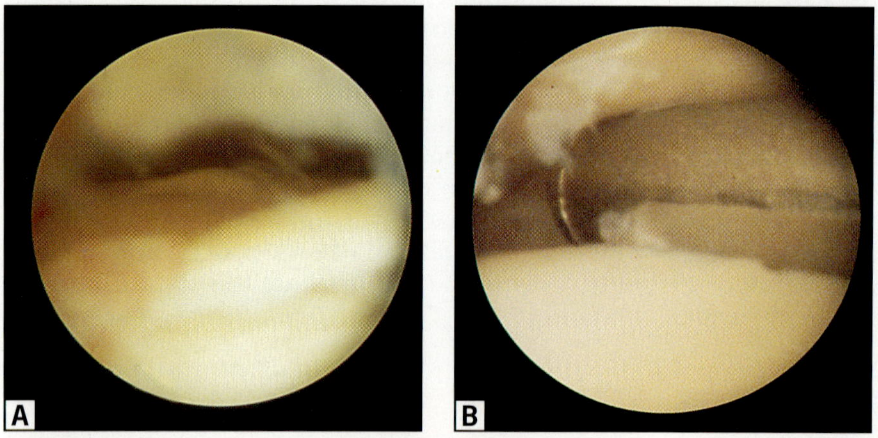

Figure 19-17. Arthroscopic debridement of osteochondral lesion of the ankle. **A**, Chrondromalacic changes and chondral flaps seen from the anterior aspect of the ankle. **B**, Debridement being performed with a small motorized instrument (2.9 mm).

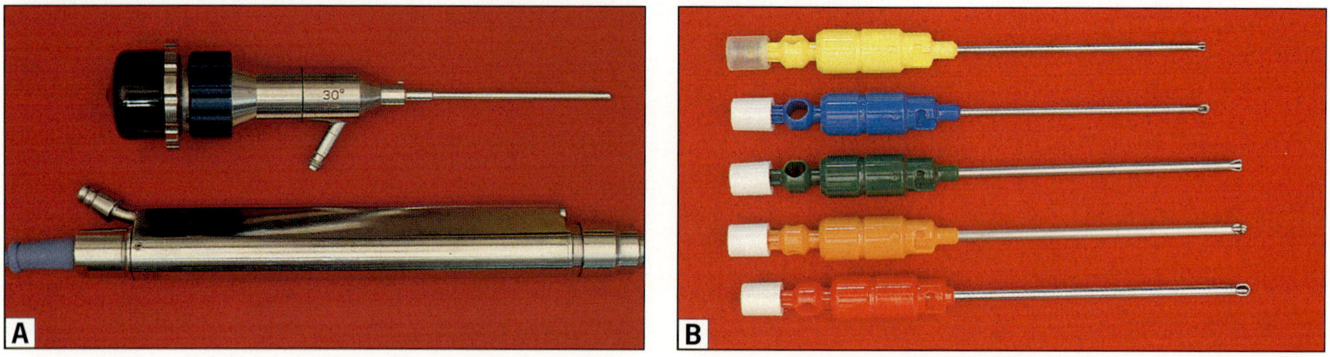

Figure 19-18. Equipment for debridement of osteochondral lesions in small joints. **A**, A small short videocamera for use in ankle or any small joint arthroscopy. **B**, Various sizes of disposable blades (full-radius, Whisker, and abrader).

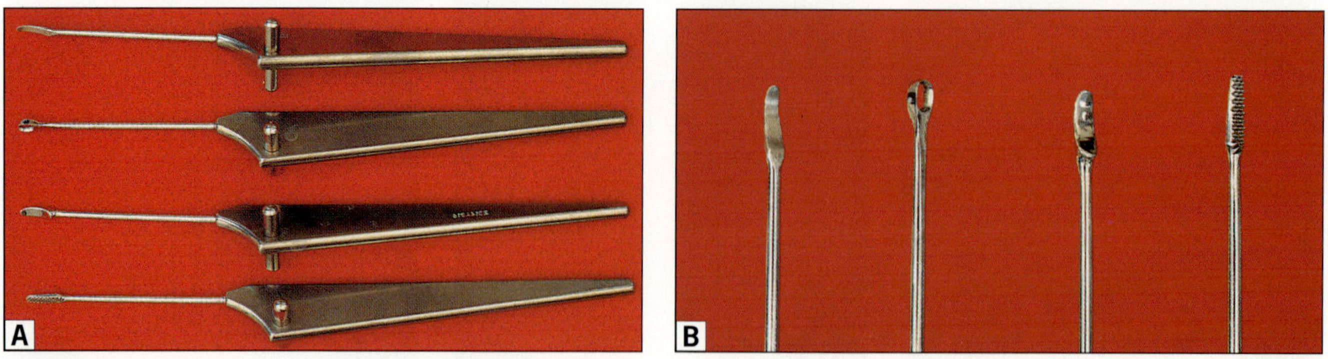

Figure 19-19. Instruments for ankle arthroscopy. **A**, Various sizes of some small-sized hand instruments (rasps, curettes, knife) for use in ankle arthroscopic surgery. **B**, Close-up of the small-sized hand instruments.

technique has its limitations because any deformities of the ankle, such as varus or valgus alignment of the ankle greater than 15°, cannot be corrected.

Like the open procedure, arthroscopic arthrodesis first requires the complete excision of the degenerated articular cartilage with the sclerotic subchondral bone. This is followed by fixation, in the neutral position, of the two articular surfaces with two transmalleolar screws. As a rule, debridement of the medial aspect is done with the arthroscope placed laterally and surgical instruments—abrader and curettes—placed medially.

Lateral debridement is done the same way with the arthroscope located medially and instruments located on the lateral side. Posterior debridement is done with the instrumentation placed posterolaterally and the scope anteriorly. An image intensifier provides the surgeon with both the proper angle for pin placement and the proper depth of penetration into the talus, avoiding damage to the subtalar joint.

Excessive removal of the subchondral bone must be avoided at all costs. At times, it might not be possible to distract the joint in an advanced case of osteoarthritis, and the tendency may be to debride too deeply in one area of the tibiotalar joint. This problem can be solved by performing a percutaneous release of the deep fibers of the deltoid ligament and the lateral ligaments as advised by Morgan [12] or by the use of fluoroscopy as advocated by Myerson [13].

Stapling

Incorrect staple placement is probably the most significant complication associated with arthroscopic repair for chronic ankle instability. Hawkins [14] noted that postoperatively, patients may experience limitations in dorsiflexion owing to a high-riding staple or a superficial position in the lateral talus secondary to postoperative migration.

One must also remember that the indications for arthroscopic repair are limited. It is important to rule out the presence of an avulsion of the ligament from the fibula. In that situation, plication of the ligament remnant with the contiguous capsule may not achieve any stability whatsoever (Fig. 19-20).

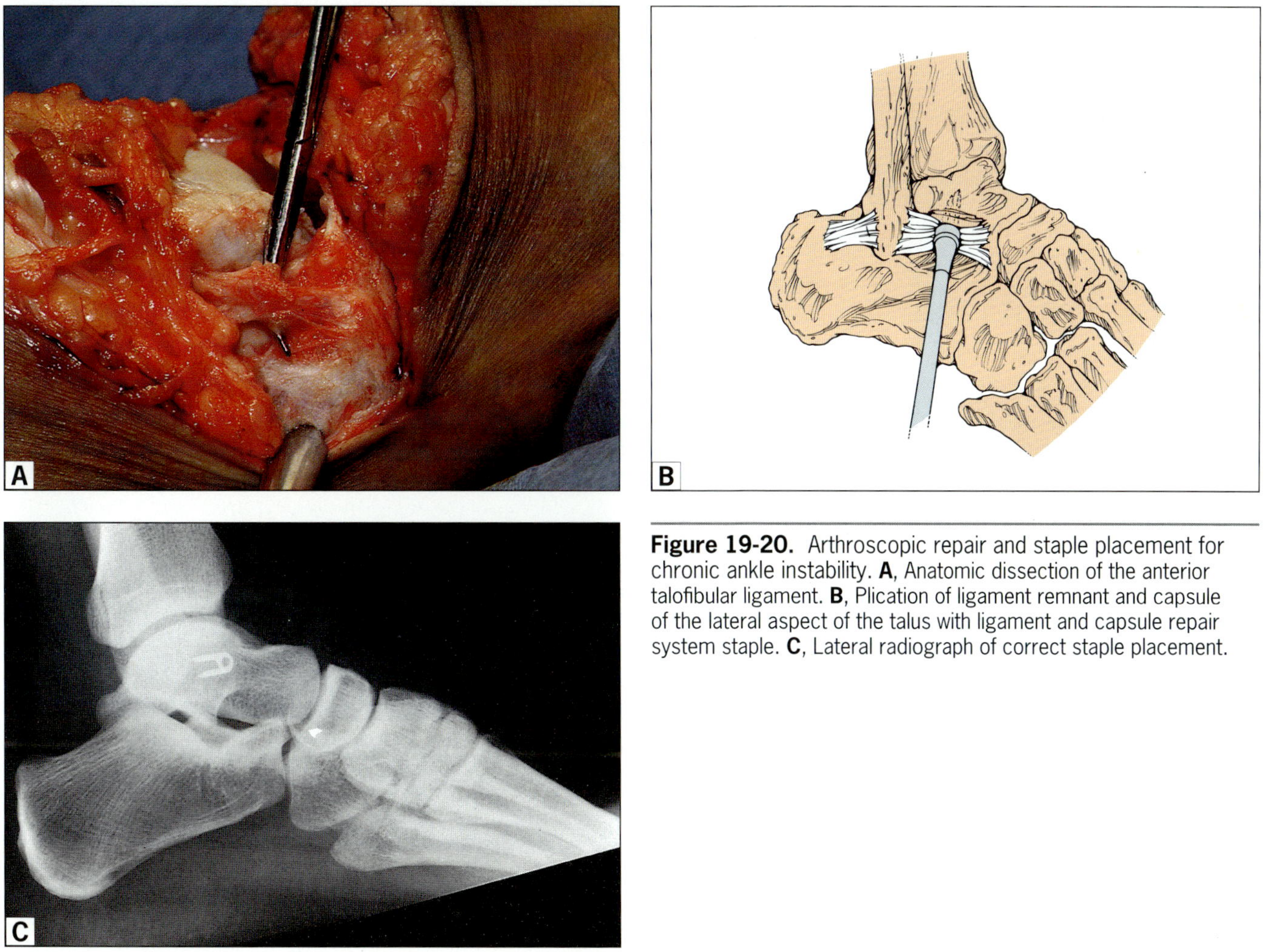

Figure 19-20. Arthroscopic repair and staple placement for chronic ankle instability. **A**, Anatomic dissection of the anterior talofibular ligament. **B**, Plication of ligament remnant and capsule of the lateral aspect of the talus with ligament and capsule repair system staple. **C**, Lateral radiograph of correct staple placement.

Conclusions

Arthroscopic surgery of the ankle is a demanding technique, and the potential for complications exists even in the hands of the most experienced arthroscopic surgeon. Many of the potential complications associated with ankle arthroscopy discussed in this chapter can be minimized or avoided by careful patient selection, a good understanding of the anatomy of the ankle, and familiarity with the various surgical procedures [15–25].

References and Recommended Reading

Recently published papers of particular interest have been highlighted as:
• Of interest
•• Of outstanding interest

1. Small NC: Complications in arthroscopy: the knee and other joints. Committee on Complications of the Arthroscopy association of North America. *Arthroscopy* 1986, 2:253–258.
2. Sherman OH, Fox JM, Snyder SJ, *et al.*: Arthroscopy—No problem: an analysis of complications in two thousand six hundred and forty cases. *J Bone Joint Surg* 1986, 68A:256–265.
3. Small NC: Complications in arthroscopic surgery performed by experienced arthroscopists. *Arthroscopy* 1988, 4:215.
4. Guhl JF: *Foot and Ankle Arthroscopy*, edn 2. Thorofare, NJ: Slack Inc.; 1993.
5. Martin DF, Baker CL, Curl WW, *et al.*: Operative ankle arthroscopy: Long-term follow-up. *Am J Sports Med* 1989, 17:16–23.
6. Barber FA, Click J, Britt BT: Complications of ankle arthroscopy. *Foot Ankle* 1990, 10:263–266.
7.•• Rodeo S, Forster R, Weiland AJ: Current concept review: neurological complications due to arthroscopy. *J Bone Joint Surg* 1993, 75A:917–926.

Prevalence and etiology of specific neurologic complications of the knee, shoulder, elbow, ankle, wrist, and hip are reviewed. Treatment of complications and ways to reduce the risk of neurologic injury during arthroscopy are discussed.

8.• Ferkel RD, Guhl JD, Heath DD: Neurological complications of ankle arthroscopy. *Arthroscopy* 1994, 10:352.

In a retrospective review of 600 patients undergoing consecutive ankle arthroscopy, 45 (7.5%) complications were noted. Fifty-six percent of those complications were neurologic.

9. Guhl JF: New concepts (distraction) in ankle arthroscopy. *Arthroscopy* 1988, 4:160–167.
10. Albert J, Reiman P, Njus G, *et al.*: Ligament strain and ankle joint opening during ankle distraction. *Arthroscopy* 1992, 8:469–473.
11.• Dowdy PA, Amendola A, Brown J, *et al.*: Noninvasive ankle distraction: Relationship between force, magnitude of distraction, and nerve conduction abnormalities. *Arthroscopy* 1994, 10:352–353.

The authors recommend using the noninvasive ankle distraction apparatus for ankle arthroscopy with up to 25 lbs of traction applied for up to 1 hour.

12. Morgan C: Arthroscopic arthrodesis. In *Operative Arthroscopy. Edited by McGinty J. New York: Raven Press; 1991, 695–701.*
13. Myerson MS, Quill G: Ankle arthrodesis: a comparison of arthroscopic and open method of treatment. *Clin Orthop* 1991, 268:84–95.
14. Hawkins RB: Arthroscopic repair for chronic lateral instability. In *Foot and Ankle Arthroscopy*, edn 2. Edited by Guhl J. Thorofare, NJ: Slack Inc.; 1993:155–160.
15. Voto SJ, Ewing JW, Fleissner PR, Jr., *et al.*: Ankle arthroscopy: Neurovascular and arthroscopic anatomy of standard and trans-Achilles tendon portal placement. *Arthroscopy* 1989, 5:41–46.
16. Parisien JS, Vangsness T, Feldman R: Diagnostic and operative arthroscopy of the ankle: an experimental approach. *Clin Orthop* 1987, 224:228–236.
17. Parisien JS: *Techniques inTherapeutic Arthroscopy.* New York: Raven Press; 1993.
18. Parisien JS: Arthroscopic treatment of osteochondral lesions of the talus. *Am J Sports Med* 1986, 14:211–217.
19. Parisien JS: Arthroscopic surgery of the ankle. In *Arthroscopic Surgery.* Edited by Parisien JS. New York: McGraw Hill; 1988:259–281.
20. Parisien JS, Feldman R: Arthroscopy of the ankle and posterior subtalar joints. In *Disorders of the Foot and Ankle.* Edited by Jahss M. New York: WB Saunders; 1991:205–235.
21. Parisien JS: Arthroscopic surgery in osteocartilaginous lesions of the ankle. In *Operative Arthroscopy* Edited by McGinty J. New York: Raven Press; 1991:727.
22. Hawkins RB: Arthroscopic treatment of sports-related anterior osteophytes in the ankle. *Foot Ankle* 1988, 9:87–90.
23. Stone JW, Guhl JF: Ankle arthroscopy. In *Current Practice in Foot and Ankle Surgery.* Edited by Pfeffer GB, Frey CC. New York: McGraw Hill; 1993:1–29.
24. Ferkel RD, Fischer SP: Progress in ankle arthroscopy. *Clin Orthop* 1989, 240:210–220.
25. Pritsch M, Horoshovshi H, Farine I: Arthroscopic treatment of osteochondral lesions of the talus. *J Bone Joint Surg* 1986, 68A:862–865.

20

CHAPTER

Endoscopic Carpal Tunnel Release

EDWARD S. BITTAR
PAUL C. DELL

In 1933, Learmonth [1] described a surgical technique for the treatment of median nerve compression neuropathy at the wrist. The technique involved transection of the anterior annular ligament by passing the blades of an open pair of scissors on either side of the transverse carpal ligament (TCL). Open transection of the TCL has been successfully used for over 60 years and has become the standard of care for the surgical treatment of carpal tunnel syndrome (CTS) [2–6]. The technique of open carpal tunnel release (CTR) has been widely used without significant alteration until recently when techniques for endoscopic carpal tunnel release (ECTR) were introduced. The proponents of ECTR suggest that the technique enables the surgeon to endoscopically visualize and transect the TCL while leaving the overlying skin, subcutaneous tissue, palmar fascia, and palmaris brevis muscle undisturbed. It has also been proposed that ECTR has the benefit of decreased postoperative morbidity, shorter postoperative recuperation time with an earlier return to full function and full work duty, and the cosmetic appeal of small incisions.

Since the first description of ECTR using a universal subcutaneous endoscope by Okutsu in 1987 [7], the technique has been extensively modified, and several systems for ECTR have become commercially available. Wider acceptance of ECTR techniques has generated controversy [8,9], primarily because of technical demands and the proposed increased risk of endoscopic surgery. This chapter surveys the available techniques and equipment for ECTR and reviews some of the controversy surrounding these innovative approaches to CTR.

TECHNIQUES

Several ECTR techniques have been described using two basic approaches: single-incision and two-incision techniques (Table 20-1). Single-incision techniques require, in all but one design, the use of a plastic blunt-ended cannula that is introduced into the carpal tunnel through a single incision made proximal to the TCL. An arthroscope can then be introduced into the cannula to visualize the TCL and monitor entry of a knife for transection of the TCL. One unique design uses a pistol-grip housing that incorporates a specially designed endoscope and blade assembly in a preassembled unit.

Two-incision designs rely on a slotted cannula system that is introduced through an incision just proximal to the TCL and exits just distal to the TCL in the palm. The slotted portion of the cannula is positioned so it is opened onto the deep surface of the TCL in the carpal tunnel. Knives are introduced through either end of the cannula and are alternated with an endoscope to visualize the transection of the TCL.

Single-Incision Method

Okutsu technique

In 1987, Okutsu [7] described the use of a universal subcutaneous endoscope (USE) system for endoscopic release of the TCL. The USE system consists of a beveled, clear plastic sheath that houses a 30°, fore-oblique arthroscope. A bullet-nosed plastic obturator allows relatively atraumatic entry into the soft-tissue compartments. The obturator is replaced by the USE system, allowing full view of the surrounding soft-tissue envelope through the transparent sheath. Release of the TCL using the USE system was described by Okutsu [10] in 1989. The obturator is introduced on the ulnar side of the palmaris longus tendon through a transverse incision 5 to 10 mm in length and 3 cm proximal to the distal palmar wrist crease. The obturator is gently inserted into the carpal tunnel. Once removed, it creates a passageway for the plastic sheath and arthroscope assembly. Transverse fibers of the TCL help to define the borders of the ligament. A retrograde knife is introduced on the ulnar side of the sheath, and transection of the TCL is accomplished under endoscopic visualization as the blade and the arthroscope are withdrawn simultaneously. Subsequent prototype designs of the sheath incorporated a gutter placed longitudinally along its length to act as a guide for the retrograde knife. Okutsu and coworkers [11] retrospectively reviewed 39 of 199 ECTR cases performed over a 5-year period from 1986 to 1991. No complications were reported in their series.

Table 20-1 Endoscopic carpal tunnel release techniques

Study	Device	Trade name and manufacturer
Single-incision		
Okutsu, *et al.* [7]	Clear plastic cannula	Not commercially available
Agee*	Pistol-grip housing	Agee Inside Job Carpal Ligament Release System (3M Health Care, St. Paul, MN)
Agee, *et al.* [12•]	Modified pistol-grip	3M Agee Carpal Tunnel Release System (3M Health Care, St. Paul, MN)
Orr	Opaque blunt-tipped plastic cannula	Uni-Cut (Acufex Microsurgical, Mansfield, MA)
Menon [15]	Opaque plastic cannula	CTS Relief Kit (Linvatec Corp., Largo, FL)
Double-incision		
Chow [16]	Slotted metal cannula	ECTRA I (Smith & Nephew Dyonics, Andover, MA)
Resnick and Miller [19]	Modified Chow technique	Not commercially available
Brown, *et al.* [20]	Slotted metal cannula system	Endotrac (Instratek, Houston, TX)
Lewicky [22]	Modified Chow technique	Not commercially available

**Paper presented at the 45th Annual Meeting of the American Society for Surgery of the Hand, Toronto, 1990.*

Agee technique

In 1990, Agee and coworkers (Paper presented at the 45th Annual Meeting of the American Society for Surgery of the Hand, Toronto, 1990) described the use of an innovative device for endoscopic release of the TCL. The 3M Agee Carpal Tunnel Release System (3M Health Care, St. Paul, MN) was originally introduced as the Agee Inside Job Carpal Ligament Release System (3M Health Care, St. Paul, MN) (Fig. 20-1A) in 1990 and incorporates a video endoscope and blade assembly into the same housing. The device has a pistol-grip handle with a trigger that actuates a blade that is housed in a plastic barrel inserted through the handle. Several prototypes were developed until the final commercially available design was available for community use. The first commercially available system, The Agee Inside Job Carpal Ligament Release System, incorporated a blade design that obscured the field of view once it was actuated (Fig. 20-1B). The original blade design did not allow visualization of the area of the ligament being transected and was therefore modified to allow the surgeon to monitor the TCL while transection was being accomplished. The Agee Inside Job Carpal Ligament Release System was on the market from 1990 through early 1991 and was voluntarily withdrawn by the manufacturer for design modifications. Modifications included in the Agee Carpal Tunnel Release System allowed the blade to be visualized endoscopically by making it periscope rather than arc from the blade assembly (Fig. 20-1C).

The advantages of this system include the use of a single transverse incision in the wrist crease between the flexor carpi radialis and flexor carpi ulnaris. Subcutaneous nerves are protected with blunt dissection while the palmar fascia of the forearm is exposed and a rectangular flap is created in the fascia based distally on the TCL. Blunt dissection of the synovial layer of tissue from the deep side of the TCL is then used to create a clear path to the carpal tunnel. Dilator probes are used to create a pathway of adequate size to accommodate the endoscopic system. The blade assembly is introduced while hugging the hook of the hamate until the distal end of the TCL is visualized. The trigger is depressed, actuating the retractable blade, and the entire system is withdrawn proximally, transecting the TCL while exiting the canal (Fig. 20-1D).

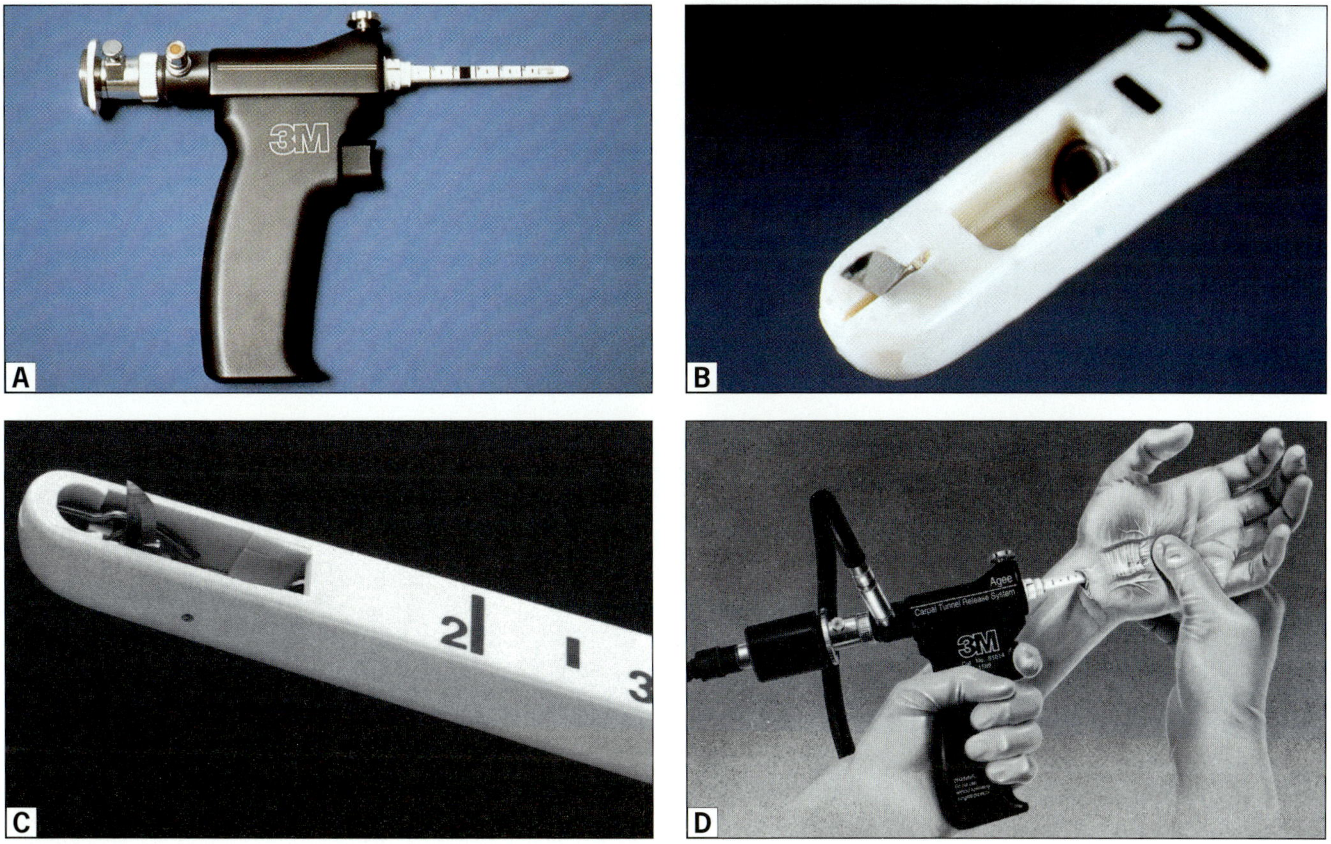

Figure 20-1. Agee technique. **A**, Agee Inside Job Carpal Tunnel Ligament Release System (3M Health Care, St. Paul, MN) with a pistol-grip handle and trigger for actuating the blade in a plastic barrel. **B**, Close-up detail of the blade assembly unit. **C**, Modified blade assembly of the 3M Agee Carpal Tunnel Release System (3M Health Care, St. Paul, MN). **D**, Surgical incision at the proximal wrist with anatomic landmarks. (Reprinted with permission of Dr. John Agee, developer of Inside Job System, and 3M Health Care, St. Paul, MN.)

The Agee Carpal Tunnel Release System is unique and requires intra-operative assembly. In the event of malfunction or breakage, the components of the system are not interchangeable with other arthroscopic equipment that is usually readily available in an operating room where arthroscopy is conventionally performed. The pistol-grip handle is heavier than other available designs and may obscure the subtle sensation of transecting individual fibers of the ligament that is reportedly possible with other systems. Multiple passes of the blade may be necessary to completely cut the ligament. The entire assembly must be reintroduced into the carpal tunnel with each pass of the blade, thereby increasing the risk of injury to the contents of the carpal tunnel because the assembly is completely withdrawn each time the blade is used.

The Agee Inside Job Carpal Ligament Release System was tested on 82 wrists in a multicenter trial that resulted in no permanent neurologic injury to patients. There were, however, neurologic injuries reported using the device in other clinical settings outside of the study [12•]. Two cases required repeat surgeries to completely transect the partially divided TCL. More recently, the 3M Agee Carpal Tunnel Release System was evaluated in a multicenter trial of over 1000 endoscopic carpal tunnel releases that resulted in no permanent device-related complications [13].

Orr technique

In 1992 the Uni-Cut (Acufex Microsurgical, Mansfield, MA) system for ECTR was introduced by Orr [14]. The single-incision system utilizes an opaque, blunt-tipped, plastic cannula with a built-in handle that is used to stabilize the device (Fig. 20-2A). The technique requires

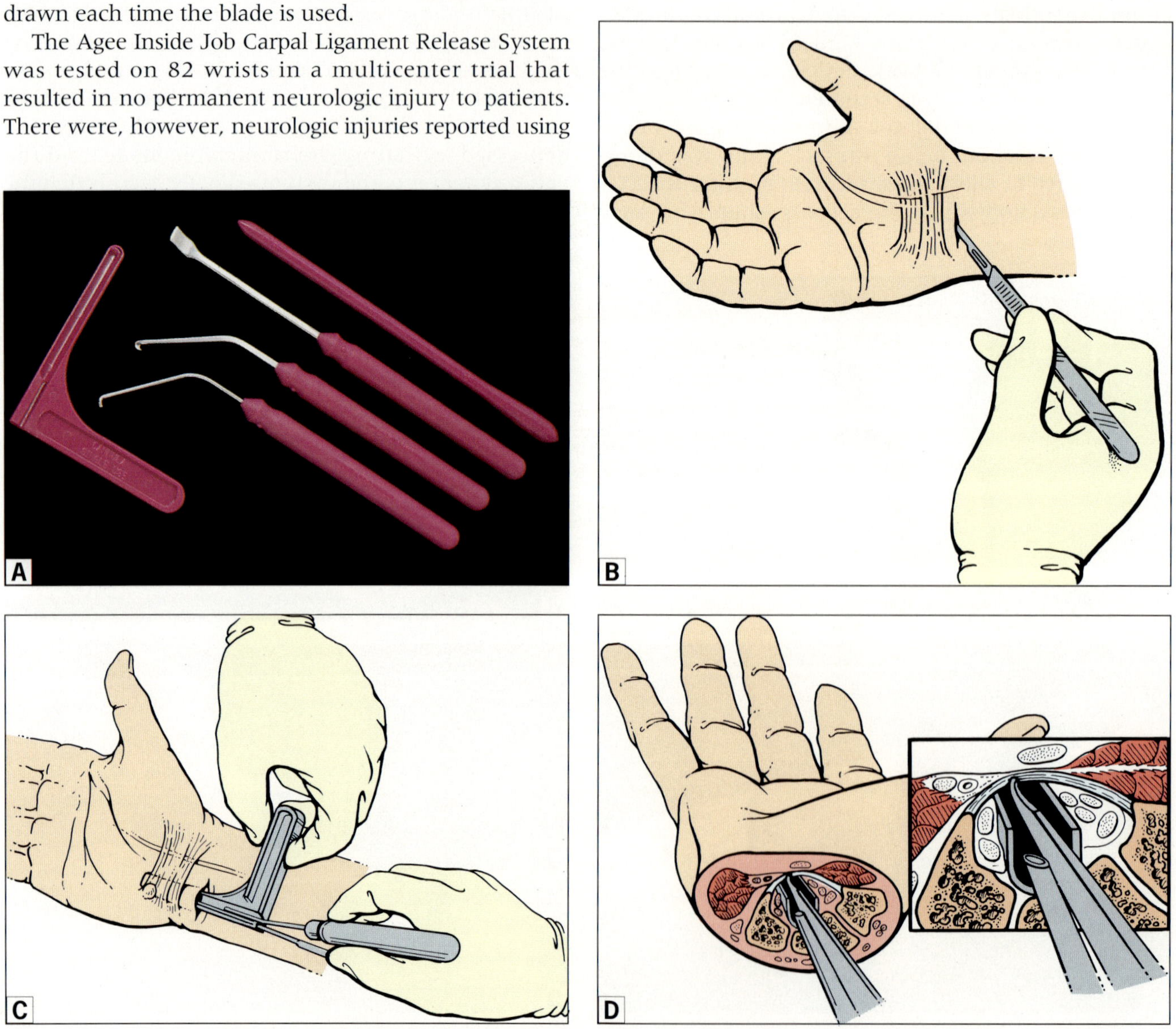

Figure 20-2. **A**, Uni-Cut Endoscopic Carpal Tunnel Release System (Acufex Microsurgical, Mansfield, MN). **B**, Transverse incision 1 cm proximal to the flexion crease of the wrist. **C**, **D**, A retrograde knife is introduced through the cannula and the transverse carpal tunnel ligament is transected from distal to proximal ends. (Reprinted with the permission of Dr. T.R. Orr and Acufex Microsurgical, Mansfield, MN.)

a transverse incision 1.2 to 1.5 cm in length and 1 cm proximal to the flexion crease of the wrist (Fig. 20-2B). Blunt dissection and preparation of the pathway is performed using a blunt elevator. The 6.5-mm end of a blunt "channeler" is used to create a clear passageway for the cannula, which is then introduced and stabilized with the handle by an assistant. The handle maintains stability of the device by maintaining the position of the cannula against the hook of the hamate. The handle also maintains alignment of the cannula with the ring finger while it is seated within the carpal canal. An arthroscope is then used to visualize the exposed deep surface of the TCL and a probe followed by a knife with a retrograde blade (Fig. 20-2C) is introduced parallel to the channel that accommodates the endoscope. The TCL is transected as the knife and endoscope are simultaneously withdrawn, leaving the cannula in the carpal tunnel (Fig. 20-2D). The 10-mm end of the channeler is then inserted into the carpal tunnel to confirm (by ease of passage) that complete transection of the TCL has been performed.

The Uni-Cut device has not yet completed multicenter testing. It has the advantages of using a single incision on the volar wrist. Conventional arthroscopy equipment can be used with the device, obviating the need to purchase additional unique equipment to accommodate the device. The device is a disposable plastic unit that has the potential disadvantage of creating small plastic shavings as the metal blade is passed over the softer plastic cannula. The endoscopic field of view is limited to the small slit in the cannula made for the endoscope. The parallel placement of the arthroscope and blade channel and the opacity of the plastic cannula also limit the field of view. The addition of a small handle provides the added advantage of stability with a single incision.

Menon technique

A single-incision ECTR technique using an opaque plastic cannula was reported by Menon in 1993 [14] (Fig. 20-3A). The commercially-available cannula (CTS Relief Kit; Linvatec Corp., Largo, FL) is introduced through an oblique incision that lies at the junction of the distal wrist crease and the radial border of the ring finger (Fig. 20-3B). Blunt and sharp dissection allows the antebrachial fascia to be entered just ulnar to the palmaris longus tendon. After dilating the opening of the fascia with an obturator followed by 5.5-mm and 7-mm dilators, the slotted cannula with the obturator inserted is introduced into the carpal tunnel until the tip of the cannula is felt just beyond the distal border of the TCL through the overlying subcutaneous tissues in the skin. The cannula has no handle and must be firmly held in line with the ring finger while hugging the side of the hook of the hamate. Once the cannula is properly positioned, a 30° arthroscope is introduced to visualize the proximal border of the TCL. A push-blade knife

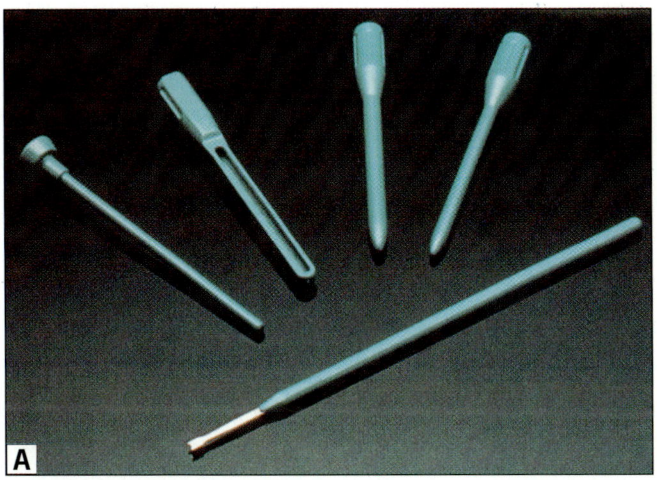

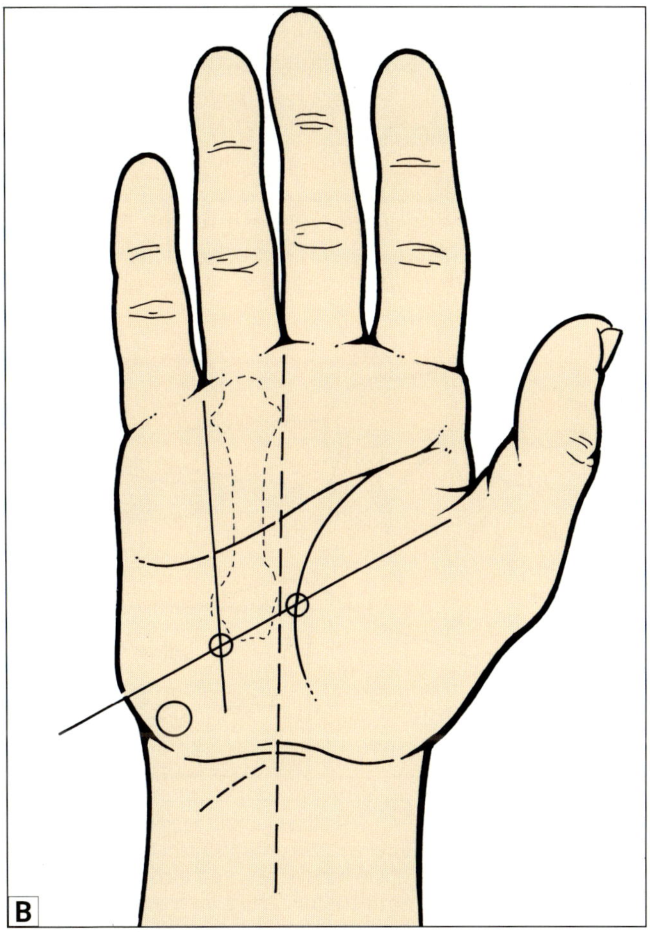

Figure 20-3. CTS Relief Kit and procedure. **A**, CTS Relief Kit (Linvatec Corp., Largo, FL) endoscopic carpal tunnel release system. **B**, Landmarks for an oblique incision proximal to the wrist crease. (*continued*)

with a concave sharp edge is then advanced into the slotted cannula and is used to transect the TCL from proximal to distal until the release of the TCL is completed (Fig. 20-3C).

Proximal to distal transection is proposed by the proponents of this technique to be safer. It is argued that cutting the distal edge of the TCL with a retrograde hook blade may inadvertently cause cutting or catching of some of the soft tissues that lie just distal to the edge of the TCL. In addition, it is argued that the concave blade can be carefully advanced to cut the last few fibers of the TCL at its distal border and leave the soft-tissue structures beyond the TCL unharmed as the advance of the blade is stopped by the closed end of the cannula. Menon [15] has proposed that the concave blade cannot be advanced distally beyond the closed end of the cannula and that the design features of the system prevent inadvertent injury to the palmar arch and digital nerves beyond the distal limit of the TCL.

The advantages of this disposable system include the ease of use and its simple design. The cannula is not round in cross-section, but has one flattened side that is slotted. The flattened side is approximated to the deep surface of the TCL and reportedly provides more torsional stability than a round cannula [15]. However, the opacity of the plastic cannula limits the field of view. It is also possible that shavings of the plastic cannula can be created by contact with the metal blade.

Two-Incision Method

Chow technique

In 1989, a two-incision technique for ECTR was described by Chow using an open-ended slotted metal cannula [16] (ECTRA I; Smith & Nephew Dyonics, Andover, MA). The original technique described by Chow involved making an entry wound on the volar wrist using a small transverse incision approximately 1 cm radial and 1 cm proximal to the pisiform bone (Fig. 20-4A). The flexor tendons were retracted radially and the ulnar neurovascular structures retracted laterally through a longitudinal incision in the deep fascia. Retraction of the ulnar neurovascular structures have since been abandoned because of the occasional reports of reversible ulnar nerve neurapraxia, presumably caused by aggressive retraction. The wrist and fingers are hyperextended on a special frame designed for that purpose as the cannula is advanced along the hook of the hamate and through the carpal tunnel (Fig. 20-4B and 20-4C). Hyperextension is used to drop the contents of the carpal canal away from the deep side of the TCL. The cannula and obturator advance until the tip of the obturator can be felt through the skin and subcutaneous tissues just beyond the distal edge of the TCL and just proximal to the palmar arch. A second small incision is made in the palm to allow the cannula and obturator to exit. A 30° arthroscope can then be introduced into the cannula from either open end (Figs. 20-4D–F). The cannula is rotated to allow the arthroscope to visualize anatomic landmarks through the slit in the cannula. Because both ends of the cannula are open, probes and blades can be interchangeably introduced through one end of the cannula while the arthroscope is seated in the opposite end. The TCL is then transected using a series of disposable blades (Fig. 20-4G) that accompany the system, including a probe blade that is used to probe the TCL and can be pushed against its free distal edge to initiate cutting of the TCL. The TCL is then cut with the retrograde blade while being visualized endoscopically through the slit in the cannula. Complete release of the TCL is appreciated endoscopically when no transverse fibers of the TCL remain intact (Figs. 20-4H and 20-4I). Both incisions are closed and a simple gauze dressing is applied allowing postoperative motion.

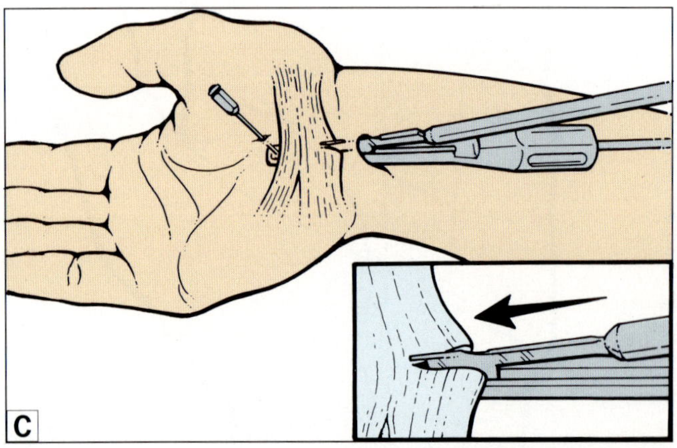

Figure 20-3. *(continued)* **C**, The obturator has been replaced by an endoscope. A needle has been used as a landmark to confirm the location of the distal edge of the transverse carpal tunnel ligament and a knife with a push-blade has begun transecting the transverse carpal ligament from the proximal edge toward the distal edge. (Reprinted with the permission of Dr. J. Menon and Linvatec Corp., Largo, FL.)

No permanent complications were reported in 1993 by Chow [17••] after 4 years of experience with ECTR in 650 wrists using the ECTRA system. In one case, however, after ECTR, persistent symptoms suggested incomplete release of the TCL and required repeat ECTR 1 year later with resolution of symptoms.

In 1994, a multicenter prospective study of 1291 cases of ECTR was completed by nine surgeons using the Chow technique and the ECTRA system. (Nagle and coworkers, Paper presented at the 48th Annual Meeting of the American Society for Surgery of the Hand, Kansas City, 1993). The transbursal technique for entry into the carpal canal, as originally described by Chow [16], was deemed too risky to nerves, vessels, and tendons within the canal and was abandoned in favor of the extrabursal approach described by Agee (Agee and coworkers, Paper presented at the

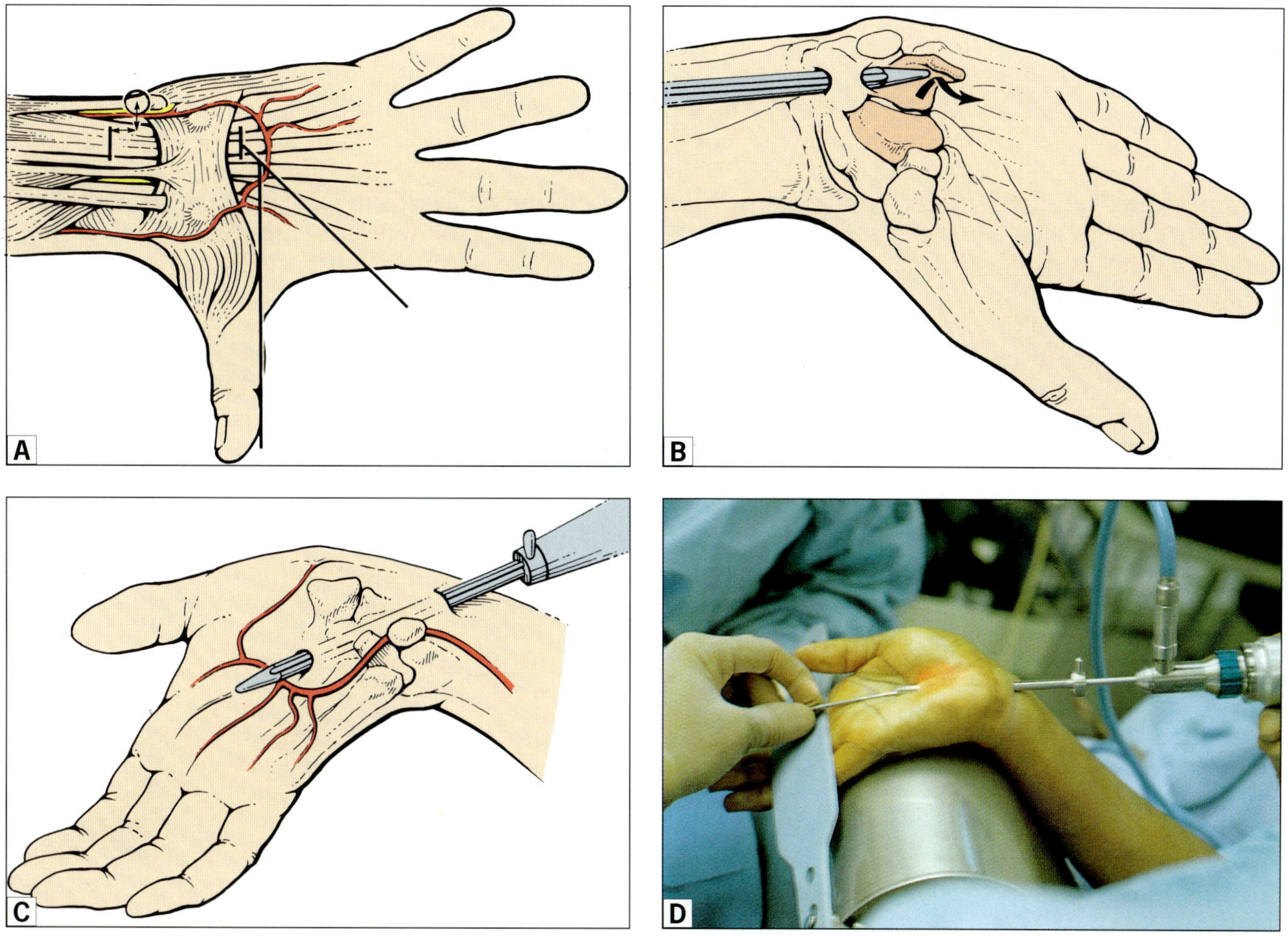

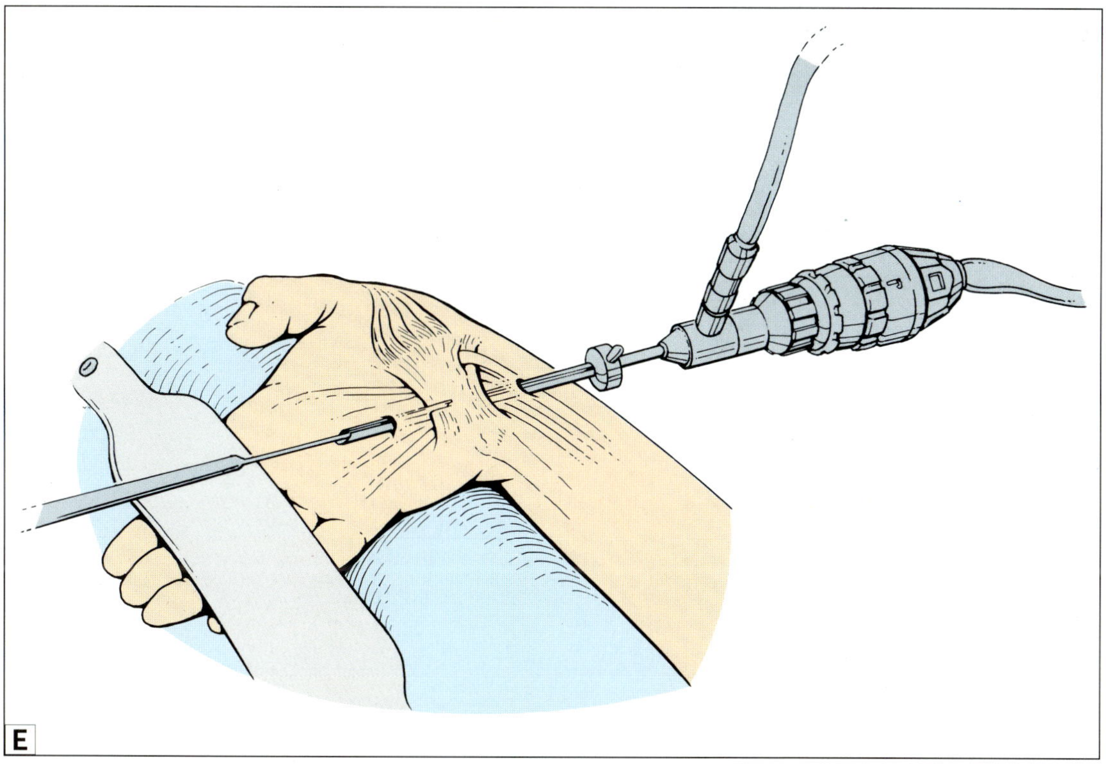

Figure 20-4. Chow ECTRA I (Smith & Nephew Dyonics, Andover, MA) endoscopic carpal tunnel release system. **A**, Surgical landmarks. **B**, Introducing the cannula and obturator through the fasciotomy site using the hook of the hamate as a guide to the ulnar recess of the carpal canal. **C**, The slotted cannula and obturator have passed through the distal palmar incision just distal to the distal edge of the transverse carpal ligament and proximal to the palmar arch. **D**, **E**, **F**, The endoscope and blades are passed on either side of the cannula, visualizing proximal and distal halves. (*continued*)

45th Annual Meeting of the American Society for Surgery of the Hand, Toronto, 1990) and North [18]. A perioperative complication rate of 1.8% was reported that included 24 of the 1291 cases. Sixteen cases of neuropraxia, five cases of incomplete release, and one case of tendon laceration were among the complications reported. The complications were almost evenly divided between cases where extrabursal and transbursal approaches were employed, but in general it was concluded that the extrabursal approach was safer and easier to use. Twenty-two late complications were also reported, including 19 recurrences of carpal tunnel syndrome and three cases of reflex sympathetic dystrophy (Nagle and coworkers, Paper presented at the 48th Annual Meeting of the Hand, Kansas City, 1993).

Resnick and Miller technique

One modification of the Chow technique includes the technique reported by Resnick and Miller in 1991 [19]. A subligamentous approach was adopted to avoid the neurovascular and tendon injuries that the authors experienced using the original Chow approach. Using the subligamentous approach, the surgeon creates a fascial flap to provide a soft-tissue window for access to the carpal tunnel. Medial retraction of the ulnar neurovascular structures and lateral retraction of the tendons is thereby avoided along with complications that accompany retraction in almost 10% of the patients.

Brown technique

In 1992, Brown and coworkers [20] reported a two-incision modification of the Chow technique using a modified cannula system (Endotrac; Instratek, Houston, TX) (Fig. 20-5). The proximal incision is followed by a volar forearm fasciotomy, as previously described for the extrabursal approach. A slotted cannula and obturator are introduced into the carpal canal without tendon or neurovascular retraction and

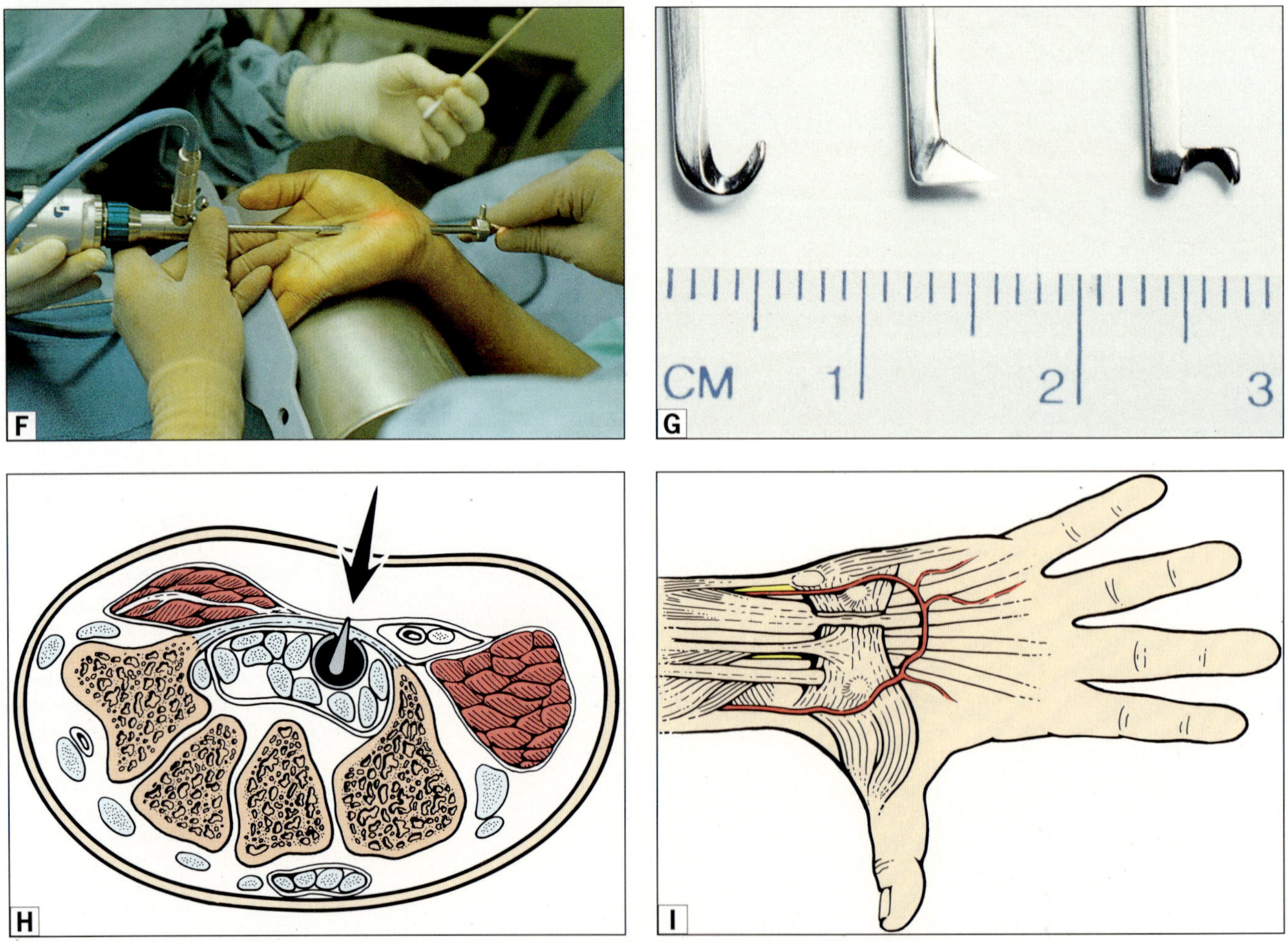

Figure 20-4. (*continued*) **G**, The three blades that accompany the system, including a probe-blade at the right and a retrograde blade on the left. **H**, Illustration of transection of the transverse carpal ligament in cross-section. **I**, Illustration of a fully transected transverse carpal ligament at its ulnar limit. (Reprinted with the permission of Dr. James Chow and Smith & Nephew Dyonics, Andover, MA.)

advanced to the exit portal region where a palmar incision is made. Use of the slotted cannula with a reportedly narrower diameter than that available with other systems was designed to reduce compression of the carpal tunnel soft-tissue contents.

The TCL is incised with a retrograde blade under endoscopic visualization. Brown and coworkers experienced fewer complications using the modified approach in 1236 endoscopic release procedures, reporting no neurovascular complications and only one tendon injury. Relief of symptoms was accomplished in 98% of patients, however, 2% of cases required a second procedure for subsequent median nerve neurolysis. Brown identified a subset of patients comprising 2% of his study population that had a thickened epineurium that required neurolysis for relief of symptoms [21•].

Lewicky technique

Lewicky reported using a guide tube modification of the Chow two-incision technique [22]. A specially designed, curved dissector is used to create a passageway to the carpal canal. The dissector is advanced through the canal and through a distal palmar incision. Once through the palmar skin incision, a length of the clear plastic tubing is attached to the end of the dissector and brought through the proximal incision in a retrograde fashion. The clear plastic tubing is left to rest in the carpal canal, preserving the passageway created by the dissector. A slotted sheath with a blunt obturator is introduced into the proximal end of the plastic tube guide. The tube guide is then drawn distally through the canal and out the distal incision with the sheath assembly

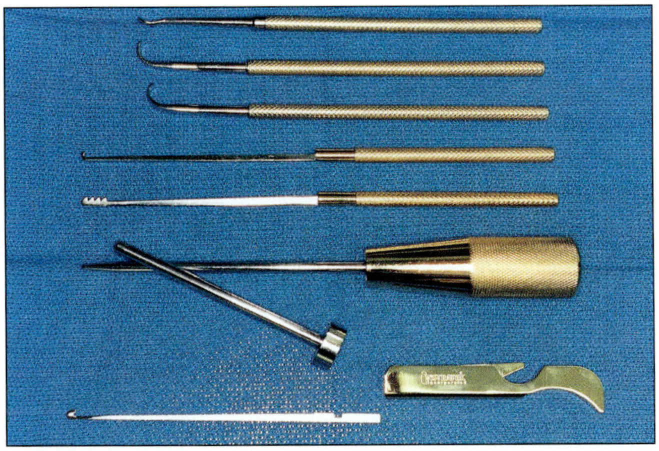

Figure 20-5. Endotrac (Instratek, Houston, TX) endoscopic carpal tunnel release system. (Reprinted with the permission of Dr. Michael G. Brown, developer of the Brown technique endoscopic carpal tunnel release system, and Instratek, Houston, TX.)

attached. It is proposed that the curved dissector eliminates some of the risk involved in creating the distal palmar incision, because the dissector can more easily locate the distal edge of the transverse carpal ligament. The remainder of the surgical technique and the guide tube system are essentially similar to the ECTRA system, as previously described.

DISCUSSION

Attendance at supervised hands-on cadaver workshops is recommended prior to clinical use of any of the ECTRA systems. Complication rates in the community setting have been higher than in prospective multicenter study group settings (Nagle and coworkers, 1993). Although all open and endoscopic techniques of CTR are not without risk because of anatomic considerations [23–25] and are not without complications [26,27], ECTR reports suggest that complications may be primarily related to endoscopic technique. Case reports of ulnar nerve transection [27,28] and incidental release of Guyon's canal [29] may suggest limitations of the ECTR technique used. Cadaveric studies of ECTR resulting in a range of 50% [30,31] to 95% [32] complete transection of the TCL using the ECTRA system may also suggest that technique alone may account for the wide variation in effectiveness of endoscopic TCL transection. Partial transection of the TCL [29] and an increase in neurovascular injury using ECTR of 1.5 to 2.5 times the rates reported for open CTR suggest that complications are technique related [33].

The second exit incision in the palm provides substantially more stability to the cannula system compared with single-incision techniques. Once the point of exit has been pierced by the cannula, a stable configuration is created and no further motion of the cannula will occur unless initiated by the surgeon. The surgeon is then free to carefully introduce equipment through either end of the cannula with fine control, which is not easily accomplished with a single-incision technique. Fine manipulation and sensibility are probably more uniformly preserved with a two-incision technique than with a single-incision technique. Additional advantages include the relative simplicity in assembly and operation of a slotted cannula technique compared with some of the design complexities of the 3M Agee Carpal Tunnel Release System.

One disadvantage of the two-incision technique is the palmar incision itself. A palmar incision reportedly causes prolonged pain, delayed postoperative recovery, and delayed return of normal grip strength and pinch strength [14]. Proponents of the two-incision technique claim that negligible morbidity occurs with a second palmar incision.

Advocates of single-incision techniques feel that the potential complication of incomplete transection of the distal portion of the TCL is more likely to occur with the two-incision approach. It is argued that the distal portion of the TCL can be inadvertently pierced by the sheath and obturator as it is being directed palmarly to create the second palmar incision. Piercing the midsubstance of the TCL slightly proximal to the distal edge would allow a small portion of the TCL to remain intact. The arthroscopic view through the slotted sheath, however, would confirm incorrectly that complete transection had been accomplished.

Conversely, the palmar arch can be inadvertently incised if the exit wound in the palm is made distal to the arch and transection includes all tissues visualized in the slot of the cannula. Single-incision techniques, however, do not provide any additional measure of protection against injury to distal neurovascular or tendinous structures.

Since 1930, open CTR techniques have provided a relatively safe and reliable means of surgically treating CTS. Endoscopic methods of CTR that are presently available share the unifying concept that they all require an endoscope to be introduced into the carpal tunnel through a portal to visualize the undersurface of the TCL while it is then transected with a blade that is also introduced into the canal. The soft-tissue dissection using ECTR is less extensive than with open techniques. The advantages of ECTR include decreased morbidity, early return to work, and early return to full function, but are tempered by the technical demands and new surgical skills required by endoscopic technique. ECTR promises to be a useful adjunct to hand surgery but requires careful attention to anatomy and endoscopic technique. Extensive cadaveric experience prior to clinical use is recommended and will undoubtedly lessen some of the dangers unique to ECTR.

REFERENCES AND RECOMMENDED READING

Recently published papers of particular interest have been highlighted as:

- • Of interest
- •• Of particular interest

1. Learmonth JR: The principle of decompression in the treatment of certain diseases of peripheral nerves. *Surg Clin North Am* 1993, 13:905–913.

2. Brain WR, Wright AD, Wilkinson M: Spontaneous compression of both median nerves in the carpal tunnel: Six cases treated surgically. *Lancet* 1947, 1:277–282.

3. Phalen GS, Gardner WJ, La Londe AA: Neuropathy of the median nerve due to compression beneath the transverse carpal ligament. *J Bone Joint Surg* 1950, 32A:109–112.

4. Phalen GS: Spontaneous compression of the median nerve at the wrist. *JAMA* 1951, 145:1128–1133.

5. Phalen GS: The carpal-tunnel syndrome. *J Bone Joint Surg* 1966, 48A:211–228.

6. Dorwart BB: Carpal tunnel syndrome: a review. *Semin Arthritis Rheum* 1984, 14:134–139.

7. Okutsu I, Ninomiya S, Takatori Y, *et al.*: Subcutaneous operation under the universal subcutaneous endoscope. *Arthroscopy* 1987, 12:77–81.

8. Jabaley ME: Commentary: single-portal endoscopic carpal tunnel release. *Contemp Orthop* 1993, 26:115–116.

9. Newmeyer WL: Editorial: thoughts on the technique of carpal tunnel release. *J Hand Surg* 1992, 17A:985–986.

10. Okutsu I, Ninomiya S, Takatori Y, *et al.*: Endoscopic management of carpal tunnel syndrome. *J Arthro Related Surg* 1989, 5:11–18.

11. Okutsu I, Ninomiya S, Takatori Y, *et al.*: Results of endoscopic management of carpal tunnel syndrome. *Orthop Rev* 1993:81–87.

12.• Agee JM, McCarroll HR, Tortosa RD, *et al.*: Endoscopic release of the carpal tunnel: a randomized prospective multicenter study. *J Hand Surg* 1992, 17A:987–995.

An excellent presentation of the single-incision endoscopic carpal tunnel release approach with accompanying results of a prospective study.

13. Agee JM, Peimer CA, Pyrek JD, *et al.*: Endoscopic carpal tunnel release: a prospective study of complications and surgical experience. In press.

14. Menon J: Endoscopic carpal tunnel release: a single-portal technique. *Contemp Orthop* 1993, 26:109–116.

15. Menon J: Endoscopic carpal tunnel release: Preliminary report. *Arthroscopy* 1994, 10:31–38.

16. Chow JC: Endoscopic release of the carpal ligament: a new technique for carpal tunnel syndrome. *Arthroscopy* 1989, 5:19–24.

17.•• Chow JC: The Chow technique of endoscopic release of the carpal ligament for carpal tunnel syndrome: Four years of clinical results. *Arthroscopy* 1993, 9:301–314.

A comprehensive review of a two-incision endoscopic carpal tunnel release technique and retrospective clinical results.

18. North ER: Endoscopic carpal tunnel release. In *Operative Repair and Reconstruction*, vol II. Edited by Gelberman, RN. Philadelphia: JB Lippincott; 1991:913–920.

19. Resnick CT, Miller BW: Endoscopic carpal tunnel release using the subligamentous two-portal technique. *Contemp Orthop* 1991, 22:269–277.

20. Brown MG, Keyser B, Rothenberg ES: Endoscopic carpal tunnel release. *J Hand Surg* 1992, 17A:1009–1011.

21.• Brown MG, Rothenberg ES, Keyser B, *et al.*: Results of 1236 endoscopic carpal tunnel release procedures using the Brown technique. *Contemp Orthop* 1993, 27:251–258.

A good review of a modified two-incision endoscopic carpal tunnel release technique outlining advantages and disadvantages.

22. Lewicky RT: Endoscopic carpal tunnel release: the guide tube technique. *Arthroscopy* 1994, 10:39–49.

23. Linburg RM, Albright JA: An anomalous branch of the median nerve. *J Bone Joint Surg* 1970, 52A:182–183.

24. Ogden JA: An unusual branch of the median nerve. *J Bone Joint Surg* 1972, 54A:1779–1781.

25. Papathanassiou BT: A variant of the motor branch of the median nerve in the hand. *J Bone Joint Surg* 1968, 50B:156–157.

26. May JW, Rosen H: Division of the sensory ramus communicans between the ulnar and median nerves: a complication following carpal tunnel release. *J Bone Joint Surg* 1981, 63A:836–838.

27. Lilly CJ, Magnell TD: Severance of the thenar branch of the median nerve as a complication of carpal tunnel release. *J Hand Surg* 1985, 10A:399–402.

28. Nath RK, Mackinnon SE, Weeks PM: Ulnar nerve transection as a complication of two-portal endoscopic carpal tunnel release: a case report. *J Hand Surg* 1993, 18:896–898.

29. Luallin SR, Toby EB: Incidental Guyon's canal release during attempted endoscopic carpal tunnel release: an anatomical study and report of two cases. *Arthroscopy* 1993, 9:382–386.

30. Lee DH, Masear VR, Meyer RD, *et al.*: Endoscopic carpal tunnel release: a cadaveric study. *J Hand Surg* 1992, 17A:1003–1008.

31. Seiler JG, Barnes K, Gelberman RH, *et al.*: Endoscopic carpal tunnel release: an anatomic study of the two-incision method in human cadavers. *J Hand Surg* 1992, 17A:996–1002.

32. Levy HJ, Soifer TB, Kleinbart FA, *et al.*: Endoscopic carpal tunnel release: an anatomic study. *Arthroscopy* 1993, 9:1–4.

33. Adams BD: Endoscopic carpal tunnel release. *J Am Academy of Orthopedic Surgeons* 1994, 2:179–184.

Index

Note: Page numbers in *italics* indicate illustrations; page numbers followed by t indicate tables.

A

Achilles tendon graft, for posterior cruciate ligament reconstruction, *101*, *102*, 102–103 *see also* Posterior cruciate ligament reconstruction
Adhesions
  of ankle, excision of, 175, *175*, *179*, *180*
  in frozen shoulder, 110, 110t, *111*
    excision of, 112–114, *113–115*, 115
  of knee, magnetic resonance imaging of, 7
Adhesive capsulitis *see* Frozen shoulder
Agee technique, for carpal tunnel release, 206t, *207*, 207–208
Aiming guides, for pin placement, in anterior cruciate ligament reconstruction, 71–72, *72*
Air extravasation, with infusion pump, 26
Allograft *see also specific types*
  disadvantages of, 103
  freezing of, 103
  meniscal *see* Meniscal allograft reconstruction
  sterilization of, 103
Anesthesia
  interscalene
    for shoulder stabilization, 118, 119
    for suture anchor capsulorrhaphy, 146
  in office arthroscopy, 13
Ankle arthrodesis
  advantages of, 185–186
  complications of *see also* Ankle arthroscopy, complications of
    prevention of, 202–203
  diagnostic arthroscopy in, 188, *189*
  disadvantages of, 186
  equipment for, 186–187, 187t, *201*, 201, *202*
  joint distention in, 186–187
Ankle arthrodesis, *continued*
  portal placement in, 188, *188*
    complications of, 194–197, *194–197*
  results of, 190
  screw fixation in, *189*, 189–190
  technique for, 186–190, *186–190*, 202–203
  traction in, 186, *187*
    complications of, 198–199, *198–200*
Ankle arthroscopy
  for adhesions, 175, *175*, *179*, *180*
  antibiotic prophylaxis for, 180, 194
  for arthrodesis, 185–191 *see also* Ankle arthrodesis
  for arthrofibrosis, 175, *175*
  for chronic ligamentous instability, 177, 182, *182*
  complications of, 193–204
    from distraction, 198–199, *198–200*
    incidence of, 193
    from incisions, 199, *200*
    infectious, 180, 194
    from instrument failure, 199, *201*
    neurological, 194
    from portal placement, 194–197, *194–197*
    retained foreign body as, 199
    sinus and fistula formation as, 199, *200*
  equipment for, *178*, 178–180, *179*, 199, *200*, *201*
  for hemophilic synovitis, 177–178
  for infectious synovitis, 177, *177*
  infusion pumps in, 22, *23*, *24*, 199, *201*
  laser, *182*, 182–183
  for nonspecific chronic synovitis, 173–174, *174*
  for ostechondral lesions, 201, *201*, *202*
  for pigmented villonodular synovitis, 175–176, *176*, *177*, *181*
  portal placement in, 178
    complications of, 194–197, *194–197*
  positioning for, 178, *178*, 203, *203*

Ankle arthroscopy, *continued*
postoperative care in, 182
for rheumatoid synovitis, 176–177, *177*
for soft-tissue impingement syndrome, 174, *174*, *180*
for synovial chondromatosis, 176, *176*
technique for, *178–182*, 178–183
Anterior acromioplasty, in frozen shoulder, 114, *115*
Anterior capsulorrhaphy *see* Capsulorrhaphy
Anterior cruciate ligament, magnetic resonance imaging of, 8
Anterior cruciate ligament reconstruction
with patellar tendon, 65–74
complications of, 78
diagnostic arthroscopy in, 66
femoral tunnel preparation in, 68–69, *69*, *70*, 71–72, *72*
graft harvest in, *67*, 67–68, *68*, *69*
graft placement in, 72–74, *72–74*
graft strength in, 51–52, 78
versus with hamstring tendons, 51–52
intercondylar notch preparation in, 66, *66*
isometry in, 72, 73
meniscal repair in, 66
morbidity in, 52, 66, 78
notchplasty in, 67, *67*, *72*
preliminary technique for, 66
versus with quadrupled semitendinosus graft, 77–78
results of, 74
supracondylar femur preparation in, 68
technique for, 66–74
tibial tunnel preparation in, 69–71, *70–73*
posterior cruciate ligament reconstruction with, 96
with quadrupled semitendinosus graft, 74–85
advantages of, 77–78
EndoButton fixation for, 78, *78*, 80, 82, *83*, 85
femoral bisocket technique for, 84–85, *85*
graft harvest in, 79, *79*
graft preparation in, 79–80, *80*, 82, *83*
graft strength in, 74–75
isometry in, 81–82, *82*
meniscal repair in, 82
notchplasty in, 80
rehabilitation after, 85, *86–87*
set-up for, 79
technique for, 79–85
tibial tunnel preparation in, 80–81, *81*
with semitendinosus and gracilis tendons, 51–61
advantages of, 51–52
closure and bracing in, 60
diagnostic arthroscopy in, 53, *53*
femoral tunnel preparation in, 57, *57*

Anterior cruciate ligament reconstruction,with semitendinosus and gracilis tendons, *continued*
graft fixation and tensioning in, 58–60, *58–60*
graft harvesting in, 54–55, *55*
graft passage in, 58, *58*
graft preparation in, 55, *56*
graft strength in, 51–52, 78
isometry in, 58
notchplasty in, 53–54, *54*
versus with patellar tendon, 51–52
rehabilitation after, 61, 61t–63t
results of, 61, *63*
set-up in, 53, *53*
short grafts in, 60, *60*
technique for, 53–60, *53–60*
tibial stump in, 54, *54*
tibial tunnel preparation in, 55–56, *56*
Anterior inferior glenohumeral ligament-labral complex
anatomy of, 144, *144*
detachment of, *134*, 134–135, *135*, 136, 143–145, 159–160 *see also* Shoulder, instability of
arthroscopic appearance of, 148, *148*, *150*, *162*
in initial acute shoulder dislocation, 118, *119*, 119, 124, 124t
pathology of, 123, 133, 159–160
repair of *see* Shoulder stabilization
Anterior labroligamentous periosteal sleeve avulsion, 134, 170, *171*
Anterior synovial impingement syndrome, of ankle, 174, *174*, 180
Anterior talofibular ligament, tears of, 177, 182, *182*, 203, *203*
Anteroposterior shoulder stability, assessment of, 128, *128*
Antibiotic prophylaxis, for ankle arthroscopy, 180, 194
Arcuate ligament complex, anatomy of, 91
Arthrex shoulder traction apparatus, for suture anchor capsulorrhaphy, 147, *147*
Arthritis
ankle, arthrodesis for, 185–191 *see also* Ankle arthrodesis
degenerative, mensicectomy and, 35–36
Arthroscope, for office arthroscopy, 13–14
Arthroscopy *see also specific joints and procedures*
laser, 29–34 *see also* Laser arthroscopic surgery
office, 11–16 *see also* Office arthroscopy
Artificial ligaments, 103
Autograft *see* Achilles tendon graft; Gracilis tendon graft; Patellar tendon graft; Semitendinosus tendon graft
Avascular necrosis, of knee, magnetic resonance imaging of, 5, *5*

B

Bankart lesion, *134*, 134–135, *135*, 136, 143–145, 159–160 *see also* Shoulder, instability of
- arthroscopic appearance of, 148, *148*, *150*, *162*
- in initial acute shoulder dislocation, 118, *119*, 119, 124, 124t
- pathology of, 123, 133, 159–160
- repair of *see* Shoulder stabilization

Biceps anchor injury, bioabsorbable tack stabilization for, 125–132 *see also* Shoulder stabilization, with bioabsorbable tack

Biceps tendon, arthroscopic appearance of, *148*

Bioabsorbable suture anchor, 146, *146*

Bioabsorbable tack, 125–132
- biodegradation profile of, 126, *126*
- complications with, 131–132
- development of, 125–126
- failure of, 132
- indications for, 126–127, *127*
- for initial acute anterior dislocation, 120–121, *121–123* *see also* Shoulder stabilization, for initial acute anterior dislocation
- insertion technique for, 127–130, *127–131*
- postoperative care with, 130–131
- properties of, 126, *126*

Bio Anchor suture anchor, 146, *146*

Blades
- full-radius, 178, *179*
- Whisker, 178, *179*, *202*

Bone bruise, magnetic resonance imaging of, 4, 94, *95*

Bone marrow injuries, magnetic resonance imaging of, 94, *95*

Bracing, after anterior cruciate ligament repair, 60

Brown technique, for endoscopic carpal tunnel release, 206t, 212–213, *213*

Buford complex, arthroscopic appearance of, 148, *148*

Bursitis, subacromial, in frozen shoulder, 109t, 109–110, 110t, *110111*

C

Cannula
- in Chow ECTRA I system, 210, *211*
- in CTS Relief Kit, 209, *209*, 210
- disposable plastic, for ankle arthroscopy, 199, *200*
- infusion pump, *19*, 19, *24*
- in Uni-Cut Carpal Tunnel Release System, *208*, 208–209

Cannulated bioabsorbable tack *see* Bioabsorbable tack

Capsular contracture, in frozen shoulder, 109, 110, 110t

Capsular laxity, in shoulder instability, 159–160

Capsulorrhaphy
- Caspari, 134, 135–140 *see also* Caspari capsulorrhaphy
- contraindications to, 135
- indications for, 135
- with staples, 145
- with suture anchors, 143–156
  - advantages of, 145
  - anchor placement in, *151*, 151–152
  - diagnostic arthroscopy in, 147–148, *148*
  - drill hole placement in, *150*, 150–151
  - equipment for, 145–146, *146*
  - glenoid rim preparation in, *149*, 149–150
  - history of, 145
  - indications for, 145
  - knot tying in, *151*, 153–154, *154*
  - portal placement for, 147
  - positioning in, 146, *147*, 149
  - postoperative care in, 154–155, *155*
  - rehabilitation in, 154–155, *155*
  - results of, 155–156, *156*
  - set-up for, 146–147, *147*
  - suture passing in, *151*, *152*, 152–153
  - technique for, 147–154, *148–155*
- transglenoid suture, 159–172
  - advantages of, 160, 171
  - anterior glenoid neck preparation in, 161, *162*, *163*
  - Bankart lesion repair in, *164–169*, 165–167
  - capsular shift in, 161–165, *163*, *164*, 168
  - complications of, 167–168
  - diagnostic arthroscopy in, 161, *161*, *162*
  - disadvantages of, 145
  - patient selection for, 172
  - postoperative management in, 167
  - results of, 170–171
  - technique for, 160–167, *162–171*
- transglenoid suture capsulorrhaphy, modifications of, 168–170, *169*, *170*

Carpal tunnel release, endoscopic, 205–214 *see also* Endoscopic carpal tunnel release

Caspari capsulorrhaphy, 133–140
- complications of, 140
- diagnostic arthroscopy in, 136
- patient selection for, 140
- portal placement in, 136, *136*
- positioning in, 135
- postoperative regimen in, 139
- results of, 139–140
- set-up in, 135–136, *136*
- technique for, 136–138, *136–139*

Chondromalacia, magnetic resonance imaging of, 3

Chondroplasty, laser *see* Laser arthroscopic surgery
Chow technique, for carpal tunnel release, 206t, 210–212, *211–212*
CO_2 laser, 30, 30t *see also* Laser arthroscopic surgery
Compartment syndromes, fluid extravasation and, 26–27
Contracture, capsular, in frozen shoulder, 109, 110, 110t
Contusion, bone, magnetic resonance imaging of, 4, 94, *95*
Coracoacromial ligament, resection of, in frozen shoulder, 114, *115*
Coracohumeral ligament, resection of, in frozen shoulder, 114, *115*
Cruciate ligaments *see under* Anterior cruciate ligament; Posterior cruciate ligament
CTS Relief Kit, 209–210, *209–210*
Cysts, meniscal, magnetic resonance imaging of, 2, *3*

D

Debridement, laser *see* Laser arthroscopic surgery
Degenerative arthritis
  mensicectomy and, 35–36
  tibiotalar, arthrodesis for *see* Ankle arthrodesis
Diabetes mellitus, frozen shoulder in, 108
Discoid meniscus, magnetic resonance imaging of, 2, *2*
Dislocation
  of knee, posterior cruciate ligament injuries in *see* Posterior cruciate ligament injuries
  of patella
    magnetic resonance imaging of, 3, *4*
    proximal extensor mechanism realignment for, 45–50, *46–49*
  of shoulder *see also* Shoulder, instability of
    pathology of, 123
    stabilization after *see* Shoulder stabilization
    tissue injury in, 144–145
Distraction, invasive/noninvasive
  in ankle arthrodesis, 186, *187*
  in ankle arthroscopy, complications from, 198–199, *198–200*
Drill injuries, in posterior cruciate ligament reconstruction, *98*, 98–99, *99*
Drill walking, prevention of, 98

E

ECTRA I system, 210–212, *211–212*
Elbow arthroscopy, infusion pumps in, 24, *25*
EndoButton fixation, for quadrupled semitendinosus graft, 78, *78*, 80, 82, *83*, 85
Endoscopic carpal tunnel release, 205–214
  advantages of, 205–206
  complications of, 213–214
  development of, 205–206
  results of, 213–214
  single-incision, 206t, 206–210
    advantages of, 214
    Agee technique for, 206t, *207*, 207–208
    disadvantages of, 213
    Menon technique for, 206t, *209*, 209–210, *210*
    Okutsu technique for, 206, 206t
    Orr technique for, 206t, *208*, 208–209
  two-incision, 206, 206t, 210–213
    advantages of, 213–214
    Brown technique for, 206t, 212–213, *213*
    Chow technique for, 206t, 210–212, *211–212*
    disadvantages of, 213–214
    Lewicky technique for, 206t, 213
    Resnick-Miller technique for, 206t, 212
Endotrac endoscopic carpal tunnel release system, 212–213, *213*
Erbium laser, 30t.34 *see also* Laser arthroscopic surgery
Excimer laser, 30t *see also* Laser arthroscopic surgery
Exercises *see also* Rehabilitation
  for frozen shoulder, 111, 111t, 114
    as conservative treatment, 111, 111t
    postmanipulation, 114

F

Femoral bisocket technique, for anterior cruciate ligament reconstruction, with quadrupled semitendinosus graft, 84–85, *85*
Fentanyl, for office arthroscopy, 13
Fistula formation, in ankle arthroscopy, 199, *200*
Fluid extravasation, with infusion pumps, 26–27
Foreign body, retained, in ankle arthroscopy, 199
Fracture
  tibial plateau, magnetic resonance imaging of, 4
  transchondral talar, arthroscopic management of, 201, *201*, *202*
Freeze drying, of allografts, 103
Frozen shoulder, 107–115
  arthroscopic diagnosis of, 109–111, *110*, *111*, 112t
    following manipulation, 112
  arthroscopic surgery of
    indications for, 111–112, 112t
    results of, 1154
    technique for, 112–114, *113–115*
  clinical presentation of, 108
  definition of, 107
  differential diagnosis of, 108
  etiology of, 107

Frozen shoulder, *continued*
exercises for
as conservative treatment, 111, 111t
postmanipulation, 114
in head trauma patients, 112
historical aspects of, 107
manipulation of
complications of, 114
exercises after, 114
indications for, 111t, 111–112
results of, 115
technique for, 112
natural history of, 108, 108t
open surgery for, 109
pathology of, 109, 109t
patient classification in, 111
physical findings in, 108
radiographic findings in, 108
rehabilitation in, 114
stages of
arthroscopic, 110t
clinical, 109t
symptoms of, 108
Full-radius blades, 178, *179*

G

Giant-cell tumor, of knee, magnetic resonance imaging of, 6–7, *7*
Glenohumeral instability *see* Shoulder, instability of
Glenohumeral ligament
arthroscopic appearance of, *148*
capsulolabral avulsion of *see also* Shoulder, instability of
anterior shoulder instability and, *134*, 134–135, *135*
arthroscopic appearance of, 148, *148*, *150*, *162*
in initial acute shoulder dislocation, 118, *119*, 119, 124, 124t
pathology of, 123, 133, 159–160
repair of *see* Shoulder stabilization
resection of, in frozen shoulder, 113, *114*
Glenoid, arthroscopic appearance of, *148*
Glenoid labrum *see* Labrum
Gracilis tendon graft
in anterior cruciate ligament reconstruction, 51–61 *see also* Anterior cruciate ligament reconstruction, with semitendinosus and gracilis tendons
ligament extender for, 60, *60*
Graft(s)
allogeneic
disadvantages of, 103
freezing of, 103
Graft(s), allogeneic, *continued*
sterilization of, 103
meniscal *see* Meniscal allograft reconstruction
tendon *see also specific types*
in cruciate ligament reconstruction *see* Anterior cruciate liagament reconstruction; Posterior cruciate ligament reconstruction
ligament extender for, 60, *60*
Guidepin placement *see* Pin placement

H

Hamstring tendons, in anterior cruciate ligament reconstruction *see under* Anterior cruciate ligament reconstruction
Head trauma, frozen shoulder and, 112
Hemophilic synovitis, 177–178
Hill-Sachs lesions, transglenoid suture capsulorrhaphy and, 168–170
Hip arthroscopy, infusion pumps in, 26, *26*
Holmium:YAG laser, 30t, 30–32, *30–33 see also* Laser arthroscopic surgery
Humeral head, arthroscopic appearance of, *148*

I

Imaging *see* Magnetic resonance imaging; Radiography
Infection, after ankle arthrodesis, antibiotic prophylaxis for, 180, 194
Infectious synovitis, of ankle, 177, *177*
Inferior glenohumeral ligament *see* Glenohumeral ligament
Inflammatory synovitis, of ankle, 176–177, *177*
Infraspinatus muscle entrapment, in transglenoid suture capsulorrhaphy, 168
Infusion pumps, *17*, 17–27
advantages and disadvantages of, 19
in ankle arthroscopy, 22, *23*, *24*, 199, *201*
cannula for, *19*, 19
complications with, 26–27
in elbow arthroscopy, 24, *25*
flow rates with, 19
guidelines for, 27
in hip arthroscopy, 26, *26*
in knee arthroscopy, 19, *20*
pressure-sensing monitors for, 19
in shoulder arthroscopy, 19–22, *21*, *22*
in wrist arthroscopy, 24, *26*
Instrumentation, for office arthroscopy, 15
Interosseous ligament tears, in ankle, laser arthroscopy for, *182*, 182–183
Interscalene anesthesia
for shoulder stabilization, 118, 119
for suture anchor capsulorrhaphy, 146

Irrigation
fluid pressure in, 18
gravity system for, 17–18, *18*
infusion pump for, 17–27 *see also* Infusion pumps
Isometry
in anterior cruciate ligament reconstruction
with patellar tendon graft, 72, 73
with quadrupled semitendinosus graft, 81–82, *82*
with semitendinosus and gracilis graft, 58
in posterior cruciate ligament reconstruction, 97–100, *98–100*

J

Joint irrigation *see* Irrigation

K

Knee
arthroscopy of
infusion pump in, 19, *20*
lasers in, 29–34 *see also* Laser arthroscopic surgery
office, 11–16 *see also* Office arthroscopy
articular cartilage lesions of, magnetic resonance imaging of, 8
avascular necrosis (osteonecrosis) of, magnetic resonance imaging of, 5, *5*
cruciate ligaments of *see under* Anterior cruciate ligament; Posterior cruciate ligament
dislocations of, posterior cruciate ligament injuries in *see* Posterior cruciate ligament injuries
intra-articular scar and adhesions in, magnetic resonance imaging of, 7
magnetic resonance imaging of, 1–8
axial views on, 3
full versus zero extension on, 3
future directions in, 8
meniscus of *see under* Meniscal
osteochondriditis dissecans of, magnetic resonance imaging of, *4*, 4–5
pigmented villonodular synovitis of, magnetic resonance imaging of, 6
synovial chondromatosis, magnetic resonance imaging of, 6
tuberculosis synovitis of, magnetic resonance imaging of, 6, *6*
tumors of, magnetic resonance imaging of, 6–7, *7*
vascular disorders of, magnetic resonance imaging of, 7, *7*
Knee brace, after anterior cruciate ligament repair, 60
Knot, Revo, in suture anchor capsulorrhaphy, 153–154, *154*
Knot pusher, for suture anchor capsulorrhaphy, 146, *146*
KTP laser, 30t *see also* Laser arthroscopic surgery
Kurasaka screw fixation, of patellar tendon graft, 74, *74*

L

Labrum
arthroscopic appearance of, *148*
injuries of, bioabsorbable tack for, 127
Labrum-anterior inferior glenohumeral ligament complex
anatomy of, 144, *144*
detachment of, *134*, 134–135, *135*, 136, 143–145, 159–160 *see also* Shoulder, instability of
arthroscopic appearance of, 148, *148*, *150*, *162*
in initial acute shoulder dislocation, 118, *119*, 119, 124, 124t
pathology of, 123, 133, 159–160
repair of *see* Shoulder stabilization
Lachman test, in anterior cruciate ligament reconstruction, with patellar tendon, 66, 74
Laser(s)
in photodynamic therapy, 34
physics of, 29–30
types of, 30t
Laser arthroscopic surgery
advantages of, 29, 32
of ankle, *182*, 182–183
complications of, 32
equipment for, 30t, 30–33, *31*, *32*
erbium laser in, 30t, 34
future of, 33–34
history of, 29–30
holmium:YAG laser in, 30t, 30–32, *30–33*
of knee, 29–34
indications for, 31, 33–34
laser types for, 30t
meniscal, 29–34
neodymium:YAG laser in, 30t, 32–33, *33*
physics of, 29–30
thulium laser in, 34
Lateral meniscal allograft reconstruction, 40–42, *41–43*
Lateral patellofemoral angle, on imaging studies, 3
Lewicky technique, for carpal tunnel release, 206t, 213
Liberator elevator, 149, *149*
Ligament(s) *see also specific ligaments*
cruciate *see* Anterior cruciate ligament; Posterior cruciate ligament

Ligament(s), *continued*
prosthetic, 103
Ligament extender, for short tendon grafts, 60, *60*
Ligament of Humphrey, anatomy of, 91
Ligament of Wrisberg, anatomy of, 91
Local anesthesia, for office arthroscopy, 13
Loose bodies, in ankle, 201

M

Magnetic resonance imaging
of knee, 1–8
of articular cartilage lesions, 8
axial views on, 3
of bone bruise, 4, 94, *95*
of chondromalacia, 3
of cruciate ligaments, 8, *8*
future directions in, 8
of intra-articular scar and adhesions, 7
of meniscal cysts, 2, *3*
of meniscal tears, 1–2, *2*
of osteochondritis dissecans, *4*, 4–5
of osteonecrosis, 5, *5*
of patellar subluxation, 3, *4*
of patellar tilt, 3
of posterior cruciate ligament injuries, 94, *95*, *96*
of synovitis, 6, *6*
of tibial plateau fracture, 4, *4*
of tumors, 6–7, *7*
of vascular conditions, 7, *7*
versus office arthroscopy, 12
of pigmented villonodular synovitis, of ankle, 176, *176*
Magnetic retrievers, 199, *201*
Marrow injuries, magnetic resonance imaging of, 94, *95*
Medial meniscal repair
with allograft, 36–40, *37–40*
in anterior cruciate ligament reconstruction with hamstring tendons, 53
Meniscal allograft reconstruction, 36–42
degenerative changes after, 36
lateral, 40–42, *41–43*
medial, 36–40, *37–40*
Meniscal cysts, magnetic resonance imaging of, 2, *3*
Meniscal-femoral ligaments, anatomy of, 91
Meniscal repair
with allograft *see* Meniscal allograft reconstruction
in anterior cruciate ligament reconstruction
with patellar tendon graft, 66
with quadrupled semitendinosus graft, 82
with semitendinosus and gracilis graft, 53
Meniscal repair, *continued*
lasers in, 33–34 *see also* Laser arthroscopic surgery
Meniscectomy
degenerative changes after, 35–36
laser, 29–34, *32*, *33* *see also* Laser arthroscopic surgery
Meniscoid lesion, of anterolateral aspect of ankle, 174
Meniscus, discoid, magnetic resonance imaging of, 2, *2*
Menon technique, for carpal tunnel release, 206t, *209*, 209–210, *210*
Midazolam, for office arthroscopy, 13
Middle glenohumeral ligament *see* Glenohumeral ligament
Mini Revo suture anchor, 146, *146*
Mitek GII suture anchor, 145, *146*
Mt. Saint Helen's maneuver, in medial meniscus allograft, 36, *37*

N

Nerve injuries, in knee dislocations, 94
Notchplasty, in anterior cruciate ligament reconstruction
with patellar tendon, 67, *67*, *72*
with quadrupled semitendinosus graft, 80
with semitendinosus and gracilis tendons, 53–54*54*

O

Office arthroscopy, 11–16
anesthesia for, 13
complications of, 15–16
equipment for, 13–14, *14*, *15*
history of, 12
indications for, 12–13
versus magnetic resonance imaging, 12
positioning for, 13, *14*, 14, *15*
postoperative care in, 15
scope of, 11–12
technique of, 15
Offset guides, for pin placement, in anterior cruciate ligament reconstruction, 71–72, *72*
Okutsu technique, for carpal tunnel release, 206, 206t
Orr technique, for carpal tunnel release, 206t, *208*, 208–209
Osteoarthritis
mensicectomy and, 35–36
tibiotalar, arthrodesis for *see* Ankle arthrodesis
Osteochondral lesions, ankle arthroscopy for, 201, *201*, *202*

Osteochondritis dissecans
of ankle, 201
of knee, magnetic resonance imaging of, *4*, 4–5
Osteonecrosis, of knee, magnetic resonance imaging of, 5, *5*

P

Pain
after bioabsorbable tack stabilization, 132
in frozen shoulder, 108
patellofemoral, after anterior cruciate ligament reconstruction, 52, 78
Patellar malalignment, magnetic resonance imaging of, 3, *3*
Patellar subluxation
magnetic resonance imaging of, 3, *4*
recurrent, assisted proximal extensor mechanism realignment for, 45–50, *46–49*
Patellar tendon
in anterior cruciate ligament reconstruction, 65–74 *see also* Anterior cruciate ligament reconstruction, with patellar tendon
in posterior cruciate ligament reconstruction, *101*, 102–103 *see also* Posterior cruciate ligament reconstruction
Patellar tilt
magnetic resonance imaging of, 3
radiographic imaging of, *46*, *47*
Patellofemoral angle, lateral, on imaging studies, 3
Patellofemoral instability, recurrent lateral, proximal extensor mechanism realignment for, 45–50, *46–49*
Patellofemoral pain, after anterior cruciate ligament reconstruction, 52, 78
Patient positioning *see* Positioning
Periarthrite scapulohumeral, 107
Peroneal nerve
ankle portal placement and, 194–195, *195*
injury of, posterior cruciate ligament injury and, 94
Perthes lesion *see* Bankart lesion
Photodynamic therapy, 34
Physical therapy *see* Rehabilitation
Pigmented villonodular synovitis
of ankle, *174*, 174–175, *175*
of knee, magnetic resonance imaging of, 6, *6*
Pin placement
in ankle arthrodesis, 189, *189*
in ankle arthroscopy, complications of, 198
in anterior cruciate ligament reconstruction
with patellar tendon graft, 69–72, *70*, *72*
with quadrupled semitendinosus graft, 81–82
with semitendinosus and gracilis graft, 55–57, *56*
Pin placement, *continued*
in Caspari capsulorrhaphy, 138, *138*
in posterior cruciate ligament reconstruction, 97–99, *98–100*
in transglenoid suture capsulorrhaphy, *164–167*, 165–167
Pneumoscrotum, with infusion pumps, 26
Popliteal artery injury, in posterior cruciate ligament reconstruction, 99
Positioning
for ankle arthrodesis, 186, *186*
for ankle arthroscopy, 178, *178*
for Caspari capsulorrhaphy, 135
for office arthroscopy, 13, *14*, 14, *15*
for shoulder stabilization, *118*, 118–119, *127*, 127–128
for suture anchor capsulorrhaphy, 146, *147*, 149
for transglenoid suture capsulorrhaphy, *160*, 160–161
Posterior cruciate ligament
curvature of, anterior cruciate tears and, 8
magnetic resonance imaging of, 8, *8*
Posterior cruciate ligament injuries
grading of, 96
history in, *92*, 93
imaging of, 94, *95*, *96*
laxity grading in, 93–94
mechanism of, *92*, 93
nonoperative treatment of
indications for, 96
morbidity in, 94–96
operative treatment of *see* Posterior cruciate ligament reconstruction
physical examination in, *93*, 93–94, *94*
Posterior cruciate ligament reconstruction, 89–103
anatomic aspects of, 90–91, *90–92*
biomechanical aspects of, 92
complications of, 103
diagnostic arthroscopy in, 96
femoral tunnel preparation in, 99–100
graft placement and fixation in, *100*, 100–101, *101*
graft selection for, *101*, 101–103, *102*
history of, 89–90
indications for, 96
isometry in, 97–100, *98–100*
limitations of, 96
neurovascular injury in, prevention of, 99, *99*
versus nonoperative management, 94–96
results of, 103
technique for, 96–103
tibial attachment visualization in, 97
tibial tunnel preparation in, 97–99, *98–100*
Posterior drawer test, in posterior cruciate ligament injury, 93–94

Posterior soft-tissue impingement syndrome, in ankle, 174, *174*
Posterolateral ligament complex, anatomy of, 91
Potassium titanyl phosphate laser, 30t *see also* Laser arthroscopic surgery
Prosthetic ligaments, 103
Proximal extensor mechanism realignment, for recurrent lateral patellofemoral instability, 45–50, *46–49*
Pumps, infusion *see* Infusion pumps

Q

Quadriceps active test, in posterior cruciate ligament injury, 93, *94*

R

Radiography
 of frozen shoulder, 108
 of posterior cruciate ligament injuries, 94
 of synovial chondromatosis of ankle, 176, *176*
Range of motion exercises *see* Rehabilitation
Rehabilitation
 after anterior cruciate ligament reconstruction
  with quadrupled semitendinosus graft, 85, *86–87*
  with semitendinosus and gracilis graft, 61, 61t–63t
 after capsulorrhaphy with suture anchors, 154–155, *155*
 after Caspari capsulorrhaphy, 139
 after frozen shoulder manipulation, 114
 after shoulder stabilization with bioabsorbable tack, 130–131
 after transglenoid suture capsulorrhaphy, 167
Resnick-Miller technique, for carpal tunnel release, 206t, 212
Revo knot, in suture anchor capsulorrhaphy, 153–154, *154*
Rheumatoid arthritis, ankle arthrodesis for, 185–191 *see also* Ankle arthrodesis
Rheumatoid synovitis, of ankle, 176–177, *177*
Rice bodies, in rheumatoid synovitis, 176
Rotator cuff, in frozen shoulder, 110

S

Sag sign, in posterior cruciate ligament injury, 93, *93*
Saphenous nerve and vein, ankle portal placement and, 194, *194*
Screw fixation
 in ankle arthrodesis, 189–190, *190*
 versus EndoButton fixation, 78
 of patellar tendon graft, 74, *74*
Screw fixation, *continued*
 in posterior cruciate ligament reconstruction, 101, *102*
 of semitendinosus and gracilis tendon graft, 58–60, *59*, *60*
Sedation, intravenous, for office arthroscopy, 13
Semitendinosus tendon graft
 in anterior cruciate ligament reconstruction *see* Anterior cruciate ligament reconstruction
 ligament extender for, 60, *60*
 in posterior cruciate ligament reconstruction, 102 *see also* Posterior cruciate ligament reconstruction
Sensory scope sheath system, 19, *20*
Sharpey's fibers, regeneration of, with femoral bisocket technique, 84
Shoulder
 anatomy of, 144, *144*
  normal arthroscopic, 148, *148*
 dislocation of *see also* Shoulder, instability of
  stabilization for *see* Shoulder stabilization
  tissue injury in, 144–145
 frozen, 107–115 *see also* Frozen shoulder
 instability of
  arthroscopic findings in, 136
  arthroscopic management of *see* Shoulder stabilization
  assessment of, 128, *128*
  Bankart repair for, 143
  after bioabsorbable tack insertion, 123, 124, 131
  capsulorrhaphy for *see* Capsulorrhaphy
  after capsulorrhaphy with suture anchors, 155–156
  after Caspari capsulorrhaphy, 140
  nonoperative treatment of, results of, 117–118
  pathology of, 123, *134*, 134–135, *135*, 136, 144–145, 159–160
  pathophysiology of, 144–145, 159–160, *160*
  after transglenoid suture capsulorrhaphy, 170–171
Shoulder arthroscopy
 for frozen shoulder *see* Frozen shoulder
 infusion pumps in, 19–22, *21*, *22*
 for instability *see* Shoulder stabilization
 office, 11–16 *see also* Office arthroscopy
Shoulder dislocation
 recurrent *see also* Shoulder, instability of
  pathology of, 123
 tissue injury in, 144–145
Shoulder guide, in transglenoid suture capsulorrhaphy, *164*, 165
Shoulder stabilization
 for anterior instability, capsulorrhaphy for *see* Capsulorrhaphy

Shoulder stabilization, *continued*
with bioabsorbable tack, 125–132
complications of, 131–132
indications for, 126–127, *127*
for initial acute anterior dislocation, 120–121, *121–123*
portal placement in, 128–130, *129*, 132
positioning for, *127*, 127–128
postoperative care in, 130–131
technique for, 127–130, *127–131*
for chronic anterior dislocation, results of, 123–124
for initial acute anterior dislocation, 117–124
bioabsorbable tack insertion in, 120–121, *121–123*
diagnostic arthroscopy in, 119, *119*
hemarthrosis in, 119
indications for, 118–119
interscalene anesthesia for, 118, 119
versus nonoperative treatment, 117–118
pathologic findings in, 121–123, 123t
positioning in, *118*, 118–119
results of, 118, 121–123
technique for, 118–121, *119–123*
techniques for, 134, 134t
Shoulder stiffness *see also* Frozen shoulder
causes of, 108
Shoulder traction
for office arthroscopy, 13, *14*, 15, *15*
for stabilization procedures, *118*, 118–119, *127*, 127–128
Shuttle Relay, in suture anchor capsulorrhaphy, 146, *146*, *151*, *152*, 152
Sinus formation, in ankle arthroscopy, 199, *200*
Sling, after capsulorrhaphy with suture anchors, 154–155, *155*
Soft-tissue impingement syndrome, of ankle, 174, *174*, *180*
Staple capsulorrhaphy, 145
Staple placement, for chronic ankle instability, 182, *182*, 203, *203*
STaR sleeve, for suture anchor capsulorrhaphy, 147, *147*
Sterilization, of allografts, 103
Subacromial bursectomy, in frozen shoulder, 114, *115*
Subacromial bursitis, in frozen shoulder, 109t, 109–110, *110*, 110t, *111*
Subluxation
patellar
magnetic resonance imaging of, 3, *4*
recurrent, proximal extensor mechanism realignment for, 45–50, *46–49*
shoulder *see also* Shoulder, instability of
pathology of, 123
stabilization of *see* Shoulder stabilization
Subluxation, shoulder, *continued*
tissue injury in, 144–145
Subscapularis bursectomy, in frozen shoulder, 113, *114*
Sulcus test, for shoulder instability, 128, *128*
Superficial peroneal nerve, ankle portal placement and, 194–195, *195*
Supralabral hole, arthroscopic appearance of, 148, *148*
Suprascapular nerve injury, in transglenoid suture capsulorrhaphy, 167
Sural nerve, ankle portal placement and, 195, *196*
Surgical table, for office arthroscopy, 14, *14*, *15*
Suture(s), for suture anchor capsulorrhaphy, 146, *146*
Suture anchors
in shoulder stabilization, 143–156 *see also* Capsulorrhaphy, with suture anchors
types of, 145–146, *146*
Suture capsulorrhaphy
with suture anchors *see* Capsulorrhaphy, with suture anchors
transglenoid *see* Capsulorrhaphy, transglenoid suture
Suture pin placement *see* Pin placement
Suture punch technique, in capsulorrhaphy *see* Caspari capsulorrhaphy
Syndesmodic disruptions, ankle, laser arthroscopy for, *182*, 182–183
Synovectomy
ankle *see also* Ankle arthroscopy
for hemophilic synovitis, 177–178
for infectious synovitis, 177
laser, *182*, 182–183
for pigmented villonodular synovitis, 176, *181*
for rheumatoid synovitis, 177, *177*
for synovial chondromatosis, 176
technique for, 201
laser *see also* Laser arthroscopic surgery
of ankle, *182*, 182–183
Synovial chondromatosis
of ankle, 176, *176*
of knee, magnetic resonance imaging of, 6
Synovial impingement syndrome, of ankle, 174, *174*, *180*
Synovitis
of ankle
hemophilic, 177–178
infectious, 177, *177*
nonspecific chronic, 173–174, *174*
pigmented villonodular, *174*, 174–175, *175*, *181*
rheumatoid, 176–177, *177*
in frozen shoulder, 109t, 109–110, *110*, 110t, *111*
of knee, magnetic resonance imaging of, 6, *6*

T

Table, for office arthroscopy, 14, *14*, *15*
Tack, bioabsorbable *see* Bioabsorbable tack
Talofibular ligament, tears of, 177, 182, *182*, 203, *203*
Talus, transchondral fracture of, arthroscopic management of, 201, *201*, *202*
Tendon(s) *see specific tendons*
Tendon grafts
  in anterior cruciate ligament repair *see* Anterior cruciate ligament reconstruction
  ligament extenders for, 60, *60*
  in posterior cruciate ligament repair *see* Posterior cruciate ligament reconstruction
Thigh holder, for office arthroscopy, 14, *14*
Thulium laser, 34 *see also* Laser arthroscopic surgery
Tibial femoral stepoff, in posterior cruciate ligament injury, 93, *93*
Tibial nerve injury, in posterior cruciate ligament reconstruction, 99, *99*
Tibial plateau fracture, magnetic resonance imaging of, 4, *4*
Tibiofibular ligament, hypertrophy of, 174, *174*
Tibiotalar arthrodesis, 185–191 *see also* Ankle arthrodesis
Traction
  in ankle arthrodesis, 186, *187*
  in ankle arthroscopy, complications from, 198–199, *198–200*
  shoulder
    for office arthroscopy, 13, *14*, 15, *15*
    for stabilization procedures, *118*, 118–119, *127*, 127–128
  for suture anchor capsulorrhaphy, 147, *147*
Tranglenoid beath pin placement, in Caspari capsulorrhaphy, 138, *138*
Transglenoid suture capsulorrhaphy, 159–172
  advantages of, 160, 171
  anterior glenoid neck preparation in, 161, *162*, *163*
  Bankart lesion repair in, *164–169*, 165–167
Transglenoid suture capsulorrhaphy, *continued*
  capsular shift in, 161–165, *163*, *164*, 168
  complications of, 167–168
  diagnostic arthroscopy in, 161, *161*, *162*
  disadvantages of, 145
  modifications of, 168–170, *169*, *170*
  patient selection for, 172
  postoperative management in, 167
  results of, 170–171
  technique for, 160–167, *162–171*
Transverse carpal ligament, transection of *see* Endoscopic carpal tunnel release
Transverse tibiofibular ligament, hypertrophy of, 174, *174*
Tuberculosis synovitis, of knee, magnetic resonance imaging of, 6, *6*
Tumors, of knee, magnetic resonance imaging of, 6–7, *7*

U

UltraSling, 154–155, *155*
Uni-Cut Endoscopic Carpal Tunnel Release System, *208*, 208–209
Universal subcutaneous endoscopy, for carpal tunnel release, 206

V

Vascular disorders, of knee, magnetic resonance imaging of, 7, *7*
Vascular injuries, in knee dislocations, 94
Videocamera, for ankle arthroscopy, *202*
Villonodular synovitis, pigmented
  of ankle, *174*, 174–175, *175*
  of knee, magnetic resonance imaging of, 6

W

Whisker blades, 178, *179*, *202*
Wrisberg discoid meniscus, magnetic resonance imaging of, 2
Wrist arthroscopy, infusion pumps in, 24, *26*